# Chiropractic Management of Chronic Hypertension:
## An Evidence-based Patient-Centered Monograph for Integrative Clinicians

Integrative, Nutritional, Botanical, and Manipulative Therapeutics
with Concepts, Perspectives, Algorithms, and Protocols for
the Safe and Effective Management of Chronic High Blood Pressure

# Alex Vasquez, D.C., N.D.

- Doctor of Chiropractic, graduate of Western States Chiropractic College. Licensed Doctor of Chiropractic, Washington (1996-2002) and Texas (2002-present)
- Doctor of Naturopathic Medicine, graduate of Bastyr University, Licensed Naturopathic Physician with Additional Prescriptive Authority in Washington (2000-2002), Licensed Naturopathic Physician in Oregon (2004-present)
- Private practice of chiropractic and naturopathic medicine in Seattle, Washington (2000-2001) and Houston, Texas (2001-2006)
- Former Adjunct Professor of Orthopedics (2000), Radiographic Interpretation (2000), and Rheumatology (2001) for the Naturopathic Medicine program at Bastyr University in Kenmore, Washington (www.bastyr.edu)
- Former Forum Consultant (2003-2007) and Former Adjunct Faculty (2004-2005), The Institute for Functional Medicine in Gig Harbor, Washington (www.functionalmedicine.org)
- Former Editor (2006-2007), *Naturopathy Digest*
- Former Columnist (2006-2007), *Nutritional Wellness*
- Author of numerous articles and letters published in *Annals of Pharmacotherapy, The Lancet, Nutritional Perspectives, British Medical Journal, Journal of Manipulative and Physiological Therapeutics, JAMA: Journal of the American Medical Association, The Original Internist, Integrative Medicine: A Clinician's Journal, Holistic Primary Care, Nutritional Wellness, Dynamic Chiropractic, Alternative Therapies in Health and Medicine, Journal of the American Osteopathic Association, Evidence-based Complementary and Alternative Medicine, Journal of Clinical Endocrinology and Metabolism*, and *Arthritis & Rheumatism*: Official Journal of the American College of Rheumatology

# OptimalHealthResearch.com

Vasquez A. <u>Chiropractic Management of Chronic Hypertension (Primary High Blood Pressure)</u>. Fort Worth, TX; Integrative and Biological Medicine Research and Consulting, LLC: 2010
10-Digit ISBN: 0-9752858-4-X
13-Digit ISBN: 9780975285848


Copyright © 2010 by Alex Vasquez. All rights reserved.

No part of this book may be reproduced, stored in a retrieval system, or transmitted by any means (electronic, mechanical, photocopying, recording, or otherwise) without written permission from the author.

See website for updated information: www.OptimalHealthResearch.com

# Preface, Introduction, and Foreword

| Section | Table of contents | Page |
|---|---|---|
| 1. | Preface, Introduction, and Foreword | 1 |
| 2. | Chiropractic Management of Chronic Hypertension | 27 |
| 3. | Wellness Promotion: Re-Establishing the Foundation for Health | 87 |
| 4. | Clinical Assessments and Concepts | 169 |
| 5. | Competencies and Self-Assessment | 235 |
| 6. | Index | 238 |

**Samples of Commonly Used Abbreviations**:
- **25-OH-D** = serum 25-hydroxy-vitamin D,
- **ACEi** = angiotensin converting enzyme inhibitor,
- **alpha-blocker** = alpha-adrenergic antagonist,
- **ARB** = angiotensin-2 receptor blocker/antagonist,
- **ARF** = acute renal failure,
- **BB** = beta blocker or beta-adrenergic antagonist,
- **CAD** = coronary artery disease,
- **CBC** = complete blood count,
- **CCB** = calcium channel blocker/antagonist,
- **CHF** = congestive heart failure,
- **COPD** = chronic obstructive pulmonary disease,
- **CPK** = creatine phosphokinase
- **CRF** = chronic renal insufficiency,
- **CVD** = cardiovascular disease,
- **DM** = diabetes mellitus,
- **ECG** or **EKG** = electrocardiogram,
- **HBP** = high blood pressure
- **HDL** = high density lipoprotein cholesterol,
- **HTN** = hypertension,
- **IHD** = ischemic heart disease,
- **MI** = myocardial infarction,
- **PRN** = from the Latin "pro re nata" meaning "on occasion" or "when necessary",
- **PVD** = peripheral vascular disease,
- **RAD** = reactive airway disease,
- **TRIGs** = serum triglycerides,
- **UA** = urinalysis,
- **US** = ultrasound.

**Dedications**: I dedicate this book to the following people in appreciation for their works, their direct and indirect support of this work, and for their contributions to the advancement of authentic healthcare.
- **To the students and practitioners of chiropractic and naturopathic medicine**, those who continue to learn so that they can provide the best possible care to their patients
- **To the researchers** whose works are cited in this text
- **To Drs Alan Gaby, Jeffrey Bland, Ronald LeFebvre, Robert Richard, and Gilbert Manso**, my most memorable and influential professors and mentors
- **To Dr Bruce Ames**[1] **and the late Dr Roger Williams**[2], for helping us to view our individuality as biochemically unique
- **To Dr Chester Wilk**[3,4] **and important others** for documenting and resisting the organized oppression of natural, non-pharmaceutical, non-surgical healthcare[5,6,7]
- **To Jorge Strunz and Ardeshir Farah,** for artistic inspiration


**Acknowledgments for Peer and Editorial Review:** Acknowledgement here does not imply that the reviewer fully agrees with or endorses the material in this text but rather that they were willing to review specific sections of the book for clinical applicability and clarity and to make suggestions to their own level of satisfaction. Credit for improvements and refinements to this text are due in part to these reviewers; responsibility for oversights remains that of the author.
- 2010 Edition of *Chiropractic Management of Chronic Hypertension*: Joseph Paun MS DC, Joe Brimhall DC, Julia Liebich DC, David Candelario OMS4 (TCOM c/o 2010), James Bogash DC, Bill Beakey, Robert Richard DO, Nick Karapasas DC
- 2009 Edition of *Chiropractic and Naturopathic Mastery of Common Clinical Disorders*: Julia Marie Liebich (NUHS DC4), Heather Kahn MD, Robert Richard DO, James Leiber DO, David Candelario (UNT-HSC TCOM DO4)
- 2007 Edition of *Integrative Orthopedics*: Barry Morgan MD, Dennis Harris DC, Richard Brown DC (DACBI candidate), Ron Mariotti ND, Patrick Makarewich MBA, Reena Singh (SCNM ND4), Zachary Watkins DC, Charles Novak MS DC, Marnie Loomis ND, James Bogash DC, Sara Croteau DC, Kris Young DC, Joshua Levitt ND, Jack Powell III MD, Chad Kessler MD, Amy Neuzil ND
- 2006 Edition of *Integrative Rheumatology*: Amy Neuzil ND, Cathryn Harbor MD, Julian Vickers DC, Tamara Sachs MD, Bob Sager BSc MD DABFM (Clinical Instructor in the Department of Family Medicine, University of Kansas), Ron Mariotti ND, Titus Chiu (DC4), Zachary Watkins (DC4), Gilbert Manso MD, Bruce Milliman ND, William Groskopp DC, Robert Silverman DC, Matthew Breske (DC4), Dean Neary ND, Thomas Walton DC, Fraser Smith ND, Ladd Carlston DC, David Jones MD, Joshua Levitt ND
- 2004 Edition of *Integrative Orthopedics*: Peter Knight ND, Kent Littleton ND MS, Barry Morgan MD, Ron Hobbs ND, Joshua Levitt ND, John Neustadt (Bastyr ND4), Allison Gandre BS (Bastyr ND4), Peter Kimble ND, Jack Powell III MD, Chad Kessler MD, Mike Gruber MD, Deirdre O'Neill ND, Mary Webb ND, Leslie Charles ND, Amy Neuzil ND

---

[1] Ames BN, Elson-Schwab I, Silver EA. High-dose vitamin therapy stimulates variant enzymes with decreased coenzyme binding affinity (increased K(m)): relevance to genetic disease and polymorphisms. *Am J Clin Nutr*. 2002 Apr;75(4):616-58  http://www.ajcn.org/cgi/content/full/75/4/616
[2] Williams RJ. Biochemical Individuality: The Basis for the Genetotrophic Concept. Austin and London: University of Texas Press; 1956
[3] Wilk CA. Medicine, Monopolies, and Malice: How the Medical Establishment Tried to Destroy Chiropractic. Garden City Park: Avery, 1996
[4] Getzendanner S. Permanent injunction order against AMA. *JAMA*. 1988 Jan 1;259(1):81-2  http://optimalhealthresearch.com/archives/wilk.html
[5] Carter JP. Racketeering in Medicine: The Suppression of Alternatives. Norfolk: Hampton Roads Pub; 1993
[6] Morley J, Rosner AL, Redwood D. A case study of misrepresentation of the scientific literature: recent reviews of chiropractic. *J Altern Complement Med*. 2001 Feb;7(1):65-78
[7] Terrett AG. Misuse of the literature by medical authors in discussing spinal manipulative therapy injury. *J Manipulative Physiol Ther*. 1995 May;18(4):203-10

**Format and Layout:** The format and layout of this book is designed to efficiently take the reader though the clinically relevant spectrum of considerations for each condition that is detailed. Important topics are given their own section within each chapter, while other less important or less common conditions are only described briefly in terms of the four "clinical essentials" of 1) definition/pathophysiology, 2) clinical presentation, 3) assessment/diagnosis, and 4) treatment/management. Each expanded section which details the more important/common conditions maintains a consistent format, taking the reader through the spectrum of primary clinical considerations: definition/pathophysiology, clinical presentations, differential diagnoses, assessments (physical examination, laboratory, imaging), complications, management, and treatment.

**References and Citations:** Major references to texts and articles are listed along with each section; these references are "recommended reading" and form the foundation for the clinical approach delineated in the text. Citations to articles, abstracts, texts, and personal communications are footnoted throughout the text to provide supporting information and to provide interested readers the resources to find additional information. Many of the cited articles are available on-line for free, and when possible I have included the website addresses so that readers can access the complete article.

**Language, Semantics, and Perspective:** As a diligent student who previously aspired to be an English professor, I have written this text with great (though inevitably imperfect) attention to detail. Individual words were chosen with care. As a diligent student who initially aspired to become an English professor, I confess to knowing, pushing, and creatively breaking several rules of grammar and punctuation. With regard to the he/she and him/her debacle of the English language, I've mixed singular and plural pronouns for the sake of being efficient and so that the images remain gender-neutral to the extent reasonable. The subtitle *The art of creating wellness while effectively managing acute and chronic musculoskeletal/health disorders* was chosen to emphasize the intentional creation of wellness rather than a limited focus on disease treatment and symptom suppression. For the 2009 printing of *Chiropractic and Naturopathic Mastery of Common Clinical Disorders*, this subtitle was slightly modified from "creating" to "co-creating" to emphasize the team effort required between physician and patient. *Managing* was chosen to emphasize the importance of treating-monitoring-referring-reassessing, rather than merely *treating*. *Disorders* was chosen to reflect the fact that a distinguishing characteristic of **life** is the ability to habitually create *organized structure* and *higher order* from chaos and *disorder*. For example, plants organize the randomly moving molecules of air and water into the organized structure of biomolecules and plant structure. Similarly, the human body creates organized structure of increased complexity from consumed plants and other foods; molecules ingested and inhaled from the environment are organized into specific biochemicals and tissue structures with distinct characteristics and definite functions. Injury and disease *result in* or *result from* a lack of order, hence my use of the word "disorders" to characterize human illness and disease. A motor vehicle accident that results in bodily injury, for example, is an example of an external chaotic force, which, when imparted upon human body tissues, results in a disruption (disorder) of the normal structure and organization that previously defined and characterized the now-damaged tissues of the body. Likewise, an autoimmune disease process that results in tissue destruction is an anti-evolutionary process that takes molecules of higher complexity and reverts them to simpler, fragmented, and non-functional forms. From the perspective of "health" as *organized structure and meaningful function* and "disease" as *the reversion to chaos,*

> **Newsletter & Updates**
> Be alerted to new integrative clinical research and updates to this textbook by signing-up for the free newsletter, sent 4-6 times per year. Contact newsletter@optimalhealthresearch.com
> or
> www.OptimalHealthResearch.com/newsletter

*destruction of structure, and the loss of function*, the task of healthcare providers is essentially to restore order, and to acutely reduce and proactively prevent/eliminate clinical-biochemical-biomechanical-emotional chaos insofar as it adversely affects the patient's life experience as an individual and our collective experience as an interdependent society.

**Integrity and Creativity:** I have endeavored to accurately represent the facts as they have been presented in texts and research, and to specifically resist any temptation to embellish or misrepresent data as others have done.[8,9] Conversely, I have not endeavored to make this book "normal" or "average" either in content nor in any intentional simplification. Rather I have allowed this text to be unique in format, content, and style, so that the personality of this text can be contrasted with that of the instructor and reader, thus enabling the learner to at least benefit from an intentionally different – though altogether honest – perspective and approach. Students using this text with the guidance of a qualified professor will benefit from the experience of "two teachers" rather than just one.

**Peer-review and Quality Control:** Peer-review is essential to help ensure accuracy and clinical applicability of health-related information. Consistent with the importance of our goals, I have employed several "checks and balances" to increase the accuracy and applicability of the information within my textbooks:

- Reliance upon authoritative references: Nearly all important statements are referenced to peer-reviewed biomedical journals or authoritative texts, such as *The Merck Manual* and *Current Medical Diagnosis and Treatment*. Each citation is provided by a footnote at the bottom of each page so that readers will know quickly and easily exactly where the information came from.
- Extensive cross-referencing: Readers will notice, if not be overwhelmed by, the number of references and citations. Many important statements have several references. Many references (especially textbooks) are referenced several times even on the same page. The purpose of this extensive referencing is three-fold: 1) to guide you to additional information, 2) to help me (the writer) stay organized, and 3) to help you and me (the practicing physicians) employ this information with confidence.
- Periodic revision: The book is updated and revised on a regular basis. New information is added; superfluous information removed. Inspired by the popular text *Current Medical Diagnosis and Treatment* which is updated every year, I want *Integrative Orthopedics* and *Integrative Rheumatology* to be accurate, timely, and in pace with the ever-growing literature on natural medicine. Any significant errors that are brought to my attention will be posted at

---

[8] **Vasquez A**. Zinc treatment for reduction of hyperplasia of prostate. *Townsend Letter for Doctors and Patients* 1996; January: 100
[9] Broad W, Wade N. Betrayers of the Truth: Fraud and Deceit in the Halls of Science. New York: Simon and Schuster; 1982

OptimalHealthResearch.com/updates; please check this page periodically to ensure that you are working with the most accurate information of which I am aware.
- <u>Peer-review</u>: The peer-review process my books takes several forms. First, colleagues and students are invited to review new and revised sections of the text before publication; every section of the book that you are holding has been independently reviewed by health science students and/or practicing clinicians from various backgrounds: allopathic, chiropractic, osteopathic, naturopathic. Second, you - the reader - are invited to provide feedback about the information in the book, typographical errors, syntax, case reports, new research, etc. If your ideas truly change the nature of the material, I will be glad to acknowledge you in the text (with your permission, of course). If your contribution is hugely significant, such as reviewing three or more chapters or helping in some important way, I will be glad to not only acknowledge you, but to also send you the next edition at a discount or courtesy when your ideas take effect. Third, I keep abreast of new literature by constantly perusing new research and advancements in the health sciences. Having been successful in three separate doctoral programs, I have learned not only to master large amounts of material but to also separate and integrate different viewpoints as appropriate. I also "field test" my protocols with patients in the various clinical arenas in which I work and also with professionals and academicians via presentations and critical dialogue. By implementing these quality control steps, I hope to create a useful text and advance our professions and our practices by improving the quality of care that we deliver to our patients. Readers with suggestions or corrections can email via the website: http://OptimalHealthResearch.com/corrections.

**How to Use This Book Safely and Most Effectively:** Ideally, these books should be read cover-to-cover within a context of coursework that is supervised by an experienced professor. For post-graduate professionals, they might consider forming a local "book club" and meeting for weekly or monthly discussions to check their understandings and share their clinical experiences to refine the application of clinical knowledge, perceptions, and skills. Virtual groups and internet forums—such as the forum hosted by the Institute for Functional Medicine at www.FunctionalMedicine.org—can provide access to an international group of professional peers where sharing of clinical experience and questions is synergistic. Throughout this book, references are amply provided and are often footnoted with hyperlinks providing full-text access. This book is intended for licensed doctorate-level healthcare professionals with graduate and post-graduate training.

**Notice:** The intention and scope of this text are to provide doctorate-level clinicians with useful information and a familiarity with available research and resources pertinent to the management of patients in a holistic primary care setting. Specifically, the information in this book is intended to be used by licensed healthcare professionals who have received hands-on clinical training and supervision at accredited chiropractic/naturopathic colleges. Additionally, information in this book should be confirmed and used in conjunction with other resources, texts, and in combination with the clinician's best judgment with the intention to "first do no harm" and second to provide effective healthcare. Information and treatments applicable to a specific *condition* may not be appropriate for or applicable to a specific *patient* in your office; this is especially true for patients with concomitant illnesses and those taking pharmaceutical medications. Throughout this text, I describe treatments—manual, dietary, nutritional, botanical, and pharmacologic—and their research support for the clinical conditions being discussed; each practitioner must determine appropriateness of these treatments for his/her individual patient and with consideration of the doctor's scope of practice, education, training, skill, and possible "off label" use of medications and treatments. This book has been carefully written and checked for accuracy by the author and professional colleagues. However, in view of the possibility of human error and new discoveries in the biomedical sciences, neither the author nor any party associated in any way with this text warrants that this text is perfect, accurate, or complete in every way, and we disclaim responsibility for harm or loss associated with the application of the material herein. With all conditions/treatments described herein, each physician must be sure to consider the balance between what is best for the patient and the physician's own level of ability, expertise, and experience. When in doubt, or if the physician is not a specialist in the treatment of a given severe condition, referral is appropriate. These notes are written with the routine "outpatient" in mind and are not tailored to severely injured patients or emergency or "playing field" or "emergency response" situations. Consult your First Aid and Emergency Response texts and course materials for appropriate information. These notes represent the author's perspective based on academic education, experience, and post-graduate continuing education and are not inclusive of every fact that a clinician may need to know. Consult other texts, references, and articles for additional information and perspectives. This is not an "entry level" book except when used in an academic setting with a knowledgeable professor who can explain the abbreviations, tests, physical exam procedures, and treatments. This book requires a certain level of knowledge from the reader and familiarity with clinical concepts, laboratory assessments, and physical examination procedures.

**Updates, Corrections, and Newsletter:** When omissions, errata, and the need for important updates become clear to me, I will post these at the website: www.OptimalHealthResearch.com/updates. Be sure to access this page periodically to ensure that you are informed of any corrections that might have clinical relevance. This book consists not only of the text in the printed pages you are holding, but also the footnotes and any updates at the website. Be alerted to new integrative clinical research and updates to this textbook by signing-up for the free newsletter at www.OptimalHealthResearch.com/newsletter or newsletter@OptimalHealthResearch.com.

**Preface to *Chiropractic and Naturopathic Mastery of Common Clinical Disorders*:** *Chiropractic and Naturopathic Mastery of Common Clinical Disorders* steps beyond the obviously musculoskeletal focus of my first three textbooks *Integrative Orthopedics*, *Integrative Rheumatology*, and *Musculoskeletal Pain: Expanded Clinical Strategies* to provide students and clinicians an evidence-based foundational approach to treating common clinical disorders such as Asthma, Hypertension, Diabetes Mellitus Type-2 and Metabolic Syndrome, and Disorders of Mood and Behavior—a section that emphasizes adult depression and anxiety. Readers of these sections will note that they differ in format from the other chapters with regard to a stronger emphasis on presenting an article-by-article review in the effort to strengthen the evidence-based nature of the clinical protocols; ultimately this is to help students and clinicians appreciate the richness (and occasional limitations) of the research supporting an integrative clinical approach. As with my previous books and all other clinical resources, clinicians should still consult other sources and texts for additional information, current updated guidelines, and changes to standards of care.

## Preface, Introduction, and Foreword

The emphasis of *Chiropractic and Naturopathic Mastery of Common Clinical Disorders* is to begin bridging the gap that continues to exist between so-called "CAM" (which includes patient's self-directed non-pharmacosurgical healthcare practices and preferences as well as integrative and mostly non-pharmacosurgical treatments utilized by trained professionals) and so-called "conventional" healthcare as is generally taught in the majority of osteopathic and allopathic medical schools. Health problems for which patients most often seek CAM treatment are listed in the illustration that follows.

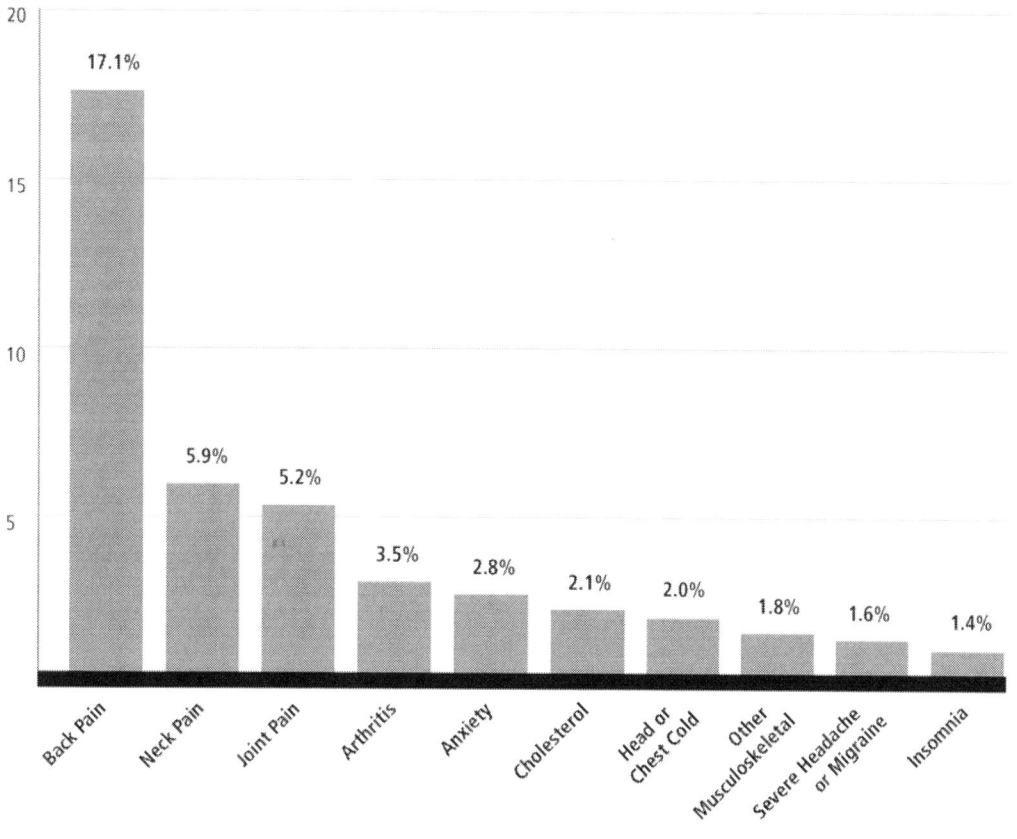

Image Credit: National Center for Complementary and Alternative Medicine, NIH, DHHS.
http://nccam.nih.gov/news/camstats/2007/graphics.htm

The following table provides a listing—in order of percentage—of the most common conditions seen in a general family practice of medicine.

| Top diagnoses | Notes and comments |
|---|---|
| 1. **Hypertension** | 5.9% of family medicine diagnoses; nearly 11 million patient visits per year. |
| 2. Diabetes mellitus | 4.1% of family medicine diagnoses; more than 7.6 million patient visits per year. |
| 3. Acute upper respiratory infection | 3.2% of family medicine diagnoses; more than 10 million patient visits per year. Most of these are caused by viral infections for which there is no direct medical treatment; most patients are treated symptomatically with decongestants and antipyretics. Complications are rare but can be serious. |
| 4. Sinusitis | 2.5% of family medicine diagnoses; more than 10 million patient visits per year. |
| 5. Acute pharyngitis | 2.3% of family medicine diagnoses; more than 4 million patient visits per year. |
| 6. Otitis media | 2.3% of family medicine diagnoses; > 4 million patient visits per year. |
| 7. Bronchitis | 1.9% of family medicine diagnoses; > 3 million patient visits per year. |
| 8. Back problems | 1.8% of family medicine diagnoses; > 3 million patient visits per year. This is a diverse group of conditions ranging from post-traumatic to benign to developmental problems such as scoliosis. Note that back pain is listed separately below. |
| 9. Hyperlipidemia | 1.7% of family medicine diagnoses; > 3 million patient visits per year. This mostly includes the lifestyle-generated dyslipidemia epidemic, with comparably fewer cases of genotropic disorders requiring pharmacotherapy. |
| 10. Urinary tract disorders | 1.6% of family medicine diagnoses; almost 3 million patient visits per year. This can include a diverse group of problems ranging from simple and self-limited urinary tract infections to sexually transmitted diseases; these are not covered in this text. |
| 11. Allergic rhinitis | 1.2% of family medicine diagnoses; > 2 million patient visits per year. A general approach to allergy treatment is included in this text. |
| 12. Back pain | 1.2% of family medicine diagnoses; > 2 million patient visits per year. |
| 13. Abdominal or pelvic symptoms | 1.1% of family medicine diagnoses; > 2 million patient visits per year. This can include a wide range of diagnoses ranging from appendicitis to dysmenorrhea. Due to the breadth and complexity, these are not covered in this text. |
| 14. Joint pain | 1.1% of family medicine diagnoses; > 2 million patient visits per year. |
| 15. Depression or anxiety | 1.1% of family medicine diagnoses; > 2 million patient visits per year. These are mostly mild cases but can also include acute situations that warrant emergency treatment including pharmacotherapy and sedation. |
| 16. Asthma | 1.1% of family medicine diagnoses; almost 2 million patient visits per year. An approach to allergy treatment is included in this text, with a section on asthma. |
| 17. Chest pain or shortness of breath | 1.1% of family medicine diagnoses; almost 2 million patient visits per year. Some of these are benign musculoskeletal pain or gastroesophageal reflux while others turn out to be life-threatening conditions such as myocardial infarction, pneumothorax, pneumonia, or—rarely—aortic dissection. These are not directly covered in this text. |
| 18. Soft tissue problems | 1% of family medicine diagnoses; 1.8 million patient visits per year. |
| 19. Acute bronchitis and bronchiolitis | 1% of family medicine diagnoses; 1.8 million patient visits per year. These include bacterial and viral infections, ranging from mild to life-threatening, especially in patients with cardiopulmonary disease. |
| 20. Skin problems | 1% of family medicine diagnoses; 1.8 million patient visits per year. Dermatology is not specifically covered in this text except for the chapter on psoriasis. Many patients will benefit from the diet and nutrition protocols described herein. |
| 21. Tendonitis | 1% of family medicine diagnoses; 1.7 million patient visits per year. |

Data are from *Essentials of Family Medicine, 5th edition* edited by Sloane PD, Slatt LM, Ebell MH, Jacques LB, Smith MA published by Lippincott Williams & Wilkins (April 1, 2007)

In *Chiropractic and Naturopathic Mastery*, I (re)introduce the Functional Medicine Matrix that I originally diagramed for the Institute for Functional Medicine (IFM) in 2003; the diagram used is updated from the original, and readers should appreciate that IFM has changed the Matrix since this version was made.

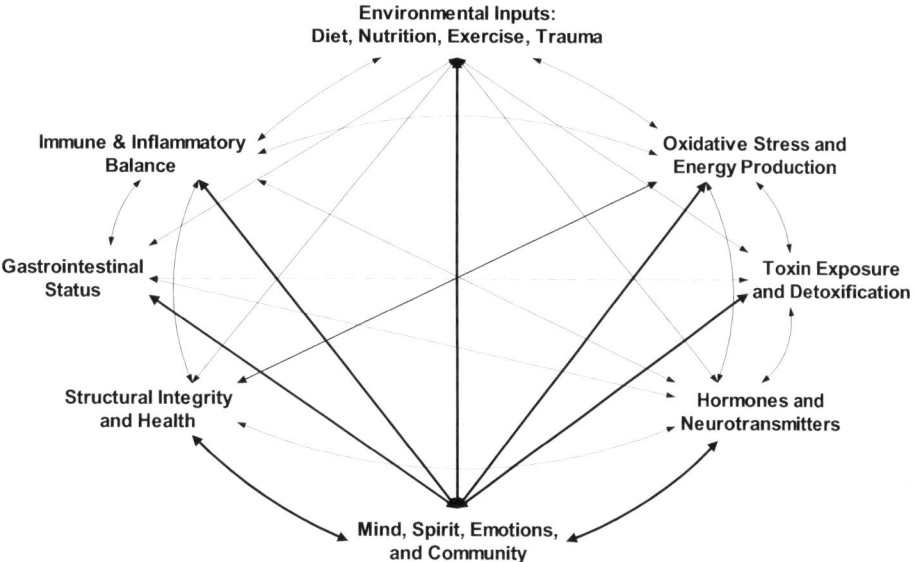

**Functional Medicine Matrix:** Updated from the original diagram by Vasquez in 2003 for the Institute for Functional Medicine (IFM). See www.FunctionalMedicine.org for updated information and additional training.

*Introduction to the Hypertension Monograph*: This monograph explores and substantiates the following positions in the ensuing discussion of hypertension in particular and *true* health and wellness promotion in general.

1. **The chiropractic profession should play a major if not dominant role in the clinical management of chronic hypertension**. At present, chiropractic care of the hypertensive patient is marginalized to an "alternative and complementary" role. The medical profession has taken a leadership position on the management of hypertension based on a wealth of drug research and the establishment of evidence-based clinical protocols and professional standards of care. In contrast, the chiropractic profession, although it has within its scope of practice the most effective treatments for hypertension, has not—until now—had a cohesive evidence-based guide for the clinical management of the hypertensive patient. This monograph serves to fill that void by providing chiropractic clinicians with ❶ an overview of the disease, ❷ its differential diagnoses and assessment (including: history, physical examination, laboratory and imaging), and ❸ clear evidence-based treatment protocols and interventional options.

   > Evidence sample from *Journal of Human Hypertension*: "Anatomical abnormalities of the cervical spine at the level of the Atlas vertebra are associated with relative ischemia of the brainstem circulation and increased blood pressure (BP). Manual correction of this mal-alignment has been associated with reduced arterial pressure." The authors used a

> double-blind, placebo-controlled design at a single center among 50 drug naïve (n=26) or washed out (n=24) patients with Stage 1 hypertension; patients were randomized to receive a National Upper Cervical Chiropractic (NUCCA) procedure or a sham procedure. Significant findings included the following, "At week 8, there were differences in systolic BP (-17 mm Hg, NUCCA versus -3 mm Hg, placebo) and diastolic BP (-10 mm Hg, NUCCA versus -2 mm Hg). … **No adverse effects were recorded. We conclude that restoration of Atlas alignment is associated with marked and sustained reductions in BP similar to the use of two-drug combination therapy.**"[10]

2. **Drug management of hypertension is by no means a panacea, leaving significant numbers of patients untreated, undertreated, or mistreated**. The expenses and adverse effects of drug management leave many patients untreated. Furthermore, according to recent peer-reviewed research, shortcomings in the medical management of hypertension place patients at risk of adverse effects, inefficacy, and unnecessary expense. Lastly, by failing to address the underlying causes of high blood pressure, and by failing to treat the constellation of comorbid conditions (e.g., insulin resistance, overweight, hyperuricemia, and nutritional deficiencies), medical suppression of elevated blood pressure cannot be viewed as optimal therapy.

> <u>Evidence sample from *New England Journal of Medicine* in 2003</u>: The data from this study show that the medical profession leaves many hypertensive patients untreated and undertreated. Specifically, profession-wide deficiencies were noted in the following areas:
> - ❶ Lifestyle modification for patients with mild hypertension: *underused*
> - ❷ Change in treatment when blood pressure is persistently uncontrolled: *underused*
> - ❸ Pharmacotherapy for uncontrolled mild hypertension: *underused*
>
> The authors wrote, "METHODS: We telephoned a random sample of adults living in 12 metropolitan areas in the United States and asked them about selected health care experiences. We also received written consent to copy their medical records for the most recent two-year period and used this information to evaluate performance on 439 indicators of quality of care for 30 acute and chronic conditions as well as preventive care. We then constructed aggregate scores. RESULTS: Participants received 54.9 percent (95 percent confidence interval, 54.3 to 55.5) of recommended care. … CONCLUSIONS: **The deficits we have identified in adherence to recommended processes for basic care pose serious threats to the health of the American public**. Strategies to reduce these deficits in care are warranted."[11]

> <u>Evidence sample from *Milbank Quarterly—A Multidisciplinary Journal of Population Health and Health Policy* in 1998</u>: The authors review pertinent literature on healthcare quality and note that among Americans only "41%–54% of patients had their hypertension controlled (mean blood pressure (150/90)." By weak criteria of HTN control, 55% of people with hypertension had blood pressure "under control" with pressures of 160/95 treated with at least one antihypertensive medication; when using more strict medical

---

[10] Bakris G, Dickholtz M Sr, Meyer PM, Kravitz G, Avery E, Miller M, Brown J, Woodfield C, Bell B. Atlas vertebra realignment and achievement of arterial pressure goal in hypertensive patients: a pilot study. *J Hum Hypertens*. 2007 May;21(5):347-52
[11] McGlynn EA, Asch SM, Adams J, Keesey J, Hicks J, DeCristofaro A, Kerr EA. The quality of health care delivered to adults in the United States. *N Engl J Med*. 2003 Jun 26;348(26):2635-45

> criteria (achievement medicated blood pressure of 140/90) only 21% of Americans were properly treated. **On average, medical care provided only 40%–55% of the appropriate treatment for HTN—note that these criteria do *not* include evidence-based nutritional interventions such as fish oil supplementation which has been shown to reduce cardiovascular mortality more effectively and cost-effectively than the "approved" drugs and medical treatments.** The authors conclude, "Studies over the past decade show that some people are receiving more care than they need, and some are receiving less. Simple averages from a number of studies indicate that 50 percent of people received recommended preventive care; 70 percent, recommended acute care; 30 percent, contraindicated acute care; 60 percent, recommended chronic care; and 20 percent, contraindicated chronic care. **These studies strongly suggest that the care delivered in the United States often does not meet professional standards.**" [12]

3. **Because hypertension is a major patient-centered and public health concern, the chiropractic profession must have an evidence-based protocol for its management**. Chronic hypertension is "disease" of epidemic and indeed pandemic proportions in America and increasingly in other nations. The lifetime incidence of high blood pressure among Americans is 90%, while on any given day, approximately one in four Americans has high blood pressure. These patients and potential patients would benefit more from integrative chiropractic care and the nutrition-based protocols in this document than they can hope to benefit from drug-only treatment. The evidence supporting the dietary and nutritional prevention and treatment of hypertension and cardiovascular disease is irrefutable. Adding to this the recent evidence that chiropractic spinal manipulation is as effective as two-drug treatment for hypertension makes the case for the chiropractic profession's assumption of a leadership role timely and of paramount importance. This document not only serves to provide individual clinicians with practical protocols, but—perhaps more importantly—this document is a call to action for the chiropractic profession. The chiropractic profession must stand and deliver the quality healthcare that our patient population needs and deserves.

> Excerpt from "The Council on Chiropractic Education's New Wellness Standard: A call to action for the chiropractic profession" [13] by Marion W Evans Jr and Ronald Rupert (Parker College of Chiropractic Research Institute) published in open-access format in *Chiropractic & Osteopathy*: Excerpt provided here in accordance with open access terms and conditions
>
> **Health Status of Spine Patients**
>
> "A review of some of the **co-morbidity issues that accompany musculoskeletal conditions** like low back pain, will demonstrate why **chiropractors need to become aggressively active in addressing patient lifestyle and other health promotion and wellness issues**. The impact of spine problems on health status has been examined through co-morbidity analysis. In 2000, Fanuele and colleagues [5] reported an

---

[12] Schuster MA, McGlynn EA, Brook RH. How good is the quality of health care in the United States? *Milbank Q*. 1998;76(4):517-63
[13] Evans MW Jr, Rupert R. The Council on Chiropractic Education's new wellness standard: a call to action for the chiropractic profession. *Chiropr Osteopat*. 2006 Oct 12;14:23 http://www.chiroandosteo.com/content/14/1/23

observational study of 17,774 patients from the 25 National Spine Network agencies or academic centers. Their goals were to quantify the impact of spinal problems on physical function and to better understand the effects of co-morbid conditions on physical function. **In their study population, 46.6% of spine patients had at least one other non-spinal condition or illness. When smoking was considered a co-morbid condition it was number one with hypertension 2nd, obesity 3rd and diabetes 4th.** Fifty-two percent of patients had a primary diagnosis of lumbosacral symptoms and 82% had experienced three or more months of pain. They concluded that society bears a heavy economic burden from patients with spinal conditions and **physicians need to recognize that spine patients have significantly more physical morbidity than the US population in aggregate**. Fanuele and colleagues stated, "It is likely that the spinal diagnosis, in itself, is mostly responsible for the significant functional disability, expressed by low physical component scores."

A study published in Pain by Von Korff and others [6] concluded that after controlling for demographic variables and for co-morbidities, chronic spinal pain was significantly associated with role disability, other pain conditions, chronic diseases and mental disorders. Their information was derived from the household face-to-face National Co-morbidity Survey Replication which was a nationally representative sample (n = 9,282) of respondents age 18 or older. Almost 20% of the US population was estimated to have chronic spinal pain in the prior 12 months with about 30% reporting lifetime prevalence of chronic spinal pain. This chronic spinal pain was more than three times higher in patients who reported other chronic pain as those without these conditions and it was twice as high in patients with a mental disorder. **Chronic physical disease associated with chronic spine pain included stroke, hypertension, asthma, COPD, irritable bowel syndrome, ulcers, HIV/AIDS, epilepsy and vision problems.** After adjusting for demographic variables the increased risk of a co-morbid chronic physical disease associated with chronic spine pain was 2.0. Among the 40 million Americans who suffer chronic spine pain, 22 million had a co-morbid physical ailment (87% with chronic spine conditions had at least one co-morbid condition). Therefore, **spine patients are in need of health education messages at a rate that may exceed that of non-spine patients**.

The association of spinal disease with smoking and obesity is also fairly well established [7,8]. Obesity is associated with more severe pain syndromes among spine patients and they suffer greater impairment in functional status [7]. As previously stated, smoking is often the most frequently found condition associated with spine disease [5,8]. These factors should be important to chiropractors as they primarily see back pain and neck pain patients [9]. The average case mix of DCs tends to include a significant amount of chronic spine patients although there is an indication that **DCs utilize certain health promotion measures with them such as; exercise recommendations, ergonomic advice and advice on dietary changes** [9]. **DCs need to place a greater emphasis on the use of common prevention and health promotion methodologies in their practices.** It is our opinion that an emphasis on wellness and health promotion is compatible with either the primary care or the "spine care model" of chiropractic and is congruent with national health initiatives and the chiropractic tradition of holism and self-reported prevention practices [9]. This will be described in more detail but should include cancer prevention dietary recommendations, proper exercise recommendations, appropriate screening procedures that are within scope of practice including, but not limited to **cardiovascular disease, hypertension, diabetes**, breast, prostate and skin cancer screening."

5. Fanuele JC, Birkmeyer NJO, Abdu WA, Tosteson T, Weinstein JN: The impact of spinal problems on the health status of patients: have we underestimated the effect? *Spine* 2000, 25(12):1509-1514
6. Von Korff M, Crance P, Lane M, Miglioretti, Simon G, Saunders K, Stang P, Brandenburg N, Kessler R: Chronic spinal pain and physical-mental comorbidity in the United States: results from the national comorbidity survey replication. *Pain* 2005, 113:331-339
7. Fanuele JC, Abdu WA, Hanscom B, Weinstein JN: Association between obesity and functional status in patients with spine disease. *Spine* 2002, 27(3):306-31
8. Scott SC, Goldberg MS, Mayo NE, Stock SR, Poîtras B: The association between cigarette smoking and back pain in adults. *Spine* 1999, 24:1090-1098
9. Christensen M, Kerkhoff D, Kollasch M: *Job analysis of chiropractic: A project report, survey analysis and summary of the practice of chiropractic within the United States*. Greeley, CO: National Board of Chiropractic Examiners; 2000:74-75

**_Bon Voyage_**: All artists, and scientists—regardless of genre—grapple with the divergent goals of 1) perfecting their work and 2) completing their work; the former is impossible, while the latter is the only means by which the effort can become useful. At some point, we must all agree that it is "good enough" and that it contains the essence of what needs to be communicated. While neither this nor any future edition of this book is likely to be "perfect", I am content with the literature reviewed, presented, and the new conclusions and implications which are described—many for the first time ever—in this text. Particularly for *Integrative Rheumatology* and *Chiropractic and Naturopathic Mastery*, each chapter aims to achieve a paradigm shift which distances us further from the simplistic pharmacocentric model and toward one which authentically empowers both practitioners and patients. With time, I will make future editions more complete and less polemical (but not less passionate). I hope you are able to implement these conclusions and research findings into your own life and into the treatment plans for your patients.

Thank you, and I wish you and your patients the best in success and health,

Alex Vasquez, D.C., N.D.
February 21, 2010

> "You work that you may keep pace with the earth and the soul of the earth.
> For to be idle is to become a stranger unto the seasons, and to step out of life's procession.
> ... Work is love made visible."            Kahlil Gibran, *The Prophet*

# Chiropractic Musculoskeletal Competence: Is Being Best Good Enough?

*Alex Vasquez, D.C., N.D.*

This article was originally published in *Dynamic Chiropractic*:
http://www.dynamicchiropractic.com/mpacms/dc/article.php?id=52085

While chiropractic doctors address a wide range of health concerns and disorders in their clinical practices, the profession as a whole and our formal training obviously emphasize musculoskeletal diagnosis and treatment; this is appropriate given that musculoskeletal disorders are a major burden to individual patients and the healthcare system as a whole.[14] Since the several of the drug interventions generally employed by allopaths appear to accelerate joint destruction[15,16,17] and result in more than 100,000 hospitalizations and well over 16,000 deaths per year[18,19,20] and since some surgical procedures for musculoskeletal pain are not more effective than placebo or conservative treatment[21,22,23], the chiropractic profession's contribution to public health by the provision of safe and effective nonpharmacologic and nonsurgical management of musculoskeletal pain is important. With these and other considerations in mind, the assessment of competence and comparative competence among front-line healthcare professionals is a worthy area of investigation.

The standardized musculoskeletal competency examination was initially developed and published by Freedman and Bernstein in their landmark study published in *Journal of Bone and Joint Surgery* in October 1998.[24] The test has been validated by a nation-wide survey of hospital residency chairpersons in orthopedics as well as internal medicine. The test consists of 25 open-ended short-answer questions which survey general orthopedic diagnoses and management on topics such as acute compartment syndrome, septic arthritis, scaphoid fracture, and lateral epicondylitis; a minimum score of 70-73% is required for passing. Just like the original study by Freedman and Bernstein, all follow-up confirmation studies assessing medical "allopathic" competence by this validated and standardized examination have shown that **medical school**

---

[14] Woolf A, Pfleger B. Burden of major musculoskeletal. conditions. *Bulletin of the World Health Organization* 2003;81:646-656 http://www.who.int/entity/bulletin/volumes/81/9/Woolf.pdf

[15] "At…concentrations comparable to those… in the synovial fluid of patients treated with the drug, several NSAIDs suppress proteoglycan synthesis… These NSAID-related effects on chondrocyte metabolism … are much more profound in osteoarthritic cartilage than in normal cartilage, due to enhanced uptake of NSAIDs by the osteoarthritic cartilage." Brandt KD. Effects of nonsteroidal anti-inflammatory drugs on chondrocyte metabolism in vitro and in vivo. *Am J Med*. 1987 Nov 20; 83(5A): 29-34

[16] "This highly significant association between NSAID use and acetabular destruction gives cause for concern, not least because of the difficulty in achieving satisfactory hip replacements in patients with severely damaged acetabula." Newman NM, Ling RS. Acetabular bone destruction related to non-steroidal anti-inflammatory drugs. *Lancet*. 1985 Jul 6; 2(8445): 11-4

[17] Vidal y Plana RR, Bizzarri D, Rovati AL. Articular cartilage pharmacology: I. In vitro studies on glucosamine and non steroidal antiinflammatory drugs. *Pharmacol Res Commun*. 1978 Jun;10(6):557-69

[18] "Conservative calculations estimate that approximately 107,000 patients are hospitalized annually for nonsteroidal anti-inflammatory drug (NSAID)-related gastrointestinal (GI) complications and at least 16,500 NSAID-related deaths occur each year among arthritis patients alone. The figures for all NSAID users would be overwhelming, yet the scope of this problem is generally under-appreciated." Singh G. Recent considerations in nonsteroidal anti-inflammatory drug gastropathy. *Am J Med*. 1998;105(1B):31S-38S

[19] Topol EJ. Failing the public health--rofecoxib, Merck, and the FDA. *N Engl J Med*. 2004 Oct 21;351(17):1707-9

[20] David J. Graham, MD, MPH, (Associate Director for Science, Office of Drug Safety, US FDA) estimated that 139,000 Americans who took Vioxx suffered serious side effects; he estimated that the drug killed between 26,000 and 55,000 people. http://www.commondreams.org/views05/0223-35.htm http://www.fda.gov/cder/drug/infopage/vioxx/vioxxgraham.pdf Accessed November 25, 2006

[21] Moseley JB, O'Malley K, Petersen NJ, Menke TJ, Brody BA, Kuykendall DH, Hollingsworth JC, Ashton CM, Wray NP. A controlled trial of arthroscopic surgery for osteoarthritis of the knee. *N Engl J Med*. 2002;347:81-8

[22] Bernstein J, Quach T. A perspective on the study of Moseley et al: questioning the value of arthroscopic knee surgery for osteoarthritis. *Cleve Clin J Med*. 2003;70(5):401, 405-6, 408-10

[23] "These findings suggest that in most cases there is no clear reason to advocate strongly for surgery apart from patient preference." Carragee E. Surgical treatment of lumbar disk disorders. JAMA. 2006 Nov 22;296(20):2485-7

[24] Freedman KB, Bernstein J. The adequacy of medical school education in musculoskeletal medicine. *J Bone Joint Surg Am*. 1998;80(10):1421-7

**preparation in musculoskeletal medicine is inadequate** and that **the vast majority of medical graduates are incompetent in basic musculoskeletal diagnosis and management**.[25,26,27,28,29] Generally, these articles have demonstrated that only 20-30% of medical graduates are competent in basic musculoskeletal knowledge; stated differently, 70-80% of medical graduates are incompetent in basic musculoskeletal knowledge, as assessed by this peer-reviewed and well-researched competency examination. These results are consistent and reproducible from different study populations and are thus probably generalizable to the medical profession as a whole.

Until recently, the question remained: "How well would *chiropractic* seniors and clinicians perform on this same test of musculoskeletal competence?" That question was partially answered in January 2007 by Humphreys *et al*[30] who administered the standardized musculoskeletal competency examination to 123 chiropractic seniors and 10 experienced clinicians. In contrast to the 20-30% success rate achieved by medical students and doctors, the chiropractic success rate at 51-64% was double *or triple* that seen among allopathic and osteopathic graduates. The chiropractic group showed a 64% success rate using minimal passing score of 70%, and a 51% success rate using minimal score of 73%. Among the 10 chiropractic clinicians, they demonstrated a 100% success rate. Thus, the performance of this small group of chiropractic doctors far outshined the results seen among 85 medical doctors working as first-year hospital residents in surgery, medicine, and orthopedics; according to Freedman and Bernstein in 1998, these medical doctors had only a 30% success rate.

While additional data from other chiropractic colleges and from larger groups of chiropractic clinicians is necessary before firm and generalized conclusions can be drawn, these results suggest that chiropractic training in musculoskeletal medicine as evaluated by a "medical" standardized and validated competency examination is clearly more thorough and more effective in ensuring minimal competence among chiropractic graduates than are the comparable educational programs utilized in allopathic medical schools. The well-documented and consistently high rate of incompetence in musculoskeletal medicine among medical graduates and clinicians is a cause for concern and has implications for state and national public health policies as well as insurance reimbursement schedules; likewise and conversely, the consistent demonstration of chiropractic superiority in this field should foster enhanced utilization of and access to chiropractic clinical services.

However, while these findings from Humphreys *et al* suggest chiropractic superiority in musculoskeletal competence, the findings also suggest that we in the chiropractic profession still have a lot of room for improvement within our own educational programs. The standardized musculoskeletal competency examination assesses only fundamental, basic, *minimal*

---

[25] Freedman KB, Bernstein J. Educational deficiencies in musculoskeletal medicine. *J Bone Joint Surg Am*. 2002;84-A(4):604-8
[26] Joy EA, Hala SV. Musculoskeletal Curricula in Medical Education: Filling In the Missing Pieces. *The Physician and Sportsmedicine*. 2004; 32: 42-45
[27] Matzkin E, Smith ME, Freccero CD, Richardson AB. Adequacy of education in musculoskeletal medicine. *J Bone Joint Surg Am*. 2005 Feb;87-A(2):310-4
[28] Schmale GA. More evidence of educational inadequacies in musculoskeletal medicine. *Clin Orthop Relat Res*. 2005 Aug;(437):251-9
[29] Stockard AR, Allen TW. Competence levels in musculoskeletal medicine: comparison of osteopathic and allopathic medical graduates. J Am Osteopath Assoc. 2006 Jun;106(6):350-5
[30] Humphreys BK, Sulkowski A, McIntyre K, Kasiban M, Patrick AN. An examination of musculoskeletal cognitive competency in chiropractic interns. J Manipulative Physiol Ther. 2007 Jan;30(1):44-9

competence; it is a very weak "standard", and the chiropractic profession should set its sights for the attainment of mastery and excellence, not the achievement of minimal competence. To foster the achievement of this goal and high educational standards in general, I publicized a list of more than 50 competencies and 100 questions[31] which are reflective of modern integrative chiropractic orthopedics[32] and which surpass the elementary competence reflected by the standardized musculoskeletal competency examination.[33] Given that the drug-surgical treatments employed by allopaths result in millions of injuries, cause more than 180,000-225,000 iatrogenic deaths per year in America (range: 493-616 iatrogenic medical deaths per day), and cost more than $136 billion per year in drug-induced adverse effects[34,35], the chiropractic profession should not be satisfied with succeeding at the goal of parity with the medical profession. We are capable of far better than that, and our patients deserve the best that we can give them.

# Affirmation and Re-Birth of the Chiropractic Profession: Setting New Standards in Office-Based Musculoskeletal Care and Health Promotion

*Alex Vasquez, D.C., N.D.*

This article was originally published in two parts in *Dynamic Chiropractic*
http://www.dynamicchiropractic.com/mpacms/dc/article.php?id=52120
http://www.dynamicchiropractic.com/mpacms/dc/article.php?id=52136

## Introduction
Musculoskeletal disorders are the leading cause of pain, suffering, disability, direct and indirect healthcare expenses, and lost productivity in America as well as the rest of the world.[36] Furthermore, patients presenting with musculoskeletal pain may suffer from any of one or more causative disorders ranging from *benign* to *life-threatening*, including myofascial dysfunction, nutritional deficiencies, metastatic cancer, occult infections, acute compartment syndrome, and cauda equina syndrome.[37] It is therefore obvious that all primary healthcare professions must ensure competence in musculoskeletal diagnosis and treatment among their graduates.[38] Anything less than this presents a disservice to individual patients and a clear and present danger to the general public. Furthermore, the interventions employed for alleviation of musculoskeletal pain should be safe, effective, and cost-effective in order to optimize safety and effectiveness for patients while minimizing iatrogenesis and the financial burden on the

---

[31] For samples of suggested competencies, see http://optimalhealthresearch.com/competencies.html and download the PDF document of more than 100 questions and competencies.
[32] **Vasquez A.** Integrative Orthopedics, Second Edition 2007. http://optimalhealthresearch.com/orthopedics.html
[33] Hammer W. Test Yourself on Med School Musculoskeletal Education. **Naturopathy Digest** http://www.naturopathydigest.com/archives/2006/may/hammer.php
[34] "Recent estimates suggest that each year more than 1 million patients are injured while in the hospital and approximately 180,000 die because of these injuries. Furthermore, drug-related morbidity and mortality are common and are estimated to cost more than $136 billion a year." Holland EG, Degruy FV. Drug-induced disorders. Am Fam Physician. 1997 Nov 1;56(7):1781-8, 1791-2
[35] "These total to 225,000 deaths per year from iatrogenic causes." Starfield B. Is US health really the best in the world? JAMA. 2000 Jul 26;284(4):483-5
[36] Woolf A, Pfleger B. Burden of major musculoskeletal. conditions. *Bulletin of the World Health Organization* 2003;81:646-656 http://www.who.int/entity/bulletin/volumes/81/9/Woolf.pdf
[37] **Vasquez A.** Integrative Orthopedics, Second Edition 2007. http://optimalhealthresearch.com/orthopedics.html
[38] For samples of suggested competencies, see http://optimalhealthresearch.com/competencies.html and download the PDF document of more than 100 questions and competencies.

healthcare system. In consideration of these important issues, this article will briefly compare and contrast chiropractic and allopathic musculoskeletal competence, and then compare and contrast natural/chiropractic interventions with those commonly employed by allopaths; citations will direct interested readers to additional information.

**Comparative Assessment of Musculoskeletal Competence**
Several research studies published in respected peer-reviewed medical journals have sought to quantify and qualify the level of musculoskeletal competence among the primary healthcare professions, with the majority of these studies having been performed among allopathic/medical students and clinicians. In 1998, Freedman and Bernstein[39] published a landmark study in *Journal of Bone and Joint Surgery* wherein they administered a validated musculoskeletal competency examination to 85 recent medical graduates who had begun their hospital residency; **82% of these medical doctors failed to demonstrate basic competency on the examination**, leading the authors to conclude, "We therefore believe that medical school preparation in musculoskeletal medicine is inadequate." They repeated their study in 2002, and this time the examination questions, which had previously been validated by orthopedic specialists, were validated by directors of internal medicine departments; their conclusions stated, "According to the standard suggested by the program directors of internal medicine residency departments, **a large majority of the examinees once again failed to demonstrate basic competency in musculoskeletal medicine on the examination. It is therefore reasonable to conclude that medical school preparation in musculoskeletal medicine is inadequate.**"[40] In their 2004 review published in *Physician and Sportsmedicine*, Joy and Van Hala[41] describe the musculoskeletal training of allopathic physicians as "woefully inadequate" and note that among a sample of 85 recent medical graduates, "…the average time spent in rotations or courses devoted to orthopedics during medical school was only 2.1 weeks. One third of these examinees graduated without *any* formal training in orthopedics." In February 2005, Matzkin et al[42] administered a standardized test of musculoskeletal competency to 334 medical students, residents, and staff physicians; the conclusion from their study reads as follows: **"Seventy-nine percent of the participants failed the basic musculoskeletal cognitive examination. This suggests that training in musculoskeletal medicine is inadequate in both medical school and nonorthopaedic residency training programs."** Later in 2005, Schmale[43] showed that when a standardized musculoskeletal examination was administered "…**less than 50% of fourth-year [medical] students showed competency**… These results suggested that the curricular approach toward teaching musculoskeletal medicine at this medical school was insufficient..." In 2006, a small study of 54 osteopathic students showed that approximately 30% of these students had achieved competence in musculoskeletal medicine as assessed by virtually the same standardized test used in the previously cited studies.[44] Finally, in early 2007, Humphreys et al[45] administered the previously

---

[39] Freedman KB, Bernstein J. The adequacy of medical school education in musculoskeletal medicine. *J Bone Joint Surg Am*. 1998;80(10):1421-7
[40] Freedman KB, Bernstein J. Educational deficiencies in musculoskeletal medicine. *J Bone Joint Surg Am*. 2002;84-A(4):604-8
[41] Joy EA, Hala SV. Musculoskeletal Curricula in Medical Education: Filling In the Missing Pieces. *Physician and Sportsmedicine*. 2004; 32: 42-45
[42] Matzkin E, Smith ME, Freccero CD, Richardson AB. Adequacy of education in musculoskeletal medicine. *J Bone Joint Surg Am*. 2005 Feb;87-A(2):310-4
[43] Schmale GA. More evidence of educational inadequacies in musculoskeletal medicine. *Clin Orthop Relat Res*. 2005 Aug;(437):251-9
[44] Stockard AR, Allen TW. Competence levels in musculoskeletal medicine: comparison of osteopathic and allopathic medical graduates. *J Am Osteopath Assoc*. 2006 Jun;106(6):350-5
[45] Humphreys BK, Sulkowski A, McIntyre K, Kasiban M, Patrick AN. An examination of musculoskeletal cognitive competency in chiropractic interns. *J Manipulative Physiol Ther*. 2007 Jan;30(1):44-9

utilized standardized competency examination to a sample of 123 **senior chiropractic students from a single college to find that 51% of these students were competent in musculoskeletal care by this standard**. Remarkably, **the pass-rate for a group of 10 chiropractic doctors was 100% on this same examination that was consistently failed by allopathic students/doctors** and, according to a small study, osteopathic students. Thus, while additional data with larger, controlled, and more representative groups is needed, **the best available current evidence indicates that generally only 20-30% of allopathic seniors and graduates are competent in musculoskeletal medicine, while the comparable rate of competence among chiropractic seniors and clinicians ranges from 52-100%**. Again, more data is needed, but based upon results obtained from the administration of a standardized interprofessionally peer-reviewed test of musculoskeletal competence, chiropractic students and doctors far outshine their allopathic and osteopathic counterparts. Thus, to say that "chiropractors are just as good as medical doctors" in the musculoskeletal arena is an inaccurate undervaluation of the chiropractic profession's education, professionalism, and potential. According to the studies evaluating musculoskeletal competence, chiropractors are not "just as good" as allopaths; chiropractors appear to be "better."

## Comparative Assessment of Clinical Outcomes

The clinical management of musculoskeletal disorders is complicated and compromised by the overuse of pharmacosurgical treatments that often do more harm than good. Non-steroidal anti-inflammatory drugs are advocated as first-line treatment by the allopathic profession despite clear evidence that such drugs accelerate joint destruction[46,47,48,49] and result in more than 100,000 hospitalizations and more than 16,000 deaths per year.[50] Selective cyclooxygenase-2 inhibiting drugs ("coxibs") received the most aggressive marketing campaigns in American history to rocket their sales into the high-profit stratosphere[51] despite clear evidence of inefficacy, exorbitant expenses, and health risks including but not limited to interstitial nephritis[52], acute cholestatic hepatitis[53], toxic epidermal necrolysis[54] and predictable adverse cardiovascular events (including hypertension, stroke, myocardial infarction, and sudden death) that affected more than 160,000 Americans[55] and killed up to 55,000 Americans.[56] Arthroscopic surgery for osteoarthritis of the knee might be considered a hazard to the general public insofar as its benefits do not exceed

---

[46] "At...concentrations comparable to those... in the synovial fluid of patients treated with the drug, several NSAIDs suppress proteoglycan synthesis... These NSAID-related effects on chondrocyte metabolism ... are much more profound in osteoarthritic cartilage than in normal cartilage, due to enhanced uptake of NSAIDs by the osteoarthritic cartilage." Brandt KD. Effects of nonsteroidal anti-inflammatory drugs on chondrocyte metabolism in vitro and in vivo. *Am J Med*. 1987 Nov 20; 83(5A): 29-34

[47] "The case of a young healthy man, who developed avascular necrosis of head of femur after prolonged administration of indomethacin, is reported here." Prathapkumar KR, Smith I, Attara GA. Indomethacin induced avascular necrosis of head of femur. *Postgrad Med J*. 2000 Sep; 76(899): 574-5

[48] "This highly significant association between NSAID use and acetabular destruction gives cause for concern, not least because of the difficulty in achieving satisfactory hip replacements in patients with severely damaged acetabula." Newman NM, Ling RS. Acetabular bone destruction related to non-steroidal anti-inflammatory drugs. *Lancet*. 1985 Jul 6; 2(8445): 11-4

[49] Vidal y Plana RR, Bizzarri D, Rovati AL. Articular cartilage pharmacology: I. In vitro studies on glucosamine and non steroidal antiinflammatory drugs. *Pharmacol Res Commun*. 1978 Jun;10(6):557-69

[50] "Conservative calculations estimate that approximately 107,000 patients are hospitalized annually for nonsteroidal anti-inflammatory drug (NSAID)-related gastrointestinal (GI) complications and at least 16,500 NSAID-related deaths occur each year among arthritis patients alone. The figures for all NSAID users would be overwhelming, yet the scope of this problem is generally under-appreciated." Singh G. Recent considerations in nonsteroidal anti-inflammatory drug gastropathy. *Am J Med*. 1998;105(1B):31S-38S

[51] "Monsanto Co. and Pfizer Inc. said prescriptions for their anti-arthritis drug, Celebrex, totaled 7.4 million in the first six month of sales -- making it the most successful U.S. drug launch ever." Monsanto, Pfizer celebrate Celebrex. St. Louis Business Journal. July 20, 1999 http://www.bizjournals.com/stlouis/stories/1999/07/19/daily5.html

[52] Markowitz GS, Falkowitz DC, Isom R, Zaki M, Imaizumi S, Appel GB, D'Agati VD. Membranous glomerulopathy and acute interstitial nephritis following treatment with celecoxib. *Clin Nephrol*. 2003;59(2):137-42

[53] Grieco A, Miele L, Giorgi A, Civello IM, Gasbarrini G. Acute cholestatic hepatitis associated with celecoxib. *Ann Pharmacother*. 2002;36(12):1887-9

[54] Berger P, Dwyer D, Corallo CE. Toxic epidermal necrolysis after celecoxib therapy. *Pharmacotherapy*. 2002 Sep;22(9):1193-5. See also: Friedman B, Orlet HK, Still JM, Law E. Toxic epidermal necrolysis due to administration of celecoxib (Celebrex). *South Med J*. 2002;95(10):1213-4

[55] Topol EJ. Failing the public health--rofecoxib, Merck, and the FDA. *N Engl J Med*. 2004 Oct 21;351(17):1707-9

[56] David J. Graham, MD, MPH, (Associate Director for Science, Office of Drug Safety, US FDA) estimated that 139,000 Americans who took Vioxx suffered serious side effects; he estimated that the drug killed between 26,000 and 55,000 people. http://www.commondreams.org/views05/0223-35.htm http://www.fda.gov/cder/drug/infopage/vioxx/vioxxgraham.pdf Accessed November 25, 2006

those produced by placebo surgery[57,58] yet the procedure exposes patients to risk of anesthesia and other drugs while burdening patients, employers, insurers, and the American government with billions of dollars in annual costs.[59] Similarly, the comparative cost-effectiveness of surgery for lumbar disc herniation has not been established, and long-term results from this procedure are not dramatically different from non-surgical treatment.[60] Generally speaking, drug/surgical treatments cause more than 180,000-225,000 iatrogenic deaths per year (range: 493-616 iatrogenic medical deaths per day in America), millions of injuries, and cost more than $136 billion per year in drug-induced adverse effects.[61,62] These are probably serious underestimations of iatrogenic injury/death and unnecessary expense, since medical errors are common and are often unreported.[63,64,65,66]

Regarding cost-effectiveness, safety, patient satisfaction, and treatment outcomes for conservatively managed musculoskeletal conditions, the chiropractic profession fares well and often better than the allopathic/medical profession.[67,68,69,70,71,72] The dietary and nutritional interventions commonly used by chiropractic doctors for the supportive and direct treatment of musculoskeletal pain and inflammation are well substantiated by basic and clinical research published in peer-reviewed biomedical journals; see the following reviews for additional citations.[73,74,75] Consistent with chiropractic philosophy, the nutritional therapeutics employed by

---

[57] Moseley JB, O'Malley K, Petersen NJ, Menke TJ, Brody BA, Kuykendall DH, Hollingsworth JC, Ashton CM, Wray NP. A controlled trial of arthroscopic surgery for osteoarthritis of the knee. *N Engl J Med.* 2002;347:81-8

[58] Bernstein J, Quach T. A perspective on the study of Moseley et al: questioning the value of arthroscopic knee surgery for osteoarthritis. *Cleve Clin J Med.* 2003;70(5):401, 405-6, 408-10

[59] Gina Kolata. A Knee Surgery for Arthritis Is Called Sham. *The New York Times*, July 11, 2002

[60] "These findings suggest that in most cases there is no clear reason to advocate strongly for surgery apart from patient preference." Carragee E. Surgical treatment of lumbar disk disorders. *JAMA*. 2006 Nov 22;296(20):2485-7

[61] "Recent estimates suggest that each year more than 1 million patients are injured while in the hospital and approximately 180,000 die because of these injuries. Furthermore, drug-related morbidity and mortality are common and are estimated to cost more than $136 billion a year." Holland EG, Degruy FV. Drug-induced disorders. Am Fam Physician. 1997 Nov 1;56(7):1781-8, 1791-2

[62] "These total to 225,000 deaths per year from iatrogenic causes." Starfield B. Is US health really the best in the world? JAMA. 2000 Jul 26;284(4):483-5

[63] "Medical errors in pediatric patients are significantly underreported in incident report systems, particularly by physicians." Taylor JA, Brownstein D, Christakis DA, Blackburn S, Strandjord TP, Klein EJ, Shafii J. Use of incident reports by physicians and nurses to document medical errors in pediatric patients. *Pediatrics.* 2004 Sep;114(3):729-35 http://pediatrics.aappublications.org/cgi/content/full/114/3/729

[64] Osmon S, Harris CB, Dunagan WC, Prentice D, Fraser VJ, Kollef MH. Reporting of medical errors: an intensive care unit experience. *Crit Care Med.* 2004 Mar;32(3):727-33

[65] "UE incidence is strongly underreported by staff in comparison with observers." Capuzzo M, Nawfal I, Campi M, Valpondi V, Verri M, Alvisi R. Reporting of unintended events in an intensive care unit: comparison between staff and observer. *BMC Emerg Med.* 2005 May 27;5(1):3 http://www.biomedcentral.com/1471-227X/5/3

[66] "Health care professionals rarely document disclosure of iatrogenic events to patients and surrogates... The low rate of incidence report filing, however, suggests that, even when health care providers do discuss errors with patients, they do not disclose those conversations to the institution." Lehmann LS, Puopolo AL, Shaykevich S, Brennan TA. Iatrogenic events resulting in intensive care admission: frequency, cause, and disclosure to patients and institutions. *Am J Med.* 2005 Apr;118(4):409-13

[67] Manga P, Angus D, Papadopoulos C, et al. *The Effectiveness and Cost-Effectiveness of Chiropractic Management of Low-Back Pain*. Richmond Hill, Ontario: Kenilworth Publishing; 1993

[68] Meade TW, Dyer S, Browne W, Townsend J, Frank AO. Low-back pain of mechanical origin: randomised comparison of chiropractic and hospital outpatient treatment. *BMJ.* 1990;300(6737):1431-7

[69] Meade TW, Dyer S, Browne W, Frank AO. Randomised comparison of chiropractic and hospital outpatient management for low-back pain: results from extended follow up. *BMJ.* 1995;311(7001):349-5

[70] Legorreta AP, Metz RD, Nelson CF, Ray S, Chernicoff HO, Dinubile NA. Comparative analysis of individuals with and without chiropractic coverage: patient characteristics, utilization, and costs. *Arch Intern Med.* 2004;164:1985-92. This article documented reduced healthcare expenses among patients with chiropractic coverage compared to patients lacking such coverage, suggesting that chiropractic access may reduce overall healthcare costs and utilization of more dangerous drug and surgical treatments. Further, population-wide adverse effects associated with chiropractic care were not discovered.

[71] Rosner AL. Evidence-based clinical guidelines for the management of acute low-back pain: response to the guidelines prepared for the Australian Medical Health and Research Council. *J Manipulative Physiol Ther.* 2001;24(3):214-20

[72] Oliphant D. Safety of spinal manipulation in the treatment of lumbar disk herniations: a systematic review and risk assessment. *J Manipulative Physiol Ther.* 2004;27:197-210

[73] **Vasquez A**. Reducing Pain and Inflammation Naturally. Part 1: New Insights into Fatty Acid Biochemistry and the Influence of Diet. *Nutritional Perspectives* 2004; October: 5, 7-10, 12, 14 http://optimalhealthresearch.com/part1

[74] **Vasquez A**. Reducing Pain and Inflammation Naturally. Part 2: New Insights into Fatty Acid Supplementation and Its Effect on Eicosanoid Production and Genetic Expression. *Nutritional Perspectives* 2005; January: 5-16 http://optimalhealthresearch.com/part2

chiropractic doctors simultaneously alleviate pain while promoting musculoskeletal health and overall wellness. For example, vitamin D not only promotes skeletal health and eradicates low-back pain in deficient patients[76] but also improves sensorimotor/proprioceptive coordination[77] and reduces systemic inflammation[78] while also alleviating hypertension[79] and promoting psychological wellbeing[80] among its many other benefits.[81] Use of niacinamide[82], fatty acids[83], and specific botanical supplements (including willow extract[84] and proteolytic enzymes such as bromelain[85]) has been shown to alleviate pain and inflammation while promoting improved overall health and wellness.

Although their profession emphasizes musculoskeletal care, chiropractic doctors also treat nonmusculoskeletal conditions and promote overall health and wellness. Chiropractic management of chronic hypertension is so successful that it could revolutionize cardiovascular care in this country *and internationally* based on the unparalleled safety, effectiveness, and cost-effectiveness documented by Goldhamer and colleagues[86,87,88]; further, select nutritional supplements can also be used for the safe and effective *nonpharmaceutical* treatment of hypertension.[89] Research I've extensively reviewed and compiled elsewhere (*Integrative Orthopedics*) strongly suggests that integrative chiropractic wellness promotion could raise and set a new standard in healthcare, delivering safety, efficacy, and cost-effectiveness that have hitherto not been seen in America. **So why is it that a profession with so much current promise and future potential is so undervalued, underutilized, underfunded?** In order to understand and describe the limitations placed on the chiropractic profession and the limitations placed on patients who could benefit from enhanced access to chiropractic care, we have to look at limiting forces that exist *inside* and *outside* the profession.

---

[75] **Vasquez A**. Reducing pain and inflammation naturally - Part 3: Improving overall health while safely and effectively treating musculoskeletal pain. *Nutritional Perspectives* 2005; 28: 34-38, 40-42 http://optimalhealthresearch.com/part3
[76] Al Faraj S, Al Mutairi K. Vitamin D deficiency and chronic low back pain in Saudi Arabia. *Spine*. 2003 Jan 15;28(2):177-9
[77] "This suggests that vitamin D supplementation improves neuromuscular or neuroprotective function, which may in part explain the mechanism whereby vitamin D reduces falls and fractures." Dhesi JK, et al. Vitamin D supplementation improves neuromuscular function in older people who fall. *Age Ageing*. 2004;33:589-95
[78] Timms PM, Mannan N, Hitman GA, et al. Circulating MMP9, vitamin D and variation in the TIMP-1 response with VDR genotype: mechanisms for inflammatory damage in chronic disorders? *QJM*. 2002 Dec;95(12):787-96
[79] Pfeifer M, Begerow B, Minne HW, Nachtigall D, Hansen C. Effects of a short-term vitamin D(3) and calcium supplementation on blood pressure and parathyroid hormone levels in elderly women. *J Clin Endocrinol Metab*. 2001 Apr;86(4):1633-7
[80] Vieth R, Kimball S, Hu A, Walfish PG. Randomized comparison of the effects of the vitamin D3 adequate intake versus 100 mcg (4000 IU) per day on biochemical responses and the wellbeing of patients. *Nutr J*. 2004 Jul 19;3:8
[81] **Vasquez A**, Manso G, Cannell J. The clinical importance of vitamin D (cholecalciferol): a paradigm shift with implications for all healthcare providers. *Altern Ther Health Med*. 2004 Sep-Oct;10(5):28-36 http://optimalhealthresearch.com/monograph04
[82] Kaufman W. Niacinamide therapy for joint mobility. Therapeutic reversal of a common clinical manifestation of the "normal" aging process. *Conn State Med J* 1953;17:584-591
[83] Maroon JC, Bost JW. Omega-3 fatty acids (fish oil) as an anti-inflammatory: an alternative to nonsteroidal anti-inflammatory drugs for discogenic pain. *Surg Neurol*. 2006 Apr;65(4):326-31
[84] "CONCLUSION: Willow bark extract may be a useful and safe treatment for low back pain." Chrubasik S, Eisenberg E, Balan E, Weinberger T, Luzzati R, Conradt C. Treatment of low back pain exacerbations with willow bark extract: a randomized double-blind study. *Am J Med*. 2000 Jul;109(1):9-14
[85] Trickett P. Proteolytic enzymes in treatment of athletic injuries. *Appl Ther*. 1964;30:647-52. See also: Walker AF, Bundy R, Hicks SM, Middleton RW. Bromelain reduces mild acute knee pain and improves well-being in a dose-dependent fashion in an open study of otherwise healthy adults. *Phytomedicine*. 2002;9:681-6. For nonmusculoskeletal considerations, see: Gonzalez NJ, Isaacs LL. Evaluation of pancreatic proteolytic enzyme treatment of adenocarcinoma of the pancreas, with nutrition and detoxification support. *Nutr Cancer*. 1999;33(2):117-24; see also: Sakalova A, Bock PR, Dedik L, Hanisch J, Schiess W, Gazova S, Chabronova I, Holomanova D, Mistrik M, Hrubisko M. Retrolective cohort study of an additive therapy with an oral enzyme preparation in patients with multiple myeloma. *Cancer Chemother Pharmacol*. 2001 Jul;47 Suppl:S38-44
[86] Goldhamer A, et al. Medically supervised water-only fasting in the treatment of hypertension. *J Manipulative Physiol Ther* 2001 Jun;24(5):335-9
[87] Goldhamer AC, et al. Medically supervised water-only fasting in the treatment of borderline hypertension. *J Altern Complement Med*. 2002 Oct;8(5):643-50
[88] Goldhamer AC. Initial cost of care results in medically supervised water-only fasting for treating high blood pressure and diabetes. *J Altern Complement Med*. 2002 Dec;8(6):696-7
[89] Vasquez A. Nutritional Treatments for Hypertension. *Naturopathy Digest* 2006 Nov http://www.naturopathydigest.com/archives/2006/nov/vasquez.php

## Limitations from Outside

The American Medical Association (AMA) and other powerful pharmacosurgical groups conspired to destroy the chiropractic profession[90,91] the osteopathic profession[92], and the naturopathic profession, and hence limit Americans' right to choose their healthcare; the details of these events and the resulting court order are well documented and widely accessible.[93,94,95,96] There can be no doubt that these illegal actions by the AMA and its coconspirators set the chiropractic profession back considerably by measures of income, professional advancement, cultural authority, esteem, and internal cohesion. Thus, by each one of these measures, the illegal AMA conspiracy was *and continues to be* a remarkable success. Even today, the AMA is spearheading nationwide actions to further limit the practices of non-allopathic professionals[97]; this is a problem in Texas, for example, where the well-funded Texas Medical Association recently sued the Texas Board of Chiropractic Examiners to enforce restrictions in the scope of chiropractic practice.[98] Medical journals and associations continue to defame the chiropractic profession even when the scientific bases for such defamatory actions are unfounded.[99,100,101] Insurance companies and so-called "health maintenance organizations" limit chiropractic reimbursement and coverage and thereby restrict patients' access to care and the individual practitioner's ability to survive and thrive. Since a profession can never exceed the average success of each its members, different groups collectively succeed in restricting *the profession* by restricting *the practices of individual doctors*. Defamation and marginalization of the profession undermines attempts to gain federal and private funding for better faculty, facilities, and research, and lack of these resources promotes additional devaluation and marginalization; thus a vicious cycle is created.

## Limitations from Inside

The intensity of the AMA's conspiracy forced early chiropractors to adopt the use of non-medical jargon so that chiropractic practice would not be misconstrued as "practicing medicine without a

---

[90] Getzendanner S. Permanent injunction order against AMA. *JAMA*. 1988 Jan 1;259(1):81-2 http://www.optimalhealthresearch.com/archives/wilk-ama-judgement.pdf
[91] Wilk CA. Medicine, Monopolies, and Malice: How the Medical Establishment Tried to Destroy Chiropractic. Garden City Park: Avery, 1996
[92] The osteopathic profession—labeled as "cultists" by the American Medical Association, which stated in 1953 that "…all voluntary associations with osteopaths are unethical"—was likewise faced with extinction, until merger with allopathic medicine was the only remaining strategy—a strategy which the medical profession believed would eventually destroy the osteopathic profession. In his review of osteopathic history, Gevitz* writes, "…the M.D.'s gradually came to believe that the only way to destroy osteopathy was through the absorption of D.O.'s, much as the homeopaths and eclectics had been swallowed up early in the century." Even today, the AMA continues to list osteopathic medicine under "alternative medicine"** even though several osteopathic medical colleges have consistently provided training that is superior to most "conventional" medical schools.*** See the following references: *Gevitz N. The D.O.'s: Osteopathic Medicine in America. Johns Hopkins University Press; 1991; pages 100-103. **American Medical Association. Report 12 of the Council on Scientific Affairs (A-97) Full Text http://www.ama-assn.org/ama/pub/category/13638.html on February 15, 2005. *** Special report. America's best graduate schools. Schools of Medicine. The top schools: primary care. *US News World Rep*. 2004 Apr 12;136(12):74
[93] Spivak JL. The Medical Trust Unmasked. Louis S. Siegfried Publishers; New York: 1961
[94] Trever W. In the Public Interest. Los Angeles; Scriptures Unlimited; 1972. This is probably the most authoritative documentation of the illegal actions of the AMA up to 1972; contains numerous photocopies of actual AMA documents and minutes of official meetings with overt intentionality of destroying Americans' healthcare options so that the AMA and related organizations would have a monopoly in national healthcare.
[95] Wolinsky H, Brune T. The Serpent on the Staff: The Unhealthy Politics of the American Medical Association. GP Putnam and Sons, New York, 1994
[96] Carter JP. Racketeering in Medicine: The Suppression of Alternatives. Norfolk: Hampton Roads Pub; 1993
[97] "In an effort to marshal the medical community's resources against the growing threat of expanding scope of practice for allied health professionals, the AMA has formed a national partnership to confront such initiatives nationwide… The committee will use $25,000…" Daly R, American Psychiatric Association. AMA Forms Coalition to Thwart Non-M.D. Practice Expansion. *Psychiatric News* 2006 March; 41: 17 http://pn.psychiatryonline.org/cgi/content/full/41/5/17-a?eaf Accessed November 25, 2006
[98] Physicians Ask Court to Protect Patients From Illegal Chiropractic Activities. http://www.texmed.org/Template.aspx?id=5259
[99] Terrett AG. Misuse of the literature by medical authors in discussing spinal manipulative therapy injury. *J Manipulative Physiol Ther* 1995;18:203-10
[100] Morley J, Rosner AL, Redwood D. A case study of misrepresentation of the scientific literature: recent reviews of chiropractic. *J Altern Complement Med*. 2001 Feb;7(1):65-78
[101] Wenban AB. Inappropriate use of the title 'chiropractor' and term 'chiropractic manipulation' in the peer-reviewed biomedical literature. *Chiropr Osteopat*. 2006 Aug 22;14:16 http://www.chiroandosteo.com/content/14/1/16

license", thereby saving chiropractors from the medical witch-hunt that generally aimed to jail the practitioner and burn his/her practice and reputation at the stake.[102] Rejection of medical concepts and terminology eventually morphed from "anti-medical" to "anti-scientific" in some chiropractic colleges and organizations, such that a sizable and vocal faction of chiropractic graduates entered practice with a disdain for words and phrases like diagnosis, treatment, spinal manipulation, and lab tests; these graduates were lead to believe that the chiropractic profession did nothing more than "analyze" and "adjust" the spine and that using lab tests and nutritional supplements made them "too medical." Thankfully, authentic chiropractic holism (represented schematically by the Triad of Health; see graphic) is being revitalized in individual practitioners and the profession. Obviously, we as a profession can waste no time or attention on antiscientific dogmatists who retard the advancement of our profession under the guise of a limited and self-serving interpretation of "chiropractic philosophy" which often devolves into a kind of "chiropractic evangelism" based on the belief that the "adjustment cures all." Anyone who advocates that the chiropractic profession is concerned only with the spine—*to the exclusion of the rest of the body and other factors that affect health*—has misunderstood, misrepresented, and limited our profession.

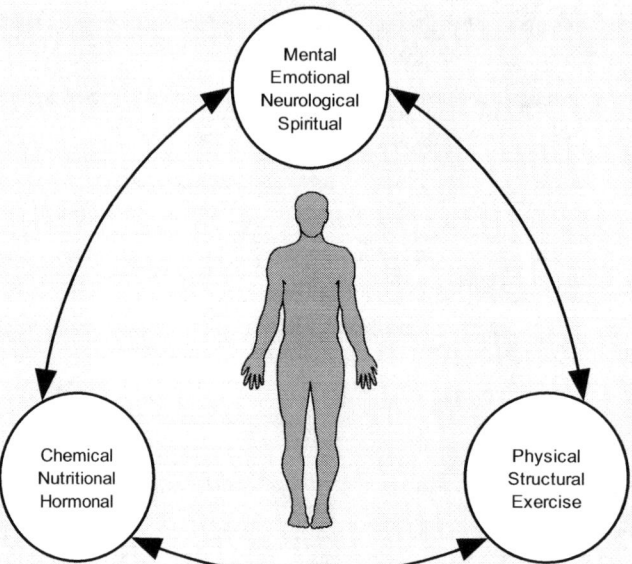

Illustration from Vasquez A. *Integrative Orthopedics, Second Edition: 2007.* Used with permission.

## The Rebirth of the Chiropractic Profession

The time has come for the chiropractic profession to reaffirm and reunite with its original holistic identity. DD Palmer wrote "The human body represents the actions of three laws—spiritual, mechanical, and chemical—united as one triune. As long as there is perfect union of these three, there is health."[103] The chiropractic profession has been holistic and "integrative" since its very inception.[104]

---

[102] Seaman D. A Cure for the Curse of Chiropractic, Part One. *Dynamic Chiropractic*. January 29, 2007, Volume 25, Issue 03 http://www.chiroweb.com/archives/25/03/16.html
[103] Palmer DD. *The Science, Art, and Phiosophy, of Chiropractic*. Portland, OR; Portland Printing House Company, 1910: page 107
[104] Beckman JF, Fernandez CE, Coulter ID. A systems model of health care: a proposal. *J Manipulative Physiol Ther*. 1996 Mar-Apr; 19(3): 208-15

Four of the biggest threats to the American public health are 1) skyrocketing medical costs (resulting in bankruptcy and healthcare inaccessibility[105]), 2) nationwide shortage of physicians (further contributing to increased costs and inaccessibility), 3) lifestyle diseases such as obesity, diabetes, and hypertension, and 4) medical iatrogenesis (conservatively estimated to be the fourth-sixth leading cause of death in America[106]). Increased utilization of chiropractic services would have a salutary effect on each and every one of these problems. The 2007 definition of the chiropractic profession clearly affirms and articulates our holistic tenets, and our practices should reflect this diagnostic and therapeutic diversity: "Doctors of Chiropractic are physicians who consider man as an integrated being and give special attention to the physiological and biochemical aspects including structural, spinal, musculoskeletal, neurological, vascular, psychological, nutritional, visceral, emotional and environmental relationships..."[107]

The American public has made its position very clear: they want nonmedical and nonsurgical healthcare options; they prefer safe and effective natural treatments over expensive and often hazardous drugs and surgery. **The chiropractic profession is uniquely positioned to take on an empowered role in the American healthcare system. Chiropractic doctors should embrace their holistic heritage and provide the American people with the safe and effective integrative healthcare it demands and deserves. Public demand is on our side.[108] The research is on our side. The days of "submission for survival" are past. The time for action, reaffirmation, and authentic and assertive empowerment has arrived.**

---

[105] Himmelstein DU, Warren E, Thorne D, Woolhandler S. Illness and injury as contributors to bankruptcy. *Health Aff* (Millwood). 2005 Jan-Jun;Suppl Web Exclusives:W5-63-W5-73

[106] "Even if the lower confidence limit of 76000 fatalities was used to be conservative, we estimated that ADRs could still constitute the sixth leading cause of death in the United States, after heart disease (743460), cancer (529904), stroke (150108), pulmonary disease (101077), and accidents (90523); this would rank ADRs ahead of pneumonia (75719) and diabetes (53894)." Lazarou J, Pomeranz BH, Corey PN. Incidence of adverse drug reactions in hospitalized patients: a meta-analysis of prospective studies. *JAMA*. 1998;279:1200-5

[107] American Chiropractic Association. Preface: Master Plan Definitions. http://www.amerchiro.org/level2_css.cfm?T1ID=10&T2ID=117 Accessed Feb 11, 2007

[108] Eisenberg DM, Davis RB, Ettner SL, Appel S, Wilkey S, Van Rompay M, Kessler RC.Trends in alternative medicine use in the United States, 1990-1997: results of a follow-up national survey. *JAMA*. 1998;280:1569-75

## Foreword

In this publication, Dr. Vasquez encourages and challenges doctors of chiropractic to re-imagine their roles in the delivery of health care services. In particular, he focuses on the care of patients with chronic hypertension, recognizing that high blood pressure is merely an indicator of underlying functional disorders and not a discrete disease entity.

Why chronic hypertension? As Dr. Vasquez notes, heart disease and vascular disorders cause tremendous losses in quality of life for a large segment of the population and are the primary causes of death in our society. Chronic high blood pressure is both *a cause of* and *an indicator of* vascular dysfunction and disease. For the most part, these health problems are self-inflicted, meaning that they are the result of how we live, what we eat, and how we view health care in general. Similarly, Dr. Vasquez submits that patients with vascular problems as indicated by chronic hypertension can be managed through dietary changes and exercise almost always more effectively and safely than by conventional drug-based therapies.

Why chiropractic doctors? Doctors of chiropractic have traditionally and consistently viewed their patients as whole beings, and the chiropractic management of patient concerns has been directed toward optimizing function and performance rather than simply eliminating disease symptoms. Lifestyle advice and dietary counseling are consistent with the philosophy and scope of chiropractic practice, because they address the cause and not just the symptoms of the underlying disorder. Dr. Vasquez artfully contends that chronic hypertension is a clinical finding of vascular dysfunction that is best managed with exercise and dietary measures, and that chiropractic doctors are uniquely positioned to provide such management. I wholeheartedly agree with him.

Clinical evaluation and management of patients with chronic hypertension should and can be done by chiropractic doctors, and Dr. Vasquez's text shows how this can be accomplished. The benefits of this protocol extend beyond reduced hypertensive morbidity and mortality to include alleviation of comorbid conditions such as depression, migraines, and back pain and enhanced vitality and sense of wellbeing. I commend Dr. Vasquez's excellent work and encourage the profession to embrace and apply his recommendations.

Joseph Brimhall, D.C.
President, University of Western States
January 2010

# Hypertension (HTN)
# High Blood Pressure (HBP)

**Description & Pathophysiology**:
- The emphasis of this section will, of course, be the integrative management of so-called "primary" or "idiopathic" hypertension (HTN), which is generally considered "idiopathic" from an outdated medical perspective that previously and currently failed to appreciate and integrate the research that has clarified the numerous causes of and contributors to HTN. From the allopathic medical perspective, >90-95% of HTN is considered idiopathic and thus by definition "of no known cause" and therefore appropriate for treatment with drugs. **Medically managed patients with HTN generally take two or more antihypertensive drugs from the time of diagnosis until the end of their lives; these drugs commonly cause adverse effects, are relatively devoid of collateral benefits, and do not address the underlying causative physiologic imbalances. Patients managed with nutritional and lifestyle modifications must likewise remain compliant with the prescribed health-promoting treatment-diet-lifestyle, but they generally experience clinically and statistically meaningful collateral benefits**; for example, ❶ **correction of vitamin D deficiency can alleviate hypertension**[1] and musculoskeletal pain[2] while improving mood[3,4]; ❷ **fish oil supplementation slightly lowers blood pressure** but tremendously and safely lowers cardiovascular mortality and all-cause mortality[5] while also improving mental health[6] and alleviating pain and inflammation[7,8]; ❸ **CoQ-10 is very effective for the treatment of HTN**[9] while also restoring lost renal function[10,11], alleviating migraine headaches[12], and helping to control asthma.[13] The exemplary nutritional interventions listed in the previous sentence are virtually devoid of adverse effects when employed with a modicum of competence and are widely available. If the routine outpatient medical treatment of HTN

---

[1] "A short-term supplementation with vitamin D(3) and calcium is more effective in reducing SBP than calcium alone. Inadequate vitamin D(3) and calcium intake could play a contributory role in the pathogenesis and progression of hypertension and cardiovascular disease in elderly women." Pfeifer M, Begerow B, Minne HW, Nachtigall D, Hansen C. Effects of a short-term vitamin D(3) and calcium supplementation on blood pressure and parathyroid hormone levels in elderly women. *J Clin Endocrinol Metab*. 2001 Apr;86(4):1633-7
[2] "Findings showed that 83% of the study patients (n = 299) had an abnormally low level of vitamin D before treatment with vitamin D supplements. After treatment, clinical improvement in symptoms was seen in all the groups that had a low level of vitamin D, and in 95% of all the patients (n = 341). CONCLUSIONS: Vitamin D deficiency is a major contributor to chronic low back pain in areas where vitamin D deficiency is endemic." Al Faraj S, Al Mutairi K. Vitamin D deficiency and chronic low back pain in Saudi Arabia. *Spine*. 2003;28:177-9
[3] Vieth R, Kimball S, Hu A, Walfish PG. Randomized comparison of the effects of the vitamin D3 adequate intake versus 100 mcg (4000 IU) per day on biochemical responses and the wellbeing of patients. *Nutrition Journal* 2004, 3:8 http://www.nutritionj.com/content/3/1/8
[4] Lansdowne AT, Provost SC: Vitamin D3 enhances mood in healthy subjects during winter. *Psychopharmacology* (Berl) 1998, 135:319-323
[5] GISSI-Prevenzione Investigators. Dietary supplementation with n-3 polyunsaturated fatty acids and vitamin E after myocardial infarction: results of the GISSI-Prevenzione trial. Gruppo Italiano per lo Studio della Sopravvivenza nell'Infarto miocardico. *Lancet*. 1999 Aug 7;354(9177):447-55
[6] Peet M, Stokes C. Omega-3 fatty acids in the treatment of psychiatric disorders. *Drugs*. 2005;65(8):1051-9
[7] Maroon JC, Bost JW. Omega-3 fatty acids (fish oil) as an anti-inflammatory: an alternative to nonsteroidal anti-inflammatory drugs for discogenic pain. *Surg Neurol*. 2006 Apr;65(4):326-31
[8] "Many of the placebo-controlled trials of fish oil in chronic inflammatory diseases reveal significant benefit, including decreased disease activity and a lowered use of anti-inflammatory drugs." Simopoulos AP. Omega-3 fatty acids in inflammation and autoimmune diseases. *J Am Coll Nutr*. 2002 Dec;21(6):495-505
[9] Singh RB, Niaz MA, Rastogi SS, Shukla PK, Thakur AS. Effect of hydrosoluble coenzyme Q10 on blood pressures and insulin resistance in hypertensive patients with coronary artery disease. *J Hum Hypertens*. 1999 Mar;13(3):203-8
[10] Singh RB, Khanna HK, Niaz MA. Randomized, double-blind placebo-controlled trial of coenzyme Q10 in chronic renal failure: discovery of a new role. *J Nutr Environ Med* 2000;10:281-8
[11] Singh RB, Kumar A, Naiz MA, Singh RG, Gujrati S, Singh VP, Singh M, Singh UP, Taneja C, AND Rastogi SS. Randomized, Double-blind, Placebo-controlled Trial of Coenzyme Q10 in Patients with Endstage Renal Failure. *J Nutr Environ Med* 2003; 13 (1): 13–22
[12] Rozen TD, Oshinsky ML, Gebeline CA, Bradley KC, Young WB, Shechter AL, Silberstein SD. Open label trial of coenzyme Q10 as a migraine preventive. *Cephalalgia* 2002;22(2):137-41
[13] Gvozdjáková A, Kucharská J, Bartkovjaková M, Gazdíková K, Gazdík FE. Coenzyme Q10 supplementation reduces corticosteroids dosage in patients with bronchial asthma. *Biofactors*. 2005;25(1-4):235-40

were to shift away from synthetic chemical drugs that function by interfering with normal physiology (e.g., beta-adrenergic *blockers*, calcium channel *blockers*, ACE *inhibitors*, angiotensin-2 receptor *blockers*, etc) and toward the favor of natural treatments—diet optimization, body weight optimization, and evidence-based nutritional supplementation—that promote normalization of blood pressure by helping restore balance to the body's physiology (i.e., by facilitating the restoration of homeostasis) then meaningful authentic progress in the otherwise never-ending "fight against hypertension" would be made. (For more discussion, see "Thinking Outside the (Pill) Box" in the section of addenda and articles at the end of this document.)

> **Antihypertensive Drugs Function by Blocking Normal Function**
>
> "All antihypertensive [drugs]… produce their effects by interfering with normal mechanisms of blood pressure regulation."
>
> Benowitz NL. "Antihypertensive Agents." In Katzung BG (editor). Basic and Clinical Pharmacology. Tenth Edition. New York: McGraw Hill Medical; 2007, p159

- Increased risk for cardiovascular mortality begins with blood pressures that are still well within the accepted normal range; therefore blood pressure that is consistent with **an official diagnosis of hypertension—blood pressure consistently greater than 140 mm Hg systolic and/or greater than 90 mm Hg diastolic**—is clearly worthy of treatment if part of the clinical goal is—*as it should be*—to reduce unnecessary morbidity and early mortality. Benowitz[14] wrote, "**Starting at 115/75 mm Hg, cardiovascular risk doubles with each increment of 20/10 mm Hg throughout the blood pressure range.**" Thus, based on this data, from a *wellness* perspective proactive integrative clinicians would define HTN as > 115/75 mm Hg. Data from the Framingham study showed that sustained BP > 140/90 induces left ventricular hypertrophy.[15] A reduction of systolic BP (sBP) of -5 mm Hg correlates with a -7% reduction in cardiovascular mortality[16]; thus patients must be encouraged to take HTN and its effective treatment seriously, since even small numerical changes in BP can have impressive effects on the risk for cardiovascular complications.

- Sustained HTN accelerates the development of cardiovascular disease (CVD) and end-organ damage by several mechanisms including promotion of endothelial damage resulting in accelerated atherosclerosis (e.g., stroke, myocardial infarction, peripheral vascular disease), direct pressure (e.g., retinal hemorrhages, aortic aneurysm), hyperplastic arteriolosclerosis and occlusive vasculopathy due to smooth muscle proliferation, fibrosis, and hyaline deposition (e.g., hypertensive nephrosclerosis), interstitial edema (e.g., cerebral edema, peripheral edema), and pathologic myocardial adaptation (e.g.,

> **"Prehypertension" is Deadly: Mortality Increases Starting at 115/75 mm Hg**
>
> "Hypertension-related diseases are the leading causes of morbidity and mortality in industrially developed societies. Surprisingly, **68% of all mortality attributed to high blood pressure (BP) occurs with systolic BP between 120 and 140 mm Hg and diastolic BP below 90 mm Hg**. Dietary and lifestyle modifications are effective in the treatment of borderline hypertension."
>
> Goldhamer AC, Lisle DJ, Sultana P, Anderson SV, Parpia B, Hughes B, Campbell TC. Medically supervised water-only fasting in the treatment of borderline hypertension. *J Altern Complement Med*. 2002 Oct;8(5):643-50

---

[14] Benowitz NL. "Antihypertensive Agents." In Katzung BG (editor). Basic and Clinical Pharmacology. Tenth Edition. New York: McGraw Hill Medical; 2007, 159

[15] Kumar V, Abbas AK, Fausto N (Editors). Robbins and Cotran Pathologic Basis of Disease. Seventh Edition. Philadelphia: Elsevier; 2005, 587

[16] Nahas R. Complementary and alternative medicine approaches to blood pressure reduction: An evidence-based review. *Can Fam Physician*. 2008 Nov;54(11):1529-33 http://www.cfp.ca/cgi/content/full/54/11/1529

hypertrophic cardiomyopathy, hypertensive heart disease, congestive heart failure). Hyperplastic arteriolosclerosis causes hypertensive nephrosclerosis, characterized by renal ischemia which triggers release of renin and increased formation of angiotensin-2 which exacerbates renal ischemia and systemic hypertension.[17]

> **Hypertension costs more than 12% of healthcare expenditures: more than $185 billion per year in the US**
>
> "In 1998, the **direct costs of hypertension** in the USA were calculated to be **12.6%** of health care expenditures (**$185 billion**)... A similar figure was found based on analysis of the 1996 Medical Expenditure Panel Survey (i.e., **$177 billion**)."
>
> Tarride JE, Lim M, DesMeules M, Luo W, Burke N, O'Reilly D, Bowen J, Goeree R. A review of the cost of cardiovascular disease. Can J Cardiol. 2009 Jun;25(6):e195-202

- HTN is the single most important risk factor for the development of CVD. On a population-wide basis, achieving the target of ≤ 140 mmHg systolic would result in a 28-44% reduction in stroke and a 20-35% reduction in ischemic heart disease (IHD). In describing these benefits for the United Kingdom (population ~60 million in 2005), Tomson and Lip[18] noted that control of HTN would prevent approximately 42,800 strokes and 82,800 IHD events per year. In the United States (population ~300 million in 2005), **65% of adults are overweight or obese** (generally a direct result of *overconsumption malnutrition* and physical inactivity), and the number of deaths attributable to obesity is 280,184 yearly. At least 11 million Americans have type-2 diabetes mellitus, while **50 million Americans have HTN**.[19]

- HTN is important clinically for several reasons. First, as previously noted, HTN is a treatable and therefore avoidable contributor to cardiovascular disease (CVD) and other forms of end-organ damage—stroke, myocardial infarction, congestive heart failure, peripheral vascular disease, renal failure, and hypertensive retinopathy. Second, HTN as a clinical manifestation is often (always) a sign of underlying dysfunction or disease; thus **the finding of HTN is a sign to the clinician that one or more underlying physiologic imbalances are present and in need of detection and corrective interventional attention**. Third, HTN is not merely a disease; it is a business (leading diagnosis in Family Medicine practices[20]), and an industry (direct costs approach $200 billion per year in the United States). Among allopathic/osteopathic Family Medicine physicians, HTN is the single most common cause for patient visits; it is the most common single clinical diagnosis in Family Medicine practice. For the medical profession and pharmaceutical industry, antihypertensive medications and services are a major source of revenue. Direct annual medical expenses related to HTN exceed $185 billion per year in the United States. Most patients treated exclusively with drugs require *multiple drugs* for adequate BP control.[21]

- The prevalence of HTN among hunter-gatherer societies is virtually zero.[22] Contrasting the absence of CVD noted in *physically active* societies that consume *natural diets* against the pandemics of HTN and CVD seen in Westernized/industrialized nations, O'Keefe and

---

[17] Kumar V, Abbas AK, Fausto N (Editors). Robbins and Cotran Pathologic Basis of Disease. Seventh Edition. Philadelphia: Elsevier; 2005, 1007-8
[18] Tomson J, Lip GY. Blood pressure demographics: nature or nurture…genes or environment? BMC Med. 2005 Jan 7;3:3 http://www.biomedcentral.com/1741-7015/3/3
[19] Cordain L, Eaton SB, Sebastian A, Mann N, Lindeberg S, Watkins BA, O'Keefe JH, Brand-Miller J. Origins and evolution of the Western diet: health implications for the 21st century. Am J Clin Nutr. 2005 Feb;81(2):341-54 http://www.ajcn.org/cgi/content/full/81/2/341
[20] Sloane PD, Slatt LM, Ebell MH, Jacques LB, Smith MA (Eds). Essentials of Family Medicine, 5th Edition. Lippincott Williams & Wilkins, 2007
[21] Domino FJ (editor in chief). The 5-Minute Clinical Consult. 2010. 18th Edition. Philadelphia; Wolters Kluwer: 2009, 656-7
[22] Eaton SB, Shostak M, Konner M. The Paleolithic Prescription. New York: Harper and Row Publishers; 1988, 49

Cordain[23] wrote, "The lifetime incidence of hypertension [among Americans] is an astounding 90%, and the metabolic syndrome is present in up to 40% of middle-aged American adults. **Cardiovascular disease remains the number 1 cause of death**, accounting for 41% of all fatalities, and the prevalence of heart disease in the United States is projected to double during the next 50 years."

- In industrialized nations, the prevalence of HTN in adults is approximately 1 per 4-5 (20-25%) with the vast majority of these considered "idiopathic", "chronic", and "recalcitrant" from the dominant allopathic medical perspective. Integrative clinicians who appreciate the broad range of causes of and synergistic contributors to systemic hypertension do not generally appreciate the disease as *idiopathic* nor *chronic* nor *recalcitrant* but rather find it *understandable* and *highly amenable* to the numerous interventions—sometimes specific for each patient (e.g., food allergens)—supported by publications in peer-reviewed biomedical journals. The high prevalence of primary hypertension seen in industrialized/Westernized societies does not necessarily imply that the people in these societies are as a group genetically defective and therefore "in need of medical intervention" but perhaps rather that the industrialized/Westernized lifestyle is inherently adverse to the preservation of human health and longevity.[24]

- The obligations imposed upon clinicians in the management of hypertension are those of ❶ assessment for urgent situations and end-organ damage, ❷ differential diagnosis and comprehensive assessment, and ❸ effective treatment, which may occasionally necessitate referral to a specialist for recalcitrant cases, additional testing, or liability defense/dispersal. Because hypertension—like diabetes and hemochromatosis—is generally asymptomatic especially in its early stages and in milder cases, doctors (derived from the Latin *docere*, which means "to teach"[25]) have the responsibility ❹ to instruct patients on the nature of their disorder, its effects and treatment, and the consequences of nontreatment. Patients have the responsibility to comply with the treatment plan, implement an effective alternate plan, or absorb the consequences, most commonly including stroke, accelerated atherosclerosis (and resultant arterial occlusion leading to organ hypoperfusion [e.g., erectile dysfunction, peripheral arterial disease, mesenteric ischemia]), myocardial infarction, heart failure, aneurysm, nephropathy (and its attendant need for dialysis or transplant), vision loss, and the resultant disability and suffering associated with each of these. Finally, ❺ doctors must pre-schedule patients for follow-up office visits to monitor treatment adherence and therapeutic effectiveness.

**Clinical Presentations**:
- Clearly the vast majority of clinical presentations of HTN are silent, discovered only when the clinician finds elevated blood pressure on routine examination. This underscores the importance of hypertension screening among asymptomatic patients. The second and remaining group of clinical presentations of HTN includes those of end-organ damage: nephropathy, retinopathy, cardiomyopathy, and the consequences of HTN-accelerated CVD

---

[23] O'Keefe JH Jr, Cordain L. Cardiovascular disease resulting from a diet and lifestyle at odds with our Paleolithic genome: how to become a 21st-century hunter-gatherer. *Mayo Clin Proc*. 2004 Jan;79(1):101-8 http://www.mayoclinicproceedings.com/content/79/1/101.full.pdf

[24] Price WA. Nutrition and Physical Degeneration: A Comparison of Primitive and Modern Diets and Their Effects. Santa Monica; Price-Pottinger Nutrition Foundation: 1945

[25] Prakash R, Misra R, Misra R. Doctors as Teachers. *Psychiatric News* 2002; 37: 37 http://www.pn.psychiatryonline.org/content/37/9/37.1.full

including stroke, myocardial infarction, aortic dissection, and rupture of an enlarged (generally >5.5 cm) abdominal aortic aneurysm.
- Typical clinical presentations of the hypertensive patient can range from incidental to catastrophic and include the following:
    - Asymptomatic
    - Headache
    - Altered mental status
    - Congestive heart failure presenting with fatigue, lower extremity edema, or dyspnea
    - Myocardial infarction or sudden death due to accelerated CVD complicated by cardiac hypertrophy (i.e., supply-demand mismatch)
    - Retinopathy presenting as vision impairment
    - Accelerated complications of diabetes mellitus
    - Hypertensive nephropathy presenting with renal insufficiency: azotemia, edema, malignant hypertension, anuria/oliguria
    - Incidental finding during presentation and evaluation for another concern such as routine examination, injury, or infection

**Major Differential Diagnoses**: Characteristics of secondary hypertension include therapeutic recalcitrance, onset at an early age (< 30y) or an advanced age (>50y), and the typical features of the causative disorder, such as hypokalemia with hyperaldosteronism, and depression or musculoskeletal pain with hypovitaminosis D. Listed below are some of the more common primary causes of hypertension with a brief sketch of their classic clinical characteristics, including physical examination and laboratory findings.

- Aortic coarctation: Classic presentation includes upper extremity hypertension with lower extremity hypotension/hypoperfusion/claudication in a child or young adult; secondary activation of the renin-angiotensin system due to renal hypoperfusion exacerbates the HTN and complicates this *focal* anatomic disorder by adding a *systemic* neurohormonal component. Diagnosed by imaging the aorta such as with computed tomography (CT), magnetic resonance imaging/angiography (MRI/MRA), or echocardiogram (echo) or ultrasound (US).
- Cocaine: Acute and chronic uses of cocaine cause acute and chronic elevations in blood pressure. Drug cessation is the key to treatment; urine drug testing is appropriate for patients suspected of undisclosed drug use or noncompliance with cessation.
- Cushing's disease/syndrome: Excess glucocorticoids whether endogenous or exogenous promote sodium retention directly and by causing hyperinsulinemia via induction of peripheral insulin resistance. Useful tests include measurements of serum ACTH, urinary/salivary cortisol in addition to looking for the clinical characteristics of striae, sarcopenia, abdominal obesity, etc.
- Estrogen, oral contraceptives: As a group of various hormones, estrogens generally tend to promote sodium and water retention, which promotes volume overload and the development of HTN. For women with "estrogen dominance" due to endogenous production or exogenous administration of estrogens, supplementation with pyridoxine 50-250 mg/d (always with magnesium 600-1,200 mg/d or to bowel tolerance) and/or

progesterone can frequently offset the HTN-inducing effects of estrogens; a more comprehensive anti-estrogen protocol is outlined in chapter 4 of *Integrative Rheumatology*.[26]

- Ethanol: Excess ethanol consumption raises blood pressure and makes HTN more difficult to treat.
- Hypercalcemia: Easily diagnosed by routine laboratory testing; may be caused by hyperparathyroidism, malignancy, or rarely by nutritional excesses of calcium and/or vitamin D. Most hypercalcemia (80-90%) is due to hyperparathyroisim or malignancy; the most common cause of hypercalcemia in the outpatient setting is hyperparathyroidism, while in the hospital setting the most common cause is malignancy.[27]
- Insulin resistance and hyperinsulinemia: Insulin promotes renal retention of sodium which leads to water retention and the subsequent volume overload and systemic hypertension which logically follow in sequence. This explains the well proven and replicable benefit of low-carbohydrate diets in treating "idiopathic" HTN in the general population.
- Nonsteroidal anti-inflammatory drugs (NSAIDs): NSAIDs in general and COX-2 inhibitors (coxibs) in particular reduce endogenous production of vasodilating prostacyclin and thus cause pharmacologic/iatrogenic renal artery constriction, which leads to varying degrees of HTN via activation of the rennin-angiotensin system. This explains, in part, the increased cardiovascular mortality due to overutilization of coxibs such as rofecoxib/Vioxx, withdrawn from the US market in 2005 by the US FDA due to its causation of increased cardiovascular deaths.
- Pheochromocytoma: Exceedingly rare in contrast to the frequency with which it is mentioned in textbooks and seen in clinical practice; classic presentation is episodic HTN, headache, and diaphoresis; diagnosed with increased urinary catecholamines or vanillylmandelic acid with CT/MRI; treatment is surgical excision of the adrenal/extra-adrenal mass.
- Preeclampsia: A syndrome seen in pregnant women after week 20 of gestation consisting of hypertension, proteinuria, edema, and/or hypoperfusion; this syndrome can accelerate rapidly and cause life-threatening complications for the mother and/or fetus. Evidence suggests that the incidence of preeclampsia can be reduced via increased intake of aspirin, ascorbate, calcium, tocopherol(s), and magnesium while fully developed and recalcitrant cases require drug therapy and emergency interventions.[28]
- Primary hyperaldosteronism (Conn's syndrome): Caused by a unilateral adrenal adenoma or bilateral adrenal hyperplasia; typical finding is HTN with hypokalemia, rarely with slight hypernatremia; diagnosis is by increased urine or serum aldosterone, or by the more specific elevated aldosterone:renin ratio.
- Renal artery (renovascular) stenosis: Classically caused by fibromuscular dysplasia in young adult women (<25y) and by atherosclerosis in older adults (>50y); elevation in creatinine following administration of an ACE-inhibitor (angiotensin converting enzyme inhibitor) is a typical scenario for renal artery stenosis in medical school exams. Diagnosis is by renal ultrasound or arteriography; treatment is with stent placement, angioplasty, surgical repair, with or without chronic drug treatments.
- Renal disease: Renal disease can both *lead to* and *result from* HTN; chronic HTN causes renal parenchymal damage, and parenchymal damage (whether due to HTN or another cause such

---

[26] **Vasquez A**. Integrative Rheumatology. IBMRC 2006, 2007 and all future editions. http://optimalhealthresearch.com/rheumatology.html
[27] Bent S, Gensler LS, Frances C. Saint-Frances Guide: Clinical Clerkship in Outpatient Medicine. 2nd Edition. Philadelphia; Wolters Kluwer: 2008, 490
[28] Domino FJ (editor in chief). The 5-Minute Clinical Consult. 2010. 18th Edition. Philadelphia; Wolters Kluwer: 2009, 1062

as glomerulonephritis, pyelonephritis, polycystic kidneys, etc) leads to water retention and activation of the renin-angiotensin-aldosterone system thus promoting a vicious cycle. The clinical picture typically includes edema, elevated BUN and creatinine, and in severe cases anemia due to insufficient erythropoietin and osteomalacia due to insufficient formation of 1,25-dihydroxyvitamin D3.

- <u>Sleep apnea</u>: Obstructive sleep apnea (OSA) is a risk factor for HTN, and treatment for OSA with continuous positive airway pressure (CPAP) can produce small-modest reductions in BP that are proportionate to the severity of the HTN and compliance with treatment.
- <u>Systemic sclerosis and scleroderma</u>: HTN in general and treatment-resistant HTN in particular are seen in systemic sclerosis and scleroderma.
- <u>Thyroid disease, including both hyperthyroidism and hypothyroidism</u>: Assess clinically (e.g., pulse rate, physical exam, weight loss/gain, Achilles reflex return speed, body temperature), and with laboratory testing: serum TSH, free T4, free T3 and/or total T3; strongly consider testing reverse T3 when assessing for functional hypothyroidism. Some integrative clinicians hold that the ratio of total T3 to reverse T3 should be >10:1.
- <u>Tobacco use</u>: Tobacco smoke constituents cause arterioconstriction which promotes HTN. Constituents and free radicals in tobacco smoke are more pathogenic than nicotine, while the latter in isolation indeed causes adverse cardiovascular effects.
- <u>Upper cervical spine dysfunction/subluxation</u>: A remarkable clinical trial published in *Journal of Human Hypertension* in 2007 by Bakris et al[29] showed that **correction of upper cervical spine subluxation by chiropractic spinal manipulation causes "marked and sustained reductions in BP [blood pressure] similar to the use of two-drug combination therapy."**
- <u>Vitamin D deficiency</u>: Vitamin D deficiency is common in the general population—often up to 90-100% of subjects in large population-based studies—and causes intracellular hypercalcinosis[30] via elevated PTH levels and contributes to chronic HTN[31] via endothelial dysfunction, systemic inflammation, insulin resistance, and activation of the renin-angiotensin-aldosterone system.[32] **Correction of vitamin D deficiency can cause a reduction in elevated blood pressure equal to or greater than that which can be achieved by single-drug oral antihypertensive medication**[33] while also providing numerous collateral benefits (including reductions in depression, pain, and risks for autoimmune and malignant diseases) at lower cost and greater safety than can be achieved with pharmaceutical drugs.[34,35]

---

[29] Bakris G, Dickholtz M Sr, Meyer PM, Kravitz G, Avery E, Miller M, Brown J, Woodfield C, Bell B. Atlas vertebra realignment and achievement of arterial pressure goal in hypertensive patients: a pilot study. *J Hum Hypertens*. 2007 May;21(5):347-52

[30] **Vasquez A**. Intracellular Hypercalcinosis: A Functional Nutritional Disorder with Implications Ranging from Myofascial Trigger Points to Affective Disorders, Hypertension, and Cancer. *Naturopathy Digest* 2006 Previously published in-print and on-line at http://www.naturopathydigest.com/archives/2006/sep/vasquez.php and included at the end of this chapter.

[31] **Vasquez A**. Nutritional Treatments for Hypertension. *Naturopathy Digest* 2006. Previously published in-print and on-line at http://www.naturopathydigest.com/archives/2006/nov/vasquez.php and included at the end of this chapter.

[32] Pilz S, Tomaschitz A, Ritz E, Pieber TR; Medscape. Vitamin D status and arterial hypertension: a systematic review. *Nat Rev Cardiol*. 2009 Oct;6(10):621-30

[33] "A short-term supplementation with vitamin D(3) and calcium is more effective in reducing SBP than calcium alone. Inadequate vitamin D(3) and calcium intake could play a contributory role in the pathogenesis and progression of hypertension and cardiovascular disease in elderly women." Pfeifer M, Begerow B, Minne HW, Nachtigall D, Hansen C. Effects of a short-term vitamin D(3) and calcium supplementation on blood pressure and parathyroid hormone levels in elderly women. *J Clin Endocrinol Metab*. 2001 Apr;86(4):1633-7

[34] **Vasquez A**, Manso G, Cannell J. The clinical importance of vitamin D (cholecalciferol): a paradigm shift with implications for all healthcare providers. *Altern Ther Health Med*. 2004 Sep-Oct;10(5):28-36 http://optimalhealthresearch.com/cholecalciferol.html

[35] Faloon B. Millions of Needless Deaths. *Life Extension Magazine*. 2009 January http://lef.org/magazine/mag2009/jan2009_Millions-of-Needless-Deaths_01.htm

**Clinical Assessments**:
- **History/subjective**: As stated previously, **most patients with HTN are asymptomatic** and only become symptomatic as a result of severe HTN which is causing end-organ compromise, such as renal insufficiency, cerebral edema, or transient myocardial ischemia. The clinical history should include inquiry about chest pain, shortness of breath, family history of CVD or DM, morning occipital headaches, new stressors, tobacco/caffeine use, and current medications/drugs including antihypertensives, nonsteroidal antiinflammatory drugs (NSAIDs), estrogens, ethanol, cocaine, sympathomimetics and decongestants. During this standard *history of the present illness* which all clinicians are taught to master before graduation from their respective colleges, astute clinicians have already begun the psychographic assessment (described hereafter as "BVG-LOC profiling") which will enable them to couch the treatment objectives and details in a manner tailored for that particular patient. In this context, the patient's BVG-LOC profile (i.e., personal profile of beliefs, values, goals, and locus of control) must be appreciated by the clinician since each aspect is essential to the understanding needed by the clinician in order to address or "speak to" the patient in such a way as to improve treatment compliance—these concepts are discussed more under the section *Clinical Management* below.
- **Physical Examination/Objective**:
  - Physical examination and vital signs: A screening physical examination is necessary (with details emphasized below) along with documentation of findings and vital signs, including blood pressure, pulse rate, breathing rate, temperature, pain level; weight and body mass index should be noted. Auscultation of the heart, lungs, carotid and renal arteries is performed; and cranial nerves are screened. Deep tendon reflexes are checked for hyperreflexia, and the Achilles reflex return is assessed for any delay that might indicate hypothyroidism[36], a well-documented cause of HTN and dyslipidemia.
  - Blood pressure measurement: Screening for HTN should be performed at least once every two years starting at 18 years of age. The blood pressure cuff must be at heart level and properly fitted to the patient; the patient should be relaxed and seated for 5 minutes prior to blood pressure measurement. The two measurements upon which the diagnosis of HTN is being considered should occur on different visits at least 3 days apart; if the blood pressure is >160/100 mm Hg on any one visit, then a presumptive diagnosis of HTN can be made and treatment initiated. Blood pressure ≥120/80 -140/90 is considered "prehypertension" and is observed for progression without drug treatment[37] but is obviously a prime opportunity to intervene with nutritional and lifestyle interventions. Blood pressure ≥140/90-160/100 is considered "stage 1 hypertension" and in the medical model is initially treated with one drug—generally a thiazide—while blood pressure ≥160/100-210/120 ("stage 2 hypertension") is often treated initially with a two-drug combination, with one of those drugs generally being a thiazide. Blood pressures ≥210/120 are worthy of urgent or emergency treatment, based on the absence or presence of symptoms or organ damage, respectively, in an emergency hospital setting.

---

[36] Degowin RL. *DeGowin and DeGowin's Diagnostic Evaluation. Sixth Edition*. New York: McGraw Hill: 1994, 900. For a more recent citation, see Khurana AK, Sinha RS, Ghorai BK, Bihari N. Ankle reflex photomotogram in thyroid dysfunctions. *J Assoc Physicians India*. 1990 Mar;38(3):201-3
[37] Le T, Dehlendorf C, Mendoza M, Ohata C. First Aid for the Family Medicine Boards. New York: McGraw-Hill Medical; 2008, 50

- o Cardiopulmonary examination: Auscultation for rate, rhythm, rales/crackles; localize the cardiac point of maximal impulse (PMI) for evidence of lateral displacement or increased intensity which could indicate cardiomegaly or left ventricular hypertrophy.
- o Body mass index (BMI) for assessing current BMI and predicting amount and duration of weight loss: Given that the average citizen of industrialized nations is overweight, nearly all patients can benefit from developing a specific goal-oriented and time-oriented plan for the achievement of weight optimization. **Contrasting current BMI with optimal BMI** clarifies the **amount of weight** that needs to be lost and provides an estimate of the **duration of the weight loss program**, given that adherent patients can lose an average of 4-8 lbs (~9-15 kg) per month. Although some patients can achieve highly significant improvements in various parameters such as glycemic control and blood pressure without significant weight loss, the fact remains that obesity is a **risk factor** and often the **primary determinant** for CVD as well as osteoarthritis, many types of cancer, and significant but immeasurable (and generally unspoken) suffering associated with low self esteem, inefficacy, social isolation, and depression. Patients have a myriad of reasons and rationalizations for maintaining their overweight status quo—every excuse from being "big boned" to "big framed" to "I've always been big" to "Everyone in my family is big" to "I don't have time to take care of myself" to "I don't know how to cook" to "I simply cannot [eat right, exercise, say no to candy, give up wheat, give up ice cream, drink coffee without sugar and cream]." Clinicians need to anticipate this resistance and have a diverse array of techniques—ranging from patient to insistent, from gentle to confrontational, from emotional to intellectual—to use *as appropriate to the individual patient's needs* to coax, inspire, lead, or push the patient who will benefit from weight loss. Elevated BMI correlates with numerous biochemical risk factors for CVD—progressively elevated levels of blood glucose, insulin, triglycerides, increasing severity of insulin resistance, with progressively lower levels of beneficial high-density lipoprotein (HDL) cholesterol—and an increased risk for cardiovascular death, psychosocial problems including low self-esteem, reduced academic performance, impaired interpersonal relationships including *for example* being a target for prejudice.[38] Elevated BMI is a preventable and treatable condition; physicians should not ignore this problem simply because it is common or difficult for some patients to acknowledge and effectively address.

> **Weight Loss Provides Numerous Psychosocial and Physical Benefits**
>
> "With a substantial weight loss of 35 kg and 42% loss of excessive weight, and correction of disturbed metabolic parameters, they significantly improved in general well-being, health distress, and perceived attractiveness, approaching halfway the values of a normal-weight reference group. ... In physical activity, they bypassed the reference group. Days of sick leave decreased to the level of the reference group. Improvements in HRQL paralleled the rate of weight loss."
>
> Mathus-Vliegen EM, de Weerd S, de Wit LT. Health-related quality-of-life in patients with morbid obesity after gastric banding for surgically induced weight loss. *Surgery*. 2004 May;135(5):489-97

---

[38] Costa GB, Horta N, Resende ZF, et al. Body mass index has a good correlation with proatherosclerotic profile in children and adolescents. *Arq Bras Cardiol*. 2009 Sep;93(3):261-7 http://www.scielo.br/pdf/abc/v93n3/en_a10v93n3.pdf

## BODY MASS INDEX interpretation

- Underweight: Under 18.5
- **Normal: 18.5-24**
- Overweight: 25-29
- Obese: 30 and over
- Severe obesity: > 40
- Morbid obesity: >40.0–49.9

### WEIGHT in pounds

| HEIGHT | 100 | 110 | 120 | 130 | 140 | 150 | 160 | 170 | 180 | 190 | 200 | 210 | 220 | 230 | 240 | 250 |
|---|---|---|---|---|---|---|---|---|---|---|---|---|---|---|---|---|
| 5'0" | 20 | 21 | 23 | 25 | 27 | 29 | 31 | 33 | 35 | 37 | 39 | 41 | 43 | 45 | 47 | 49 |
| 5'1" | 19 | 21 | 23 | 25 | 26 | 28 | 30 | 32 | 34 | 36 | 38 | 40 | 42 | 43 | 45 | 47 |
| 5'2" | 18 | 20 | 22 | 24 | 26 | 27 | 29 | 31 | 33 | 35 | 37 | 38 | 40 | 42 | 44 | 46 |
| 5'3" | 18 | 19 | 21 | 23 | 25 | 27 | 28 | 30 | 32 | 34 | 35 | 37 | 39 | 41 | 43 | 44 |
| 5'4" | 17 | 19 | 21 | 22 | 24 | 26 | 27 | 29 | 31 | 33 | 34 | 36 | 38 | 39 | 41 | 43 |
| 5'5" | 17 | 18 | 20 | 22 | 23 | 25 | 27 | 28 | 30 | 32 | 33 | 35 | 37 | 38 | 40 | 42 |
| 5'6" | 16 | 18 | 19 | 21 | 23 | 24 | 26 | 27 | 29 | 31 | 32 | 34 | 36 | 37 | 39 | 40 |
| 5'7" | 16 | 17 | 19 | 20 | 22 | 23 | 25 | 27 | 28 | 30 | 31 | 33 | 34 | 36 | 38 | 39 |
| 5'8" | 15 | 17 | 18 | 20 | 21 | 23 | 24 | 26 | 27 | 29 | 30 | 32 | 33 | 35 | 36 | 38 |
| 5'9" | 15 | 16 | 18 | 19 | 21 | 22 | 24 | 25 | 27 | 28 | 30 | 31 | 32 | 34 | 35 | 37 |
| 5'10" | 14 | 16 | 17 | 19 | 20 | 22 | 23 | 24 | 26 | 27 | 29 | 30 | 32 | 33 | 34 | 36 |
| 5'11" | 14 | 15 | 17 | 18 | 20 | 21 | 22 | 24 | 25 | 26 | 27 | 28 | 30 | 32 | 33 | 35 |
| 6'0" | 14 | 15 | 16 | 18 | 19 | 20 | 22 | 23 | 24 | 26 | 27 | 28 | 30 | 31 | 33 | 34 |
| 6'1" | 13 | 15 | 16 | 17 | 18 | 20 | 21 | 22 | 24 | 25 | 26 | 28 | 29 | 30 | 32 | 33 |
| 6'2" | 13 | 14 | 15 | 17 | 18 | 19 | 21 | 22 | 23 | 24 | 26 | 27 | 28 | 30 | 31 | 32 |
| 6'3" | 12 | 14 | 15 | 16 | 17 | 19 | 20 | 21 | 22 | 24 | 25 | 26 | 27 | 29 | 30 | 31 |
| 6'4" | 12 | 13 | 15 | 16 | 17 | 18 | 19 | 21 | 22 | 23 | 24 | 26 | 27 | 28 | 29 | 30 |

- Auscultation for bruits: Use the stethoscope bell over the carotid arteries (atherosclerosis) and renal arteries (renovascular hypertension due to atherosclerosis or fibromuscular dysplasia). Occasionally, an aortic bruit may be heard, particularly in cases of malformation or dissection.
- Neurologic examination: Observation for facial symmetry, inquiry about headache and mental status, and quick screening for symmetric and normal extremity muscle strength and reflexes may be sufficient for "low index" cases of mild hypertension in middle-aged patients without concomitant disease, particularly dyslipidemia or diabetes mellitus. However, as the number and severity of risk factors accumulate, the case becomes progressively worthy of a "high index" examination to establish a comprehensive assessment of baseline status and to screen for underlying causes or contributors to the HTN, as well as for other risk factors for CVD and complications from HTN. Situations indicating the appropriateness of a more thorough examination include younger or older patients in whom the HTN is more likely to be secondary to an underlying cause, patients with comorbidities or increased risk for complications, patients with more severe hypertension, and in patients with possible or impending complications from chronic HTN. All patients deserve a thorough exam, whether for the assessment of baseline status, complications, contributions, or for the reassurance (for both doctor and patient) that is attained after a competent professional evaluation reveals no abnormalities.

- Eye and fundoscopic examination: Look for cotton-wool spots, retinal/flame hemorrhages, arteriovenous nicking, and papilledema; manifestations of diabetic retinopathy may also be seen if DM is concomitant. Patients with DM are referred for ophthalmological evaluation at the time of diagnosis and annually/biannually thereafter depending on severity and compliance with and effectiveness of treatment.
- Inspection for diagonal ear lobe crease: Numerous studies have shown that the diagonal ear lobe crease is one of the easiest and most sensitive (~75%) and specific (~80%) physical examination findings to correlate with advanced atherosclerosis and cardiovascular disease.[39,40]
- Examination of the extremities: Assess pulse strength, arm:leg blood pressure differences[41] (ankle:brachial index should be > 1), lower extremity edema, capillary refill/perfusion and trophic changes consistent with peripheral vascular disease.
- Renal disease survey: Generally, no physical examination finding correlates specifically with renal disease. Renal diseases are the most common causes of secondary hypertension; perform serum BUN and creatinine; check urine albumin:creatinine ratio on a random urine sample; obtain renal US imaging, or CT if necessary.

**Clinical Pearls for Managing the Patient with Declining GFR**
- When the GFR = 60, modify dosages or withdraw certain drugs. Treat the causative problem and/or begin specialist co-management.
- When the GFR = 30, the patient needs to consult a nephrologist.
- When the GFR = 15, the patient needs a transplant or dialysis.

- **Laboratory Assessments**:
  - Chemistry/metabolic panel: Attention is given in particular to glucose, BUN, creatinine, calcium, and potassium. Glomerular filtration rate (GFR) can be estimated by the Cockcroft-Gault equation and should be used by clinicians to monitor renal function in patients at risk for renal insufficiency, namely patients with HTN, diabetes mellitus, advanced age, and known renal disease. **Estimated GFR = (140 - age) x weight (kg) / (72 x serum creatinine); in women, multiply this result by .85.** GFR values consistently less than 60 for 3 months are consistent with chronic kidney disease and approximately 50% loss of renal function; at this level of impaired renal function, drug doses need to be modified. Hypercalcemia is a rare cause of HTN and requires evaluation for underlying cause, such as hyperparathyroidism, hyperthyroidism, malignancy (especially multiple myeloma, lymphoma, or cancer of the breast, lung, or kidney), granulomatous diseases such as sarcoidosis, vitamin D or vitamin A excess, adverse drug effect (especially lithium or thiazide diuretics), Paget disease of bone, adrenal insufficiency, or genotropic metabolic disorder such as familial hypocalciuric hypercalcemia.
  - Urinalysis (UA): Test for hematuria, proteinuria, and glucosuria; random albumin:creatinine ratio is indicated in diabetic patients to assess for microalbuminuria.

---

[39] Edston E. The earlobe crease, coronary artery disease, and sudden cardiac death: an autopsy study of 520 individuals. *Am J Forensic Med Pathol*. 2006 Jun;27(2):129-33

[40] Motamed M, Pelekoudas N. The predictive value of diagonal ear-lobe crease sign. *Int J Clin Pract*. 1998 Jul-Aug;52(5):305-6

[41] Ankle-brachial index test. http://www.webmd.com/heart-disease/ankle-brachial-index-test Referenced January 2010

- o  **Thyroid testing**: Thyroid testing should be comprehensive and include TSH, free T4, free or total T3 and reverse T3, and *preferably* antithyroid antibodies. Treat as indicated.
- o  **Other cardiovascular risk factors**: Lipids, homocysteine, high-sensitivity c-reactive protein (hsCRP) can also be assessed.
- o  **Uric acid**: Many years ago uric acid was generally included in the standard chemistry/metabolic panel; these days it has to be ordered as a separate test. For at least a decade, "a strong, specific, stepwise, independent association of increasing serum uric acid and cardiac morbidity and mortality" has been noted[42], and recent research has shown that inhibition of uric acid production with allopurinol prevents fructose-induced urate-mediated metabolic disturbances that contribute to CVD, HTN, and the metabolic syndrome.[43] The roles of fructose and uric acid are discussed in greater detail in the following section on *Treatment Considerations*.
- o  **Serum 25-hydroxy-vitamin D**: In our review by Vasquez, Manso, and Cannell[44] in 2004, we fulfilled our promise of creating a "paradigm shift" that summarized new applications for the clinical use of vitamin D beyond its application in patients with osteoporosis or malabsorption to include the mandate for empiric treatment or laboratory assessment of all patients seen in clinical practice. The goal with vitamin D supplementation is to get serum 25-hydroxy-vitamin D levels into the optimal range, as defined in the illustration. As the cardioprotective role of vitamin D becomes more clear, the peer-reviewed medical research increasingly advocates that "**vitamin D supplementation should be prescribed to patients with hypertension and 25-hydroxyvitamin D levels below target values.**"[45]

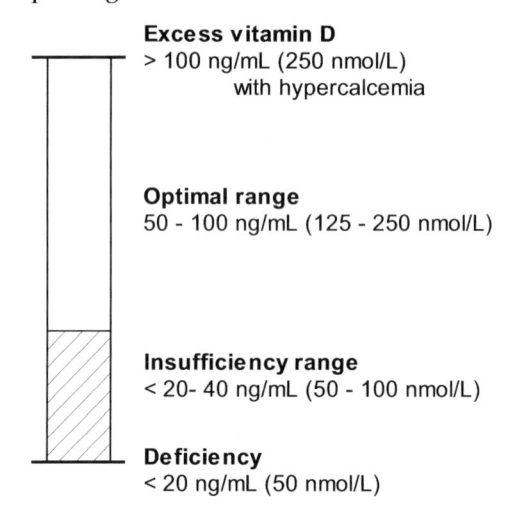

    **Excess vitamin D**
    > 100 ng/mL (250 nmol/L) with hypercalcemia

    **Optimal range**
    50 - 100 ng/mL (125 - 250 nmol/L)

    **Insufficiency range**
    < 20- 40 ng/mL (50 - 100 nmol/L)

    **Deficiency**
    < 20 ng/mL (50 nmol/L)

    **Interpretation of serum 25(OH) vitamin D levels.** Modified from Vasquez et al, *Alternative Therapies in Health and Medicine* 2004 and Vasquez A. *Musculoskeletal Pain: Expanded Clinical Strategies* (Institute for Functional Medicine) 2008.

- o  **Urine pH**: Urine pH can easily be monitored in-office or at home with the use of simple pH strips. A urine pH of 7.0-8 is desirable as an indicator of dietary compliance and avoidance of the acidogenic Western diet, which is generally HTN-inducing due to its content of sodium, chloride, simple sugars and insufficiency of magnesium, potassium, calcium, and phytonutrients. Urine alkalinization is generally benign in patients without renal disease; patients susceptible to urinary tract infections (UTIs) might experience an increased frequency of UTIs and may need to improve hygiene, supplement with

---

[42] Alderman M. Uric acid in hypertension and cardiovascular disease. *Can J Cardiol* 1999 Nov;15 Suppl F:20F-2F
[43] News release from American Heart Association's 63rd High Blood Pressure Research Conference. High-sugar diet increases men's blood pressure; gout drug protective. Abstract P127. Sept. 23, 2009. http://americanheart.mediaroom.com/index.php?s=43&item=829 Accessed December 19, 2009
[44] **Vasquez A**, Manso G, Cannell J. The clinical importance of vitamin D (cholecalciferol): a paradigm shift with implications for all healthcare providers. *Altern Ther Health Med*. 2004 Sep-Oct;10(5):28-36 http://optimalhealthresearch.com/cholecalciferol.html
[45] Pilz S, Tomaschitz A, Ritz E, Pieber TR; Medscape. Vitamin D status and arterial hypertension: a systematic review. *Nat Rev Cardiol*. 2009 Oct;6(10):621-30

- additional ascorbic acid to prevent urine from becoming excessively alkaline, and/or correct gastrointestinal dysbiosis.
  - <u>Serum fasting insulin</u>: Insulin promotes renal retention of sodium which leads to water retention and the subsequent volume overload and systemic hypertension which logically follow in sequence. Consider testing fasting serum insulin in patients likely to have hyperinsulinemia and insulin resistance; this can be used to tailor treatment, monitor benefit and compliance, and as a teaching aid for patients requiring or requesting additional details and insight.
  - <u>Tests for lead accumulation</u>: In the United States, a consistent correlation has been found between body burden of lead and HTN, even when blood lead levels are well below the current US occupational exposure limit guidelines (40 microg/dl).[46] In studying the effects of lead on HTN in humans, Schwartz and Stewart[47] contrasted blood lead, dimercaptosuccinic acid (DMSA)-chelatable lead, and tibial lead to find that blood lead was the assessment that most strongly correlated with HTN; they concluded, "**Systolic blood pressure was elevated by blood lead levels as low as 5 microg/dl.**" Thus, clinicians might first measure blood lead levels, which do not measure total body burden but rather the lead that is mobile or *in transit* within the body and which appears to have the best correlation with HTN; normal blood lead results could then be challenged with DMSA-provoked heavy metal testing. For heavy metal testing, this author's preference is to use DMSA-provoked measurement of urine toxic metals. After a minimal dose of DMSA (e.g., in the range of 50-100 mg) to screen for hypersensitivity, patients take oral DMSA 10 mg/kg as a single oral dose in the morning on an empty stomach after emptying the bladder and send a sample from the next urination for laboratory analysis. Follow laboratory protocol if different from these instructions. While detoxification procedures are reviewed in much greater detail in *Integrative Rheumatology*[48], use of DMSA for lead and mercury chelation/detoxification and for diagnostic purposes is generally safe and effective.[49,50,51,52,53]
  - <u>Serum aldosterone, preferably with aldosterone:renin ratio</u>: As the screening blood test for primary hyperaldosteronism, this test is indicated in any hypertensive patient with unexplained hypokalemia.
- **<u>Imaging</u>**:
  - <u>Electrocardiography (ECG, EKG)</u>: ECG is appropriate for patients at increased risk for coronary artery disease (CAD), myocardial infarction (MI) with CVD risk factors such as

---

[46] Nash D, Magder L, Lustberg M, Sherwin RW, Rubin RJ, Kaufmann RB, Silbergeld EK. Blood lead, blood pressure, and hypertension in perimenopausal and postmenopausal women. *JAMA*. 2003 Mar 26;289(12):1523-32  http://jama.ama-assn.org/cgi/content/full/289/12/1523
[47] "Systolic blood pressure was elevated by blood lead levels as low as 5 microg/dl." Schwartz BS, Stewart WF. Different associations of blood lead, meso 2,3-dimercaptosuccinic acid (DMSA)-chelatable lead, and tibial lead levels with blood pressure in 543 former organolead manufacturing workers. *Arch Environ Health*. 2000 Mar-Apr;55(2):85-92
[48] **Vasquez A**. Integrative Rheumatology. IBMRC 2006, 2007 and all future editions. http://optimalhealthresearch.com/rheumatology.html
[49] Bradstreet J, Geier DA, Kartzinel JJ, Adams JB, Geier MR. A case-control study of mercury burden in children with autistic spectrum disorders. *Journal of American Physicians and Surgeons* 2003; 8: 76-79   http://www.jpands.org/vol8no3/geier.pdf
[50] Crinnion WJ. Environmental medicine, part three: long-term effects of chronic low-dose mercury exposure. *Altern Med Rev*. 2000 Jun;5(3):209-23 http://www.thorne.com/altmedrev/.fulltext/5/3/209.pdf
[51] Forman J, Moline J, Cernichiari E, Sayegh S, Torres JC, Landrigan MM, Hudson J, Adel HN, Landrigan PJ. A cluster of pediatric metallic mercury exposure cases treated with meso-2,3-dimercaptosuccinic acid (DMSA). *Environ Health Perspect*. 2000 Jun;108(6):575-7 http://ehp.niehs.nih.gov/docs/2000/108p575-577forman/abstract.html
[52] Miller AL. Dimercaptosuccinic acid (DMSA), a non-toxic, water-soluble treatment for heavy metal toxicity. *Altern Med Rev*. 1998 Jun;3(3):199-207 http://www.thorne.com/altmedrev/.fulltext/3/3/199.pdf
[53] DMSA. *Altern Med Rev*. 2000 Jun;5(3):264-7 http://thorne.com/altmedrev/.fulltext/5/3/264.pdf

HTN or clinical evidence of peripheral vascular disease (PVD), congestive heart failure (CHF), or angina. The second edition of *Saint-Frances Guide: Clinical Clerkship in Outpatient Medicine*[54] states that ECG "should be ordered for most patients with hypertension."
- Upper cervical radiographs: Clinicians highly skilled in manual manipulative therapeutics might choose to radiograph the upper cervical spine as a means to determine the appropriateness and application of spinal manipulative therapy to effect "marked and sustained reductions in BP similar to the use of two-drug combination therapy."[55] Generally however, radiographs prior to spinal manipulative therapy are not advised, unless indicated by specific clinical findings or patient characteristics.
- Other imaging: CT, US, and angiographic techniques are commonly used to assess for HTN-related tumors, vascular anomalies/occlusion, and renal abnormalities. More specifically, US or CT assessment for abdominal aortic aneurysm is indicated for hypertensive patients with any history of smoking aged >65yo and patients with documented CAD/CVD.[56]

- **Biopsy/Procedure**: Generally not required except when investigating a specific pathoetiologic consideration. Angioplasty, stent placement, and aldosterone measurement in the adrenal vein to lateralize the side of an aldosterone-secreting tumor are examples of procedures used in some cases of HTN. Renal biopsy diagnoses primary renal disease if history, labs, and imaging are inconclusive.
- **Establishing the Diagnosis**: The diagnosis of hypertension is established after at least 2 measurements of blood pressure with either component greater than 140/90 mm Hg. Patients with systolic blood pressure 120-139 or diastolic blood pressure 80-89 are considered "prehypertensive"[57] and should be differentially diagnosed then treated with lifestyle and non-pharmacologic measures unless a primary cause of the hypertension is discovered. Patients with diabetes mellitus, renal disease, or CVD should have their blood pressure controlled to ≤ 130/80.

**Disease Complications**:
- The increased morbidity and mortality of HTN can manifest as any of the following:
  - Congestive heart failure presenting with fatigue, lower extremity edema, rales, dyspnea or orthopnea
  - Retinopathy and visual impairment
  - Hypertensive nephropathy presenting as azotemia, edema, recalcitrant HTN
  - Stroke—thrombotic or ischemic
  - Atrial fibrillation due to atrial enlargement
  - Myocardial infarction or sudden death due to accelerated CVD complicated by cardiac hypertrophy (i.e., supply-demand mismatch)
  - Abdominal aortic aneurysm, especially with HTN plus tobacco smoking

---

[54] Bent S, Gensler LS, Frances C. Saint-Frances Guide: Clinical Clerkship in Outpatient Medicine. 2nd Edition. Philadelphia; Wolters Kluwer: 2008, 90
[55] Bakris G, Dickholtz M Sr, Meyer PM, Kravitz G, Avery E, Miller M, Brown J, Woodfield C, Bell B. Atlas vertebra realignment and achievement of arterial pressure goal in hypertensive patients: a pilot study. *J Hum Hypertens*. 2007 May;21(5):347-52
[56] "CONCLUSIONS: In-hospital screening of AAA is very efficient among patients with coronary artery disease. Therefore, patients with CAD may be considered for routine AAA screening." Monney P, Hayoz D, Tinguely F, Cornuz J, Haesler E, Mueller XM, von Segesser LK, Tevaearai HT. High prevalence of unsuspected abdominal aortic aneurysms in patients hospitalised for surgical coronary revascularisation. *Eur J Cardiothorac Surg*. 2004 Jan;25(1):65-8
[57] Bent S, Gensler LS, Frances C. Saint-Frances Guide: Clinical Clerkship in Outpatient Medicine. 2nd Edition. Philadelphia; Wolters Kluwer: 2008, 87

**Clinical Management**: For routine outpatients, the obvious goal is to get the blood pressure down below 140/90 as quickly, safely, and cost-effectively as possible while treating any primary underlying disorders. **For patients with diabetes mellitus or any kidney disease, a lower blood pressure goal of ≤ 130/80 is indicated.** Attention to the "hierarchy of therapeutics"[58] is important here in order to prioritize the implementation of therapeutic interventions. Correction of nutritional deficiencies (e.g., vitamin D, magnesium, potassium, calcium, phytonutrients), nutritional imbalances (e.g., insulin resistance and hyperglycemia, diet-induced metabolic acidosis), and hormonal imbalances (e.g., thyroid deficiency/excess, estrogen excess, aldosterone excess) must take precedence over the simple utilization of antihypertensive drugs which suppress the manifestation of underlying dysfunction and thus allow it to perpetuate; because of the latter, pharmacotherapy often abets rather than abates chronic disease. Following the exclusion of pathologic causes of HTN, the diagnosis of HTN should be explained to the patient as a sign of internal (e.g., nutritional, hormonal, or structural) imbalance or otherwise as an opportunity to use this marker as a barometer of overall health and compliance with a health-promoting lifestyle, including optimization of diet, exercise, relationships, and nutritional intake.

| Clinical Management of HTN |
| --- |
| 1. **Assessment** for urgency and end-organ damage |
| 2. **Differential diagnosis** and comprehensive assessment |
| 3. **Effective treatment** or appropriate referral |
| 4. **Patient education** |
| 5. **Scheduled follow-up** |
| 6. **Monitor** for compliance, treatment effectiveness, adverse effects, and new complications |
| 7. **Document all of the above in the patient chart** |

- Stratification of HTN management: Factors that direct the management of HTN include severity, manifestations of associated organ damage, and the patient's general condition and comorbidities.
    - Hypertensive urgency = blood pressure >220/120 mm Hg[59] or >220/125 mm Hg[60] *without end-organ damage* and *without symptoms*: These patients are appropriately treated in the emergency department with *orally administered* medications such as nifedipine (oral, not sublingual), clonidine, and/or captopril. Patients can be discharged following normalization of blood pressure, but these patients require timely follow-up with a primary care provider. Complicating factors and concomitant disease may necessitate hospital admission.
    - Hypertensive emergency = >200/120 mm Hg *with evidence of end-organ damage* or *symptoms possibly attributable to the hypertension such as headache, blurred vision, chest pain, or shortness of breath*: Accompanying clinical manifestations may include renal failure, hematuria, proteinuria, altered mental status, papilledema, retinal vascular changes, MI, angina, stroke, aortic dissection, and pulmonary edema. Treat in intensive/critical care setting with *intravenous* antihypertensive medications such as nitroprusside, nitroglycerine,

---

[58] The "hierarchy of therapeutics" is a guiding principle of naturopathic medicine that provides a conceptual framework for the prioritization and sequencing of therapeutic interventions. This is described in chapter 1 of *Integrative Orthopedics*, *Integrative Rheumatology*, and *Chiropractic and Naturopathic Mastery of Common Clinical Disorders* and is available on-line at http://OptimalHealthResearch.com/chapter1. Another resource available in January 2010 is Chapter 3 from *Textbook of Natural Medicine, 3rd Edition*: "A Hierarchy of Healing: The Therapeutic Order. The Unifying Theory of Naturopathic Medicine" available on-line: http://www.naturalmedtext.com/storedfiles/sample_Chapter%203%20-%20A%20Hierarchy%20of%20Healing%20-%20The%20Therapeutic%20Order.pdf?CFID=6826417&CFTOKEN=33445946
[59] Bent S, Gensler LS, Frances C. Saint-Frances Guide: Clinical Clerkship in Outpatient Medicine. 2nd Edition. Philadelphia; Wolters Kluwer: 2008, 89
[60] McPhee SJ, Papadakis MA (editors). Current Medical Diagnosis and Treatment. 2009. 48th Edition. New York; McGraw Hill Medical: 401

esmolol, hydralzine, labetolol, nicardipine then transition to oral beta-blockers and ACEi (angiotensin converting enzyme inhibitor) drugs; add diuretics such as furosemide/Lasix to alleviate volume overload, pulmonary edema, HTN, and heart failure. The initial drop in blood pressure should not exceed 25% in order to prevent precipitation of organ ischemia due to reflexive arteriospasm.
  - <u>Malignant HTN</u>: Severe, intractable, and generally progressive HTN with clinical complications including renal failure, encephalopathy, or papilledema. Treat in hospital setting with intravenous antihypertensive medications (reviewed above for hypertensive emergency).
- <u>Routine recommendations that should be documented in the patient's chart</u>; these include ❶ smoking cessation, ❷ a minimum of 30 minutes of exercise per day (for patients healthy enough to exercise), ❸ weight loss/optimization, ❹ limit alcohol intake to no more than 1-2 drinks per day, ❺ restrict sodium to≤ 2,400 mg/d (i.e., ≤ 6 grams/d of sodium chloride), ❻ increase intake of fruits and vegetables, and ❼ reduce intake of total and saturated fat in order to promote weight loss and optimize serum lipids.[61] In the allopathic model, these lifestyle recommendations are used for three months before initiating drug treatment of HTN.
- <u>Tailor treatment recommendations and goals to the patient's specific psychographics and BVG-LOC profile</u>. More than 90-95% of HTN patients will be found to have no pathologic/medical cause of their HTN, thus implicating diet and lifestyle as the most responsible factors. In some situations, the resolution of the patient's HTN comes expeditiously through the simple and imperfect implementation of weight loss, diet modification, correction of nutritional deficiencies, and avoidance or reduced intake of infamous triggers such as tobacco, alcohol, and excess caffeine. **For many patients with HTN—especially when the HTN is part of a larger cluster of clinical findings such as type-2 diabetes mellitus or the metabolic syndrome (see chapter 13 of** *Chiropractic and Naturopathic Mastery of Common Clinical Disorders*)—**the successful management of their HTN will rely on the implementation of numerous changes in various aspects of "lifestyle" including diet, preparation/procurement of food, social interactions, core relationships, exercise involvement, time and money allocation, and—most importantly— changes in self image, and the establishment and** *affirmation through action* **of core values.** These issues can appear complex to the point of being "too complicated" for doctors and patients who are not personally accustomed to living consciously and for whom dispensing and consuming pills, respectively, are easier than the *consciousness raising* and the *self-disciplined and self-directed living* required to advocate and manifest a health-centered life. Complexity and convenience should not be the determinants of care. Patients with lifestyle-generated diseases should be coached in the reversal of the patterns that have caused their disease rather than being enabled to pursue these disease-promoting lifestyles while surrogate markers of metabolic-physiologic dysfunction are pharmacologically suppressed. Therapeutic lifestyle changes must be merged with the patient's beliefs (important but changeable paradigms), values (subjective-objective rules), goals (conscious and subconscious aspirations and trajectory). In order to facilitate this merger, the clinician must first understand the patient's position on these variables, then—second—deliver the

---

[61] Bent S, Gensler LS, Frances C. <u>Saint-Frances Guide: Clinical Clerkship in Outpatient Medicine. 2nd Edition</u>. Philadelphia; Wolters Kluwer: 2008, 90

treatment plan in such a way as to "speak to" the patient's beliefs, values, and goals. Many (most) patients are representative of other people in society insofar as they generally do not have declarable beliefs, values, and goals; thus, this process of the physician's gaining an understanding of the patient's unconscious psychographic details is generally not completed on the first visit and is not completed until the patient has done the requisite "homework" (perhaps facilitated by a professional therapist or lay counselor) and returned with a perceptible level of self-awareness. Clinicians who "**Seek first to understand, then to be understood**" ("Principles of Mutual Understanding" per Covey[62]) will have advantages over clinicians who steamroll patients with lifestyle impositions and a "to do" list that is foreign to the patient's inner and previous experiences.

---

### Psychographic profiling via "BVG-LOC"

- <u>Beliefs</u>: What are the fundamental beliefs and expectations that the patient has for his/her future? Is life merely "suffering and toil" or is it meant to be "a well of delight"? Patients who expect misery are generally successful in its attainment; that is, unless they are guided and provoked toward a more positive life expectancy. The clinician can correct errors in thought and information.
- <u>Values</u>: What does the patient value? "*Autonomy and independence*"—will this manifest as resistance to the clinician's advice or as a willingness to comply with treatment so as to avoid future disability? "*Strength*"—will this be resistance to the plan or disciplined adherence to the plan? "*Love*"—is this self-sacrificing 'love' for other people or is it a wholesome and healthy love that includes the self? "*My family*"—does this include avoiding disability, being alive to support and encourage family members and upcoming generations? "*Nothing really*"—what are the mental barriers and painful experiences that have resulted in this emotional numbness; what would his/her life be like if he/she were to engage in life consciously and with purpose? The clinician assigns homework for the patient to clarify—and later commit to in action—a list of personal values.
- <u>Goals</u>: What are the patient's social, physical, professional, personal, and spiritual goals? Is the current lifestyle and health/disease trajectory consistent with the attainment and extended enjoyment of these goals? Are the goals too limited, and has the patient accommodated small goals with small effort and the resulting lackluster results that reinforce self-depreciation and low self esteem, thus perpetuating a vicious cycle? Goals are a reflection of core values and one's intimate belief about what is possible and what levels of success, love, and happiness are appropriate for one's life. A person's failure to define and pursue goals is diagnostic of low self esteem and lack of psychic identity.
- <u>Locus of Control</u>: Does the patient view the world as chaotic and menacing (external locus of control), or as understandable and thus worthy of meaningful engagement (internal locus of control)? If the patient views him/herself as a victim, then compliance will be low because every and any excuse will serve as a rationalization for why he/she "couldn't" exercise, eat right, take medications or nutrients as prescribed. Patients who experience their health problems as incomprehensible and "idiopathic" are less likely to engage in purposeful health activities and are more likely to be noncompliant with treatment(s) and more passive in their willingness to rely on "doctor's orders" and drug treatments. Physicians should encourage the best self-image in and self-efficacy from patients by reminding them by either Socratic-dialectic education or direct verbalization that the patient has the power and thus the "response-ability" to strongly influence his/her health outcomes via positive health expectations and behaviors.

---

[62] Covey SR. <u>The Seven Habits of Highly Effective People</u> (first published in 1989); see also <u>The 8th Habit: From Effectiveness to Greatness</u> (published in 2004).

- <u>Patients must receive instruction on at-home blood pressure monitoring and follow-up in-office assessments</u>: At the time of diagnosis, patients are instructed of the importance of proper treatment and follow-up visits (ranging from weekly to biweekly to monthly) to facilitate compliance and monitor treatment effectiveness. HTN must never be taken lightly by the clinician or the patient as it represents and indicates a significant departure from optimal health and the failure of internal homeostatic mechanisms; more concretely, HTN is generally a silent and progressive disorder which prematurely undercuts health and vitality and which tends to culminate in unnecessary morbidity (e.g.., pain, suffering, loss of function, renal dialysis, and stroke) and early death. Patients can use office-calibrated home blood pressure monitoring equipment to self-monitor compliance, lifestyle effects, and effectiveness of treatment; patients are advised that at-home monitoring does not substitute for in-office visits and that in-office blood pressure measurements are the standard by which treatment decisions are and will be made. "White coat hypertension" (WCH) is explained as an exaggerated stress response to innocuous stimuli that has parallels in other areas of the patient's life and is therefore not an excuse for normal at-home readings; accordingly, studies have shown that patients with WCH show increased risk for cardiovascular complications.[63,64] Depending on HTN severity and the protocol being followed, patients might be seen in the office for a quick follow-up assessment once every few days, or less frequently if BP checks are occurring *reliably* at home; patients with metabolic syndrome or who are otherwise likely to be noncompliant are followed-up more frequently than medically indicated in order to promote compliance and patient-physician alliance. Following stabilization, patients are reevaluated every 3-6 months in the office; laboratory tests are routinely performed especially with any evidence of complications such as nephropathy, dyslipidemia, DM, or drug side effects.

> **Clinical Pearl**
> Serum 25-OH-cholecalciferol can be tested as a surrogate marker for compliance with nutritional supplementation (detailed later); levels should rise within one month and plateau at the optimal range within 2-3 months if dose and compliance are appropriate.
>
> Relatedly, patients should be able to recite their daily regimen of nutritional supplementation, pharmaceutical drugs, dietary prescriptions/proscriptions, and exercise-lifestyle habits.
>
> Ideally, patients might also be aware of their personal values and goals, as these are the diving forces that either support or subvert their daily behaviors.

- <u>Patients already taking antihypertensive medications are likely to require a dosage adjustment or medication discontinuation after using diet, lifestyle, and nutritional interventions.</u> Clinicians should anticipate this benefit and inform the patient and prescribing doctor appropriately. Failure to anticipate the normalization of blood pressure and to adjust medications appropriately may result in hypotension, most commonly manifested by fatigue and/or (pre)syncope.

---

[63] "CONCLUSIONS: Coronary disease may be more severe among patients with WCH than among those without." Kostandonis D, Papadopoulos V, Toumanidis S, Papamichael C, Kanakakis I, Zakopoulos N. Topography and severity of coronary artery disease in white-coat hypertension. *Eur J Intern Med.* 2008 Jun;19(4):280-4

[64] "Our findings also further stress the interest, for clinicians, of assessing the presence of a white-coat effect as a means to further identify patients at increased cardiovascular risk and guide treatment accordingly." Bochud M, Bovet P, Vollenweider P, Maillard M, Paccaud F, Wandeler G, Gabriel A, Burnier M. Association Between White-Coat Effect and Blunted Dipping of Nocturnal Blood Pressure. *Am J Hypertens.* 2009 Jul 23. [Epub ahead of print]

- <u>Drug management and comanagement of HTN may be required</u>. Drug management is appropriate in urgent situations, recalcitrant cases, patients with initial BP > 160/100, and for patients who are noncompliant with treatment, whether for reasons of insufficient money, insurmountable logistics, or—most commonly—lack of willpower and discipline to tame the appetite, make intelligent food and spending choices, and implement effectiveness in lifestyle and supplementation. Patients and clinicians can facilitate progression through the "stages of change" by appreciating the barriers and requirements that characterize the overcoming of each stage until the final stage of termination/integration is achieved.[65] In common medical practice, lifestyle interventions are minimally discussed, the process of change is not considered, and nutritional supplementation and spinal manipulation are eschewed so that drug treatment of hypertension is the allopathic standard of care.
- <u>Document everything</u>: Document all relevant clinical findings, laboratory/imaging results, treatments with rationale, patient education, and plan of scheduled follow-up, referral, and comanagment. Ensure that clinical visits include education and consent to treatment and that the "patient verbalizes understanding, and all questions are answered and concerns addressed."

**Treatment Considerations for "Primary" Hypertension**:
- <u>**Low-carbohydrate low-salt Paleo-Mediterranean Diet, with daily exercise**</u>: The health-promoting diet of choice for the majority of people is a diet based on abundant consumption of fruits, vegetables, seeds, nuts, omega-3 and monounsaturated fatty acids, and lean sources of protein such as lean meats, fatty cold-water fish, soy and whey proteins. This diet prohibits and obviates overconsumption of chemical preservatives, artificial sweeteners, and carbohydrate-dominant foods such as candies, pastries, breads, potatoes, grains, and other foods with a high glycemic load and high glycemic index. This "Paleo-Mediterranean Diet"—first detailed by Vasquez[66,67] in 2005—is a combination of the "Paleolithic" or "Paleo diet" and the well-known "Mediterranean diet", both of which are well described in peer-reviewed journals and the lay press. The Paleo-Mediterranean Diet is wholly consistent with the "polymeal"[68]—a multicomponent cardioprotective diet plan characterized by emphasis on phytonutrient-rich foods including fish, red wine, garlic, almonds, dark chocolate, and most (low-carbohydrate) fruits and vegetables—which is estimated to have the potential to lower the incidence of CVD by 76%.
    - <u>Small clinical trial: Metabolic and physiologic improvements from consuming a Paleolithic, hunter-gatherer type diet</u>: Despite the small subject size (n = 9), this study demonstrates safety and beneficial effectiveness of the Paleolithic diet in addressing several of the perturbations that characterize the metabolic syndrome and lifestyle-

---

[65] Prochaska, JO, Norcross, JC, and DiClemente, CC (1994). Changing for Good: A Revolutionary Six-Stage Program for Overcoming Bad Habits and Moving Your Life Positively Forward. NY, William Morrow and Company; 1994
[66] **Vasquez A**. The Importance of Integrative Chiropractic Health Care in Treating Musculoskeletal Pain and Reducing the Nationwide Burden of Medical Expenses and Iatrogenic Injury and Death: A Concise Review of Current Research and Implications for Clinical Practice and Healthcare Policy. *Original Internist* 2005; 12(4): 159-182
[67] **Vasquez A**. A Five-Part Nutritional Protocol that Produces Consistently Positive Results. *Nutritional Wellness* 2005 September  Available in the printed version and on-line at http://optimalhealthresearch.com/protocol   This essay was also republished in "Chiropractic and Naturopathic Mastery of Common Clinical Disorders" in 2009 http://optimalhealthresearch.com/clinical_mastery.html
[68] Franco OH, Bonneux L, de Laet C, Peeters A, Steyerberg EW, Mackenbach JP. The Polymeal: a more natural, safer, and probably tastier (than the Polypill) strategy to reduce cardiovascular disease by more than 75%. BMJ. 2004 Dec 18;329(7480):1447-50 http://www.bmj.com/cgi/reprint/329/7480/1447.pdf

induced predisposition to CVD. "Results: Compared with the baseline (usual) diet, we observed (a) **significant reductions in BP** associated with improved arterial distensibility; (b) **significant reduction in plasma insulin** vs time AUC [area under the curve], during the OGTT [oral glucose tolerance testing]; and (c) large significant reductions in total cholesterol, low-density lipoproteins (LDL) and triglycerides (-0.8, -0.7 and -0.3 mmol/l respectively). In all these measured variables, either **eight or all nine participants had identical directional responses when switched to Paleolithic type diet, that is, near consistently improved status of circulatory, carbohydrate and lipid metabolism/physiology.**"[69]

> | **Clinical benefits from a Paleolithic hunter-gatherer diet** |
> | --- |
> | ☑ **significant reductions in blood pressure**, |
> | ☑ improved arterial distensibility, |
> | ☑ **significant reduction in plasma insulin**, |
> | ☑ large significant reductions in total cholesterol, low-density lipoproteins (LDL) and triglycerides, |
> | ☑ consistently improved status of circulatory, carbohydrate and lipid metabolism/physiology. |
>
> "Conclusions: Even **short-term consumption of a paleolithic type diet improves BP and glucose tolerance, decreases insulin secretion, increases insulin sensitivity and improves lipid profiles without weight loss in healthy sedentary humans**."
>
> Frassetto LA, Schloetter M, Mietus-Synder M, Morris RC Jr, Sebastian A. Metabolic and physiologic improvements from consuming a paleolithic, hunter-gatherer type diet. *Eur J Clin Nutr*. 2009 Feb 11

o Randomized 3-month cross-over pilot study: Beneficial effects of a Paleolithic diet on cardiovascular risk factors in type 2 diabetes: Although small (n=13), this study is impressive because it shows not only the benefits of the Paleolithic diet but also its superiority over the commonly recommended "diabetic diet" which is advocated by conventional-standard-mainstream-government groups that claim to promote health and victory in the so-called war against obesity and diabetes mellitus. "Compared to the diabetes diet, the Paleolithic diet resulted in lower mean values of HbA1c (-0.4% units), triacylglycerol (-0.4 mmol/L), **diastolic blood pressure (-4 mmHg),** weight (-3 kg), BMI (-1 kg/m2) and waist circumference (-4 cm), and higher mean values of high density lipoprotein cholesterol (+0.08 mmol/L)."[70]

o The 2009 Canadian Hypertension Education Program recommendations for the management of hypertension: Part 2—therapy: These are very conventional and standard recommendations from the medical community which are included here for the sake of completeness so that doctors have a recent reference guideline from which they can move beyond in the delivery of superior clinical care. "RECOMMENDATIONS: For lifestyle modifications to prevent and treat hypertension, restrict dietary sodium to less than 2300 mg (100 mmol)/day (and 1500 mg to 2300 mg [65 mmol to 100 mmol]/day in hypertensive patients); perform 30 min to 60 min of aerobic exercise four to seven days per week; maintain a healthy body weight (body mass index 18.5 kg/m(2) to 24.9 kg/m(2)) and waist circumference (smaller than 102 cm for men and smaller than 88 cm

---

[69] Frassetto LA, Schloetter M, Mietus-Synder M, Morris RC Jr, Sebastian A. Metabolic and physiologic improvements from consuming a paleolithic, hunter-gatherer type diet. *Eur J Clin Nutr*. 2009 Feb 11. [Epub ahead of print]
[70] Jonsson T, Granfeldt Y, Ahren B, Branell UC, Palsson G, Hansson A, Soderstrom M, Lindeberg S. Beneficial effects of a Paleolithic diet on cardiovascular risk factors in type 2 diabetes: a randomized cross-over pilot study. *Cardiovasc Diabetol*. 2009 Jul 16;8(1):35. http://www.cardiab.com/content/8/1/35

for women); limit alcohol consumption to no more than 14 units [drinks] per week in men or nine units per week in women; follow a diet that is reduced in saturated fat and cholesterol, and that emphasizes fruits, vegetables and low-fat dairy products, dietary and soluble fiber, whole grains and protein from plant sources; and consider stress management in selected individuals with hypertension."[71] These guidelines would have been better if they had advised complete avoidance of grains (sources of generally acidogenic phytonutrient-poor carbohydrates) and other sources of simple carbohydrate including candies and soft drinks in general and those pseudofoods laden with high-fructose corn syrup in particular.

> **Lifestyle recommendations from the Canadian Hypertension Education Program**
> - <u>Restrict dietary sodium</u> to less than 2300 mg (100 mmol)/day (and 1500 mg to 2300 mg [65 mmol to 100 mmol]/day in hypertensive patients).
> - <u>Perform 30 min to 60 min of aerobic exercise</u> four to seven days per week.
> - <u>Maintain a healthy body weight</u> (body mass index 18.5 kg/m(2) to 24.9 kg/m(2)) and waist circumference (< 102 cm for men and < 88 cm for women).
> - <u>Limit alcohol consumption</u> to no more than 14 units per week in men or nine units per week in women.
> - <u>Follow a diet that is reduced in saturated fat and cholesterol.</u>
> - <u>Follow a diet that emphasizes fruits, vegetables and low-fat dairy products, dietary and soluble fiber, whole grains and protein from plant sources</u>.
> - <u>Consider stress management</u> in selected individuals with hypertension.
>
> Khan NA, Hemmelgarn B, Herman RJ, et al. The 2009 Canadian Hypertension Education Program recommendations for the management of hypertension: Part 2—therapy. *Can J Cardiol*. 2009 May;25(5):287-98

- o Meta-analysis: Adherence to Mediterranean diet and health status: "Greater adherence to a Mediterranean diet is associated with a significant improvement in health status, as seen by a **significant reduction in overall mortality** (-9%), mortality from **cardiovascular diseases** (-9%), incidence of or mortality from **cancer** (-6%), and incidence of **Parkinson's disease and Alzheimer's disease** (-13%). These results seem to be clinically relevant for public health, in particular for **encouraging a Mediterranean-like dietary pattern for primary prevention of major chronic diseases**."[72] The results of this meta-analysis have major implications for clinical practice and public health policy.
- **Low-carbohydrate diet, including short-term water-only fasting**: The anti-hypertensive and anti-diabetic benefits of low-carbohydrate diets and short-term fasting have been substantiated in the research literature for several decades. However, the chiropractic physician Alan Goldhamer deserves credit for the most recent revival of short-term fasting as a therapeutic tool for chronic hypertension and diabetes mellitus.

---

[71] Khan NA, Hemmelgarn B, Herman RJ, Bell CM, Mahon JL, Leiter LA, Rabkin SW, Hill MD, Padwal R, Touyz RM, Larochelle P, Feldman RD, Schiffrin EL, Campbell NR, Moe G, Prasad R, Arnold MO, Campbell TS, Milot A, Stone JA, Jones C, Ogilvie RI, Hamet P, Fodor G, Carruthers G, Burns KD, Ruzicka M, DeChamplain J, Pylypchuk G, Petrella R, Boulanger JM, Trudeau L, Hegele RA, Woo V, McFarlane P, Vallée M, Howlett J, Bacon SL, Lindsay P, Gilbert RE, Lewanczuk RZ, Tobe S; Canadian Hypertension Education Program. The 2009 Canadian Hypertension Education Program recommendations for the management of hypertension: Part 2—therapy. *Can J Cardiol*. 2009 May;25(5):287-98
[72] Sofi F, Cesari F, Abbate R, Gensini GF, Casini A. Adherence to Mediterranean diet and health status: meta-analysis. *BMJ*. 2008 Sep 11;337:a1344

- Open clinical trial: Chiropractic-supervised water-only fasting in the treatment of hypertension: In this open trial, 174 consecutive hypertensive patients were treated in an inpatient setting under clinician supervision. The treatment program began with a short prefasting period (approximately 2 to 3 days on average) during which food consumption was limited to fruits and vegetables, followed by supervised water-only fasting (approximately 10 to 11 days on average) and a refeeding period (approximately 6 to 7 days on average) introducing a low-fat, low-sodium, vegan diet. "RESULTS: Almost 90% of the subjects achieved blood pressure less than 140/90 mm Hg by the end of the treatment program. **The average reduction in blood pressure was 37/13 mm Hg,** with the greatest decrease being observed for subjects with the most severe hypertension. **Patients with stage 3 hypertension (those with systolic blood pressure greater than 180 mg Hg, diastolic blood pressure greater than 110 mg Hg, or both) had an average reduction of 60/17 mm Hg at the conclusion of treatment**. All of the subjects who were taking antihypertensive medication at entry (6.3% of the total sample) successfully discontinued the use of medication. CONCLUSION: Medically supervised water-only fasting appears to be a safe and effective means of normalizing blood pressure and may assist in motivating health-promoting diet and lifestyle changes."[73]
- Open clinical trial: Chiropractic-supervised water-only fasting in the treatment of borderline hypertension: 68 consecutive patients with borderline hypertension were treated in an inpatient setting under professional supervision. The treatment program consisted of a short prefasting period (approximately 1-2 days on average) during which food consumption was limited to fruits and vegetables followed by supervised water-only fasting (approximately 13.6 days on average). Fasting was followed by a refeeding period (approximately 6.0 days on average). The refeeding program consisted of a low-fat, low-sodium, plant-based, vegan diet. "RESULTS: Approximately 82% of the subjects achieved BP at or below 120/80 mm Hg by the end of the treatment program. **The mean BP reduction was 20/7 mm Hg,** with the greatest decrease being observed for subjects with the highest baseline BP. A linear regression of BP decrease against baseline BP showed that the estimated BP below which no further decrease would be expected was 96.0/67.0 mm Hg at the end of the fast and 99.2/67.3 mm Hg at the end of refeeding. These levels are in agreement with other estimates of the BP below which stroke events are eliminated, thus suggesting that these levels could be regarded as the "ideal" BP values. CONCLUSION: Medically supervised water-only fasting appears to be a safe and effective means of normalizing BP and may assist in motivating health-promoting diet and lifestyle changes."[74]

    > **Political Insight**
    > Alan Goldhamer—the lead author on two landmark clinical trials using supervised fasting for the impressively successful treatment of HTN—is a Doctor of Chiropractic. Despite knowing of his chiropractic credentials, journal editors required the publication to be titled "Medically supervised."

- Retrospective cost-effectiveness and clinical effectiveness analysis for short-term fasting in the treatment of hypertension and diabetes mellitus: Initial cost of care results in

---

[73] Goldhamer A, Lisle D, Parpia B, Anderson SV, Campbell TC. Medically supervised water-only fasting in the treatment of hypertension. *J Manipulative Physiol Ther* 2001 Jun;24(5):335-9 http://www.healthpromoting.com/Articles/335-339Goldhamer115263.QXD.pdf

[74] Goldhamer AC, Lisle DJ, Sultana P, Anderson SV, Parpia B, Hughes B, Campbell TC. Medically supervised water-only fasting in the treatment of borderline hypertension. *J Altern Complement Med*. 2002 Oct;8(5):643-50 http://www.healthpromoting.com/Articles/articles/study%202/acmpaper5.pdf

medically supervised water-only fasting for treating high blood pressure and diabetes: In this brief report, Dr Goldhamer again reports success with the short-term fasting program in hypertensive patients as well as diabetic patients. Here, Goldhamer reports that the **average reduction in systolic blood pressure was 30/11 mm Hg at the completion of the program and 28/11 mm Hg on follow-up.** "Weight loss averaged 26 pounds after the program and was 28 pounds below baseline on follow-up. The average cost of medical care and drugs was $5,784.00 per year in the year(s) prior to participation and $3,000.00 in the year after participation for an average reduction of $2,784.00 per subject in the first year alone. This exceeded the cost of the entire program and compound savings are expected in the years to follow."[75]

> **Clinical Pearl: lowering plasma glucose → lower insulin levels → less sodium-water retention → alleviation of hypertension**
> Treatments that lower plasma glucose levels, either via reduced intake of carbohydrates or by increasing glucose disposal (i.e., increasing insulin sensitivity) have an anti-hypertensive effect via lowering insulin levels. **Because insulin promotes sodium-water retention, any treatment that lowers glucose-insulin levels will help correct the contribution of hyperinsulinemia to hypertension.** Likewise, avoidance of dietary fructose is now known to avoid the fructose-induced elevations in serum uric acid which contribute to endothelial dysfunction, hypertension, and the metabolic syndrome.

- **Items to be avoided**: Clinicians and patients should be aware that dietary intake of food allergens, fructose, sodium chloride, and arachidonic acid can contribute to the development, perpetuation, and therapeutic recalcitrance of chronic HTN.
    - **Food allergen avoidance**: According to a clinical study of migraineurs (n = 60) published in *The Lancet*, identification and avoidance of food allergens can generally normalize blood pressure in migraine patients who have concomitant hypertension[76]; findings of this study included, "The commonest foods causing reactions were wheat (78%), orange (65%), eggs (45%), tea and coffee (40% each), chocolate and milk (37%) each), beef (35%), and corn, cane sugar, and yeast (33% each). When an average of ten common foods were avoided there was a dramatic fall in the number of headaches per month, 85% of patients becoming headache-free. The 25% of patients with hypertension became normotensive."
    - **Minimization of dietary sodium chloride**: Excess sodium (Na) promotes water retention and subsequent volume expansion, while also contributing to vasoconstriction and arterial stiffness via enhanced adrenergic reactivity and via promotion of intracellular hypercalcinosis (possibly due to enhanced sodium-calcium exchange).[77] When consumed as common table salt, the chloride (Cl) anion promotes acidosis which results in the progression of CAD/CVD morbidity and mortality and the exacerbation of HTN with increased renal losses of magnesium, potassium, and calcium. These effects justify the advice to for HTN patients to avoid dietary NaCl and also justify the use of drug diuretics that enhance Na excretion by the kidney. Clinical responsiveness to low-sodium diets ranges from clinically insignificant to a maximum reduction in the range of

---

[75] Goldhamer AC. Initial cost of care results in medically supervised water-only fasting for treating high blood pressure and diabetes. *J Altern Complement Med*. 2002 Dec;8(6):696-7 http://www.healthpromoting.com/Articles/pdf/Study%2032.pdf
[76] Grant EC. Food allergies and migraine. *Lancet*. 1979 May 5;1(8123):966-9
[77] Benowitz NL. "Antihypertensive Agents." In Katzung BG (editor). Basic and Clinical Pharmacology. Tenth Edition. New York: McGraw Hill Medical; 2007, 163

-22/-14 to -16/-9.[78] Contraindications to low-sodium diet are uncommon (e.g., hyponatremia); **low-sodium/NaCl diets should generally be a component of all antihypertensive treatment plans.** Approximately 20% of patients will show antihypertensive benefit from sodium restriction.[79] Canadian guidelines published in 2009 support the restriction of dietary sodium to less than 2300 mg (100 mmol)/day and to less than 1500-2300 mg [65 mmol to 100 mmol]/day in hypertensive patients.[80]

- **Fructose avoidance for caloric moderation and uric acid reduction,:** Production of uric acid is stimulated by ingestion of fructose (most notoriously in the form of high-fructose corn syrup, common in many processed foods and cola drinks), and uric acid directly contributes to the development of insulin resistance and HTN and other classic features of the metabolic syndrome. In a clinical trial published in September 2009, 74 adult men added fructose 200 g/d to their regular diet (typical American diet averages 50-70 g/d of fructose) for 2 weeks and experienced a +6/+3 elevation in BP, elevations in serum triglycerides and LDL cholesterol, and a more than doubling of the incidence of metabolic syndrome from approximately 20% to 50% as determined by two sets of international criteria. The authors logically concluded, "These results suggest that fructose may be a cause of metabolic syndrome. They also suggest that excessive fructose intake may have a role in the worldwide epidemic of obesity and diabetes."[81] Men in this trial who were randomized to receive allopurinol (dose unlisted) did not develop adverse effects from the increased fructose ingestion, thus clearly implicating fructose-induced hyperuricemia as the biochemical pathway involved. Clinicians should appreciate that the rapid (within 2 weeks) development of HTN and a doubling of the incidence of metabolic syndrome by the addition of fructose to the diet is of undeniably major importance as it clearly implicates high-fructose corn syrup as a major culprit in the burgeoning epidemics of HTN, type-2 diabetes mellitus, and the metabolic syndrome. In a study involving adolescents with elevated uric acid levels (serum uric acid levels > or = 6 mg/dL), allopurinol 200 mg twice daily resulted in a reduction in blood pressure of approximately -7/-5[82]; this was a proof-of-concept study (i.e., that uric acid contributes to HTN) and not necessarily an endorsement to use allopurinol for the treatment of HTN. Adverse effects due to allopurinol can include skin rash that may be followed by more severe hypersensitivity reactions such as "exfoliative, urticarial and purpuric lesions as well as Stevens-Johnson syndrome (erythema multiforme exudativum) and/or generalized vasculitis, irreversible hepatotoxicity and on rare occasions, death."[83] **Adherence to the Paleo-Mediterranean Diet in general and a low-**

---

[78] "The average fall in blood pressure from the highest to the lowest sodium intake was 16/9 mm Hg." MacGregor GA, Markandu ND, Sagnella GA, Singer DR, Cappuccio FP. Double-blind study of three sodium intakes and long-term effects of sodium restriction in essential hypertension. *Lancet*. 1989 Nov 25;2(8674):1244-7

[79] Domino FJ (editor in chief). The 5-Minute Clinical Consult. 2010. 18th Edition. Philadelphia; Wolters Kluwer: 2009, 656-7

[80] Khan NA, Hemmelgarn B, Herman RJ, Bell CM, Mahon JL, Leiter LA, Rabkin SW, Hill MD, Padwal R, Touyz RM, Larochelle P, Feldman RD, Schiffrin EL, Campbell NR, Moe G, Prasad R, Arnold MO, Campbell TS, Milot A, Stone JA, Jones C, Ogilvie RI, Hamet P, Fodor G, Carruthers G, Burns KD, Ruzicka M, DeChamplain J, Pylypchuk G, Petrella R, Boulanger JM, Trudeau L, Hegele RA, Woo V, McFarlane P, Vallée M, Howlett J, Bacon SL, Lindsay P, Gilbert RE, Lewanczuk RZ, Tobe S; Canadian Hypertension Education Program. The 2009 Canadian Hypertension Education Program recommendations for the management of hypertension: Part 2—therapy. *Can J Cardiol*. 2009 May;25(5):287-98

[81] News release from American Heart Association's 63rd High Blood Pressure Research Conference. High-sugar diet increases men's blood pressure; gout drug protective. Abstract P127. Sept. 23, 2009. http://americanheart.mediaroom.com/index.php?s=43&item=829 Accessed December 19, 2009

[82] "Allopurinol, 200 mg twice daily for 4 weeks,... For casual BP, the mean change in systolic BP for allopurinol was -6.9 mm Hg vs -2.0 mm Hg for placebo, and the mean change in diastolic BP for allopurinol was -5.1 mm Hg vs -2.4 for placebo. CONCLUSIONS: In this short-term, crossover study of adolescents with newly diagnosed hypertension, treatment with allopurinol resulted in reduction of BP." Feig DI, Soletsky B, Johnson RJ. Effect of allopurinol on blood pressure of adolescents with newly diagnosed essential hypertension: a randomized trial. *JAMA*. 2008 Aug 27;300(8):924-32

[83] Brinker AD. Allopurinol and the role of uric acid in hypertension. [letter] *JAMA*. 2009 Jan 21;301(3):270

fructose diet in particular can help reduce elevated serum uric acid levels without the use of drugs because this dietary profile is low in fructose and promotes urinary alkalinization; alkalinizing the urine via avoidance of acidogenic foodstuffs such as dairy and sodium chloride and by increased intake of fruits and vegetables (or supplemental forms of citrate and bicarbonate[84]) promotes renal excretion of uric acid, thus lessening the adverse metabolic effects of uric acid on insulin resistance and endothelial dysfunction.

> **Clinical Insight**
> Patients with lifestyle-generated diseases should be coached in the reversal of the patterns that have caused their disease rather than being enabled to pursue these disease-promoting lifestyles while surrogate markers of metabolic-physiologic dysfunction are pharmacologically suppressed.

- o **Arachidonate avoidance**: Arachidonate promotes intracellular calcium accumulation which promotes the development of HTN. Avoidance of arachidonic acid helps restore intracellular ion homeostasis and results in reduction of elevated BP. Restoration of fatty acid balance via simultaneous reduced intake of arachidonate and increased intake of oleic acid (found in olive oil), gamma-linolenic acid (found in borage seed oil, hemp seed oil, black currant seed oil, and evening primrose oil), and eicosapentaenoic acid (EPA) and docosahexaenoic acid (DHA)(both from cold-water fish oil) helps reduce intracellular hypercalcinosis that promotes chronic HTN in addition to effecting beneficial changes in inflammatory, hemorheologic, and coagulation indices.
- **Fish oil or combination fatty acid supplementation**: The cardioprotective benefits of fish oil are insufficiently represented by the minimal numerical reduction in blood pressure that is achieved with this intervention. Despite only lowering blood pressure by a few points (if at all), fish oil is safer, less expensive, and more effective than "statin" antihypercholesterolemic drug treatment for reducing total and cardiovascular mortality. Thus, combination fatty acid supplementation should be used for its cardioprotective benefits regardless of its effect on blood pressure. The combination of EPA+DHA from fish oil and GLA from borage oil (or other source) in a ratio of approximately 2:1 (e.g., daily intake of 4 grams EPA+DHA along with 2 grams GLA) appears to provide the best cardioprotective benefit based on favorable changes in serum lipids, according to a speculative prospective clinical trial by Laidlaw and Holub.[85]
- **Correction of vitamin D deficiency**: Vitamin D3 (cholecalciferol) and calcium supplementation can reduce blood pressure in cholecalciferol-deficient hypertensive patients by approximately -13/-7.[86] As I have discussed in extensive detail elsewhere, a reasonable dose of vitamin D3 for adults is in the range of 4,000-10,000 IU per day, and doctors new to vitamin D therapy should read our clinical monograph published in 2004 and

---

[84] "The treatment of uric acid stones should focus on alkalinization of the urine with citrate or bicarbonate salts." Liebman SE, Taylor JG, Bushinsky DA. Uric acid nephrolithiasis. *Curr Rheumatol Rep*. 2007 Jun;9(3):251-7

[85] "A mixture of 4 g EPA+DHA and 2 g GLA favorably altered blood lipid and fatty acid profiles in healthy women. On the basis of calculated PROCAM values, the 4:2 group was estimated to have a 43% reduction in the 10-y risk of myocardial infarction." Laidlaw M, Holub BJ. Effects of supplementation with fish oil-derived n-3 fatty acids and gamma-linolenic acid on circulating plasma lipids and fatty acid profiles in women. *Am J Clin Nutr*. 2003 Jan;77(1):37-42

[86] "A short-term supplementation with vitamin D(3) and calcium is more effective in reducing SBP than calcium alone. Inadequate vitamin D(3) and calcium intake could play a contributory role in the pathogenesis and progression of hypertension and cardiovascular disease in elderly women." Pfeifer M, Begerow B, Minne HW, Nachtigall D, Hansen C. Effects of a short-term vitamin D(3) and calcium supplementation on blood pressure and parathyroid hormone levels in elderly women. *J Clin Endocrinol Metab*. 2001 Apr;86(4):1633-7

available on-line.[87] The most important drug interaction with vitamin D is seen with hydrochlorothiazide, a commonly-used antihypertensive diuretic that promotes hypercalcemia; vitamin D therapy in patients taking hydrochlorothiazide must be implemented slowly, with professional supervision, and with weekly laboratory monitoring of serum calcium. The goal of vitamin D3 supplementation is for serum 25-OH-vitamin D levels to reach the optimal range of 50-100 ng/ml.

- **Exercise**: Current guidelines indicate that everyone should obtain 30-60 minutes of exercise 4-7 times per week unless specific contraindications exist. Patients with or at risk of CAD should receive baseline and stress/exercise ECG, perhaps with stress echocardiography if ECG abnormalities are detected.

**Excess vitamin D**
> 100 ng/mL (250 nmol/L) with hypercalcemia

**Optimal range**
50 - 100 ng/mL (125 - 250 nmol/L)

**Insufficiency range**
< 20- 40 ng/mL (50 - 100 nmol/L)

**Deficiency**
< 20 ng/mL (50 nmol/L)

Interpretation of serum 25(OH) vitamin D levels. Modified from Vasquez et al, *Alternative Therapies in Health and Medicine* 2004 and Vasquez A. *Musculoskeletal Pain: Expanded Clinical Strategies* (Institute for Functional Medicine) 2008.

- **Weight optimization**: All patients *and doctors* should maintain a healthy body weight; Canadian guidelines published in 2009 specify a body mass index 18.5-24.9 and waist circumference (<102 cm [40.2 inches] for men and <88 cm [34.6 inches] for women).[88] In most patients and clinical situations, body weight and body mass can be used as an indicator of compliance with a health-promoting diet and plan of regular *sufficiently intense* exercise. Exercise sufficiency can be assessed by the ability of the activity to produce mild breathlessness, diaphoresis, and changes in or favorable maintenance of body composition and optimal weight.

> **How to Measure Waist Circumference**
> "To measure your waist circumference, place a tape measure around your bare abdomen just above your hip bone. [Waist circumference is the distance around your natural waist (just above the navel).*] Be sure that the tape is snug (but does not compress your skin) and that it is parallel to the floor. Relax, exhale, and measure your waist."
>
> Weight and Waist Measurement: Tools for Adults. http://win.niddk.nih.gov/Publications/tools.htm Accessed February 12, 2009
> * Body Composition Tests. Accessed February 12, 2009 http://www.americanheart.org/presenter.jhtml?identifier=4489

- **Coenzyme Q-10 (CoQ-10) with doses ranging from 100-300 mg per day**: Average dietary intake of CoQ-10 is 2-5 mg/d; CoQ-10 is made endogenously, however, some patients—particularly those with migraines, asthma, hypertension, allergies, heart failure and idiopathic dilated cardiomyopathy—may have an inborn or acquired error of metabolism that prevents them

---

[87] **Vasquez** A, Manso G, Cannell J. The clinical importance of vitamin D (cholecalciferol): a paradigm shift with implications for all healthcare providers. *Altern Ther Health Med.* 2004 Sep-Oct;10(5):28-36 http://optimalhealthresearch.com/monograph04
[88] Khan NA, Hemmelgarn B, Herman RJ, Bell CM, Mahon JL, Leiter LA, Rabkin SW, Hill MD, Padwal R, Touyz RM, Larochelle P, Feldman RD, Schiffrin EL, Campbell NR, Moe G, Prasad R, Arnold MO, Campbell TS, Milot A, Stone JA, Jones C, Ogilvie RI, Hamet P, Fodor G, Carruthers G, Burns KD, Ruzicka M, DeChamplain J, Pylypchuk G, Petrella R, Boulanger JM, Trudeau L, Hegele RA, Woo V, McFarlane P, Vallée M, Howlett J, Bacon SL, Lindsay P, Gilbert RE, Lewanczuk RZ, Tobe S; Canadian Hypertension Education Program. The 2009 Canadian Hypertension Education Program recommendations for the management of hypertension: Part 2—therapy. *Can J Cardiol.* 2009 May;25(5):287-98

from making sufficient amounts of this vitally important substance. Hypertensive patients generally have lower serum CoQ-10 levels than normotensive persons. Typical blood levels of CoQ-10 range from 0.7-1 mcg/ml; however clinical benefit in CVD may require serum levels of 2-3 and up to 4 mcg/ml to attain maximal clinical benefit.[89] Testing of serum CoQ-10 levels is not necessary before starting treatment;

> **Clinical Insight**
> Because HTN and DM-obesity ("diabesity") so commonly occur together, and because effective treatments for DM commonly ameliorate HTN, clinicians treating HTN need to have knowledge of effective treatments for DM and obesity.
>
> Vasquez A. *Chiropractic and Naturopathic Mastery of Common Clinical Disorders*. 2009
> http://optimalhealthresearch.com/clinical_mastery

however patients who do not benefit as expected should have their CoQ-10 levels measured and supplementation increased to attain optimal serum levels before deciding that treatment is inefficacious. While clinical benefit may occur within the first week of supplementation, maximal improvement generally takes 4-8 weeks in order to obtain tissue saturation and beneficial changes in cell physiology. CoQ-10 is clearly one of the most powerful and broadly-beneficial nutritional supplements on the nutrition-healthcare market; research literature shows clinically meaningful benefit of CoQ-10 supplementation in patients with myocardial infarction, HTN, heart failure, renal failure, allergies, asthma, migraine, Parkinson's disease, and chronic viral infections such as HIV. CoQ-10 may interfere with coumadin/warfarin action in some patients; monitoring of INR is advised. CoQ-10 has generally been produced and studied in its form as "ubiquinone" however more current research and clinical trends suggest that the reduced form "ubiquinol" is better absorbed (x8) and is a more effective antioxidant. **In hypertensive patients, doses of 60-120 mg/d can typically lower BP by about -15/-9 mm Hg.** CoQ-10 can be safely used with antihypertensive medications and is generally safer than all antihypertensive medications.

- Review: Role of coenzyme Q10 (CoQ10) in cardiac disease, hypertension and Meniere-like syndrome: In this excellent review that covers the role of CoQ-10 in the treatment of cardiovascular diseases—heart failure, HTN, myocardial infarction, arrhythmia—and Meniere syndrome and hearing loss, Kumar et al[90] review the literature to conclude that CoQ-10 provides major clinical benefit in all of these conditions and without adverse effects. Cardioprotective properties of CoQ-10 include its role as an antioxidant, vasodilator, and membrane stabilizer in addition to its ability to decrease blood viscosity, proinflammatory cytokines, endothelial dysfunction, insulin resistance, and to promote proper diastolic and systolic function of the myocardium. Additional functions of CoQ-10 specific to its benefit in HTN appear related to the ability of CoQ-10 to antagonize aldosterone and/or angiotensin; if confirmed, these functions would support the concept that CoQ10 functions in part like an aldosterone antagonist (such as spironolactone) and/or an angiotensin 2 receptor blocker (such as losartan). **Typical blood pressure reduction with use of CoQ10 can be as high as -18/-11,** depending on dose, attained serum levels; other common nutritional deficiencies such as magnesium, potassium, and

---

[89] Kumar A, Kaur H, Devi P, Mohan V. Role of coenzyme Q10 (CoQ10) in cardiac disease, hypertension and Meniere-like syndrome. *Pharmacol Ther*. 2009 Dec;124(3):259-68

[90] Kumar A, Kaur H, Devi P, Mohan V. Role of coenzyme Q10 (CoQ10) in cardiac disease, hypertension and Meniere-like syndrome. *Pharmacol Ther*. 2009 Dec;124(3):259-68

vitamin D can also be addressed to improve efficacy. Maximal improvement might take 4-8 weeks; however, some patients will respond more quickly—within the first week—and this observation underscores the importance of frequent BP monitoring and the need to adjust doses of antihypertensive drugs as needed to avoid hypotension and its complications such as syncope.

- Randomized, double-blind, placebo-controlled trial of coenzyme Q10 in isolated systolic hypertension: Twice daily administration of 60 mg of oral CoQ-10 was given to 46 men and 37 women with isolated systolic hypertension in a 12-week randomized, double-blind, placebo-controlled trial. "RESULTS: The mean reduction in systolic blood pressure of the CoQ-treated group was 17.8 mm Hg. None of the patients exhibited orthostatic blood pressure changes. CONCLUSIONS: Our results suggest CoQ may be safely offered to hypertensive patients as an alternative treatment option."[91]

- Clinical trial with water-soluble CoQ-10: Effect of hydrosoluble coenzyme Q10 on blood pressures and insulin resistance in hypertensive patients with coronary artery disease: In this randomized double-blind placebo-controlled trial among patients receiving antihypertensive medication and with coronary artery disease (n=59: 30 in treatment group, 29 in placebo group), patients received oral coenzyme Q10 (60 mg twice daily) for 8 weeks. **In the coenzyme Q10 group, beneficial reductions were noted in systolic and diastolic blood pressures (average 168/106 reduced to 152/97 [-16/-9]),** heart rate, waist–hip ratio, fasting and 2-h plasma insulin and glucose levels, triglyceride levels and angina; CoQ-10 supplementation raised HDL-cholesterol. The authors concluded, "These findings indicate that treatment with coenzyme Q10 decreases blood pressure possibly by decreasing oxidative stress and insulin response in patients with known hypertension receiving conventional antihypertensive drugs."[92]

- Open trial using average dose of CoQ-10 225 mg/d for the treatment of essential hypertension with coenzyme Q10: This study was one of the first to use dosage adjustments to attain serum CoQ10 levels of at least 2 mcg/ml. "A total of 109 patients with symptomatic essential hypertension presenting to a private cardiology practice were observed after the addition of CoQ10 (average dose, 225 mg/day by mouth) to their existing antihypertensive drug regimen. ... A definite and gradual improvement in functional status was observed with the concomitant need to gradually decrease antihypertensive drug therapy within the first one to six months. Thereafter, clinical status and cardiovascular drug requirements stabilized with a significantly improved systolic and diastolic blood pressure. Overall New York Heart Association (NYHA) functional class improved from a mean of 2.40 to 1.36 (P < 0.001) and 51% of patients came completely off of between one and three antihypertensive drugs at an average of 4.4 months after starting CoQ10. ... In the 9.4% of patients with echocardiograms both before and during treatment, we observed a highly significant improvement in left ventricular wall thickness and diastolic function."[93]

- Open trial with low-dose CoQ-10 reduced BP -18/-12, reduced total cholesterol -9, and raised HDL +2: In this open trial with no comparative placebo group (*just like clinical*

---

[91] Burke BE, Neuenschwander R, Olson RD. Randomized, double-blind, placebo-controlled trial of coenzyme Q10 in isolated systolic hypertension. *South Med J.* 2001 Nov;94(11):1112-7
[92] Singh RB, Niaz MA, Rastogi SS, Shukla PK, Thakur AS. Effect of hydrosoluble coenzyme Q10 on blood pressures and insulin resistance in hypertensive patients with coronary artery disease. *J Hum Hypertens.* 1999 Mar;13(3):203-8
[93] Langsjoen P, Langsjoen P, Willis R, Folkers K. Treatment of essential hypertension with coenzyme Q10. *Mol Aspects Med.* 1994;15 Suppl:S265-72

*practice!*), 26 patients with essential hypertension received oral CoQ10 50 mg twice daily for 10 weeks. Major findings were as follows: systolic blood pressure (SBP) decreased from 164.5 to 146.7 mmHg and diastolic blood pressure (DBP) decreased from 98.1 to 86.1 mmHg; thus **the blood pressure reduction by CoQ-10 was -17.8/-12.** Serum total cholesterol decreased from 222.9 mg/dl to 213.3 mg/dl (P < 0.005) and HDL cholesterol increased from 41.1 mg/dl to 43.1 mg/dl (P < 0.01). In a subset of patients for whom appropriate measures were obtained, total peripheral resistance decreased from 2,283 to 1,627 dyne/sec/cm-5.[94] These anti-hypertensive results, the collateral benefits, and the absence of adverse effects make CoQ-10 appear superior to drug treatment for chronic HTN.
  - Correlational study: CoQ-10 is an independent predictor of mortality in chronic heart failure: Plasma samples from 236 patients admitted to the hospital with heart failure were assayed for LDL and total cholesterol, and total CoQ-10. "CONCLUSIONS: Plasma CoQ-10 concentration was an independent predictor of mortality in this cohort. The **CoQ-10 deficiency might be detrimental to the long-term prognosis of CHF [chronic heart failure],** and there is a rationale for controlled intervention studies with CoQ-10."[95]

- **Magnesium (Mg) dosed at 600 mg per day or to bowel tolerance**: Given the safety and low cost of magnesium, along with the high prevalence of magnesium deficiency in the general population, routine oral magnesium supplementation is warranted. The standard replacement dose for oral magnesium supplementation is 600 mg per day; some patients may tolerate less or need more, with a typical range of 200-1,800 mg/d being used in clinical practice. Insufficient doses are inefficacious, while excess doses are generally benign (causing only transient loose stools). Renal insufficiency and medication with the magnesium-retaining diuretic spironolactone indicate the need for cautious dosing and more frequent clinical and laboratory monitoring. Measurement of *intracellular* Mg levels in erythrocytes or leukocytes is more accurate than is measurement of *serum* Mg levels.

> **Key Concept**
> **Subphysiologic doses of nutrients are subtherapeutic.** In order to obtain a physiologic effect and an optimal clinical benefit from nutritional supplementation, the supplementation must be of adequate *duration, dose,* and *bioavailability* to optimally supply cellular processes. *Cofactors, co-nutrients,* and the *proper biochemical milieu* (pH in particular) are also required for optimal effectiveness of the nutritional intervention.
>
> Vasquez A. **Subphysiologic doses of vitamin D are subtherapeutic**: comment on the study by The Record Trial Group. *The Lancet* 2005. Published online May 6 http://optimalhealthresearch.com/lancet

  - Clinical trial: Oral magnesium supplementation reduces ambulatory blood pressure in patients with mild hypertension: For a 12-week period, 48 patients with mild uncomplicated hypertension were assigned either to treatment with 600 mg (25 mmol) of magnesium pidolate orally twice a day for 12 weeks + lifestyle recommendations (n=24) or to treatment with lifestyle recommendations only. "RESULTS: In the Mg(2+) supplementation group, **small but significant reductions in mean 24-h systolic and**

---

[94] Digiesi V, Cantini F, Oradei A, Bisi G, Guarino GC, Brocchi A, Bellandi F, Mancini M, Littarru GP. Coenzyme Q10 in essential hypertension. *Mol Aspects Med.* 1994;15 Suppl:s257-63
[95] Molyneux SL, Florkowski CM, George PM, Pilbrow AP, Frampton CM, Lever M, Richards AM. Coenzyme Q10: an independent predictor of mortality in chronic heart failure. *J Am Coll Cardiol.* 2008 Oct 28;52(18):1435-41

**diastolic BP levels were observed**, in contrast to control group (-5.6 vs. -1.3 mm Hg, and -2.8 vs. -1 mm Hg, respectively). These effects of Mg(2+) supplementation were consistent in both daytime and night-time periods. Serum Mg(2+) levels and urinary Mg(2+) excretion were significantly increased in the intervention group. Intracellular Mg(2+) and K(+) levels were also increased, while intracellular Ca(2+) and Na(+) levels were decreased in the intervention group. None of the intracellular ions were significantly changed in the control group. CONCLUSION: This study suggests that oral Mg(2+) supplementation is associated with small but consistent ambulatory BP reduction in patients with mild hypertension."[96] Readers should note that magnesium supplementation in this study was shown to reduce intracellular calcium and to increase intracellular potassium simultaneously with the reduction in BP. These findings are consistent with my proposal for treatment of intracellular hypercalcinosis[97] published in 2006 and with the fact that magnesium sufficiency is mandatory for the intracellular uptake of potassium; any patient with chronic hypokalemia should be tested and/or treated for magnesium insufficiency. *How do we translate "600 mg (25 mmol) of magnesium pidolate orally twice a day" into an understanding of the clinical dosage which is generally expressed in milligrams of elemental Mg?* The physiologic action of magnesium supplements depends upon their content of magnesium ion. Magnesium pidolate is the magnesium salt of pidolic acid (pyroglutamic acid), which is only 8.7% Mg by weight. Thus, "600 mg (25 mmol) of magnesium pidolate orally twice a day" provides 1,200 mg of magnesium pidolate which provides 8.7% of 600 mg of elemental magnesium, which is only 104 mg of elemental Mg per day. Given that the standard replacement dose for Mg is 600 mg per day of elemental Mg, we see that the dose used in this study was suboptimally therapeutic (only 17% of the standard dose of Mg) and that therefore the clinical results are less impressive than those which would have been obtained if the study subjects had used a more substantial amount of Mg.

- **Acetyl-L-carnitine and L-carnitine**: Acetyl-L-carnitine (ALC) first made its impression on clinicians when it was found to be effective treatment for Alzheimer's disease; later research found application for this nutrient in the treatment of hepatic coma, Peyronie's disease, male sexual dysfunction, various types of peripheral neuropathy, dysthymia, fibromyalgia, and various types of physical and mental fatigue. Common therapeutic doses are 1,500-3,000 mg per day of either or both of ALC and/or L-carnitine), taken orally, between meals; clinicians should appreciate that amino acid therapy is generally administered between meals to avoid problems arising from competitive blockade among amino acids as they are absorbed/utilized. L-carnitine and ALC can be administered together; use of one does not necessarily preclude use of the other. For example in the study by Cavallini et al[98] among aging men, L-carnitine 2 g/day plus acetyl-L-carnitine 2 g/day proved significantly more effective than testosterone in improving nocturnal penile tumescence and International Index of Erectile Function score.

---

[96] Hatzistavri LS, Sarafidis PA, Georgianos PI, Tziolas IM, Aroditis CP, Zebekakis PE, Pikilidou MI, Lasaridis AN. Oral magnesium supplementation reduces ambulatory blood pressure in patients with mild hypertension. *Am J Hypertens*. 2009 Oct;22(10):1070-5
[97] **Vasquez A**. Intracellular Hypercalcinosis: A Functional Nutritional Disorder with Implications Ranging from Myofascial Trigger Points to Affective Disorders, Hypertension, and Cancer. *Naturopathy Digest* 2006  Previously published in-print and on-line at http://www.naturopathydigest.com/archives/2006/sep/vasquez.php and included at the end of this chapter.
[98] Cavallini G, Caracciolo S, Vitali G, Modenini F, Biagiotti G. Carnitine versus androgen administration in the treatment of sexual dysfunction, depressed mood, and fatigue associated with male aging. *Urology*. 2004 Apr;63(4):641-6

- Review: Carnitine Insufficiency Caused by Aging and *Overnutrition* Compromises Mitochondrial Performance and Metabolic Control: "…we hypothesized that carnitine insufficiency might contribute to mitochondrial dysfunction and obesity-related impairments in glucose tolerance. Consistent with this prediction whole body carnitine diminution was identified as a common feature of insulin resistant states such as advanced age, genetic diabetes and diet-induced obesity."[99] This impressive study documented that carnitine deficiency is noted in patients with obesity and insulin resistance.
- Clinical trial: Ameliorating Hypertension and Insulin Resistance in Subjects at Increased Cardiovascular Risk. Effects of Acetyl-L-Carnitine Therapy: In a previous trial, acetyl-L-carnitine infusion acutely ameliorated insulin resistance in type-2 diabetics. In this sequential off-on-off pilot study, the authors prospectively evaluated the effects of 24-week oral acetyl-L-carnitine (1 g twice daily) therapy on the glucose disposal rate (GDR), assessed by hyperinsulinemic euglycemic clamps, and components of the metabolic syndrome in nondiabetic subjects at increased cardiovascular risk. "Acetyl-L-carnitine increased GDR from 4.89+/-1.47 to 6.72+/-3.12 mg/kg per minute (P=0.003, Bonferroni-adjusted) and improved glucose tolerance in patients with GDR </=7.9 mg/kg per minute, whereas it had no effects in those with higher GDRs. ... **Systolic blood pressure decreased from 144.0 to 135.1 mm Hg and from 130.8 to 123.8 mm Hg in the lower and higher GDR groups, respectively… Acetyl-L-carnitine safely ameliorated arterial hypertension**, insulin resistance, impaired glucose tolerance, and hypoadiponectinemia in subjects at increased cardiovascular risk. Whether these effects may translate into long-term cardioprotection is worth investigating."[100]
- Randomized placebo-controlled double-blind crossover study: Effect of combined treatment with alpha-Lipoic acid (400 mg/d) and acetyl-L-carnitine (1,000 mg/d) on vascular function and blood pressure in patients with documented coronary artery disease: The authors note that mitochondria produce reactive oxygen species that may contribute to vascular dysfunction, and that both oxidative stress and mitochondrial dysfunction can be ameliorated by alpha-Lipoic acid and acetyl-L-carnitine. Among 36 subjects with coronary artery disease, active treatment for 8 weeks increased brachial artery diameter by 2.3%, consistent with reduced arterial tone. "Active treatment **decreased systolic blood pressure** for the whole group and had a significant effect in the subgroup with blood pressure above the median (151 to 142 mm Hg) and in the subgroup with the metabolic syndrome (139 to 130 mm Hg)."[101] Although this study used low-modest doses of acetyl-carnitine and lipoic acid, it showed that antihypertensive benefits were greatest in patients with systolic blood pressure >135 mm Hg—blood pressure was reduced by approximately -9/-5—and in patients with metabolic syndrome—blood pressure was reduced by approximately -7/-3. More

---

[99] Noland RC, Koves TR, Seiler SE, Lum H, Lust RM, Ilkayeva O, Stevens R, Hegardt FG, Muoio DM. Carnitine Insufficiency Caused by Aging and Overnutrition Compromises Mitochondrial Performance and Metabolic Control. *J Biol Chem*. 2009 Jun 24. [Epub ahead of print]
[100] Ruggenenti P, Cattaneo D, Loriga G, Ledda F, Motterlini N, Gherardi G, Orisio S, Remuzzi G. Ameliorating Hypertension and Insulin Resistance in Subjects at Increased Cardiovascular Risk. Effects of Acetyl-L-Carnitine Therapy. *Hypertension*. 2009 Jul 20
[101] McMackin CJ, Widlansky ME, Hamburg NM, Huang AL, Weller S, Holbrook M, Gokce N, Hagen TM, Keaney JF Jr, Vita JA. Effect of combined treatment with alpha-Lipoic acid and acetyl-L-carnitine on vascular function and blood pressure in patients with coronary artery disease. *J Clin Hypertens* (Greenwich). 2007 Apr;9(4):249-55

significant results probably would have been obtained with higher doses, but these results are still statistically and clinically significant.

- **L-Arginine**: L-arginine (Arg) is the amino acid precursor for the formation of vasodilating nitric oxide (NO) produced via the action of endothelial nitric oxide synthase. A significant number of hypertensive patients have impaired conversion of Arg into NO, and a subset of these patients benefit from oral Arg supplementation. As usual, amino acid supplementation is delivered between meals (empty stomach) to facilitate absorption, and coadministration of simple carbohydrate can facilitate insulin-mediated cellular amino acid uptake. Recently, asymmetric dimethylarginine (ADMA) has been identified as an independent cardiovascular risk factor; per the excellent review by Böger[102], clinicians should appreciate that ADMA—formed from degradation of methylated proteins and an endogenous competitive inhibitor of NO synthase (NOS)—is a vasoconstrictor found in elevated levels among patients with hypercholesterolemia, atherosclerosis, hypertension, chronic renal failure, chronic heart failure, hyperthyroidism, hyperhomocysteinemia and folate deficiency. As expected, administration of Arg has demonstrated antihypertensive benefit, particularly among patients with high ADMA levels; indeed, elevated ADMA may identify which patients are likely to respond to Arg supplementation via a more favorable Arg:ADMA ratio. Laboratory testing for ADMA is available now from some research centers (such as Baylor[103]) and will surely become more widely available in the future. The predictable clinical take-home messages are that ❶ intravenous Arg administration generally produces a greater response than does oral administration, ❷ the hypotensive benefits of Arg supplementation are short-lived, ❸ the hypotenstive benefits of Arg are more consistently seen in the groups expected to have high ADMA levels as previous listed, and ❹ younger patients (with less atherosclerosis and arterial calcification) are more likely to respond. **Clinicians should appreciate that the cardioprotective benefits of Arg extend beyond and are not entirely dependent upon its antihypertensive benefit; other benefits include decreased platelet aggregation and adhesion, decreased monocyte adhesion, antiproliferative effects on vascular smooth muscle, and improved endothelium-dependent vasodilation which can occur locally and systemically without an accompanying hypotensive effect.** Very importantly, concomitant administration of the amino acid N-acetyl-cysteine (NAC) appears to enhance the cardioprotective efficacy of Arg according to recent research.[104] Aside from the possibility of promoting reactivation of herpes simplex outbreaks, Arg is remarkably safe and is commonly used in immunonutrition formulas as a life-saving treatment in critically ill patients; Zhou and Martindale[105] recently noted, "The numerous potential beneficial effects of arginine in the critically ill patient include: 1) stimulation of immune function via its influence on lymphocyte, macrophage, and dendritic cells; 2) improved wound healing; 3) increased net nitrogen balance; 4) **increased blood flow to key vascular beds**; and 5) decreased clinical infections and length of hospital stay." The doses employed have ranged

---

[102] Böger RH. Asymmetric dimethylarginine, an endogenous inhibitor of nitric oxide synthase, explains the "L-arginine paradox" and acts as a novel cardiovascular risk factor. *J Nutr*. 2004 Oct;134(10 Suppl):2842S-2847S http://jn.nutrition.org/cgi/content/full/134/10/2842S
[103] Institute of Metabolic Disease at Baylor Research Institute. Asymmetric dimethylarginine (ADMA). http://www.baylorhealth.edu/imd/researchtests/asymmetric.htm Accessed December 2009
[104] Martina V, Masha A, Gigliardi VR, et al. Long-term N-acetylcysteine and L-arginine administration reduces endothelial activation and systolic blood pressure in hypertensive patients with type 2 diabetes. *Diabetes Care*. 2008 May;31(5):940-4 http://care.diabetesjournals.org/content/31/5/940.long
[105] "The numerous potential beneficial effects of arginine in the critically ill patient include: 1) stimulation of immune function via its influence on lymphocyte, macrophage, and dendritic cells; 2) improved wound healing; 3) increased net nitrogen balance; 4) increased blood flow to key vascular beds; and 5) decreased clinical infections and length of hospital stay." Zhou M, Martindale RG. Arginine in the critical care setting. *J Nutr*. 2007 Jun;137(6 Suppl 2):1687S-1692S http://jn.nutrition.org/cgi/content/full/137/6/1687S

widely from 1,200 mg/d to 30,000 mg/d, (i.e., 1.2-30 g/d) and have included both oral and intravenous administration. Of course, Arg can be used with other dietary and nutritional interventions and with drug treatments with the caveat that common sense is employed to minimize the risk of hypotension by not drastically implementing too many treatments all at once.

- o Open clinical trial: The effects of sustained-release L-arginine on blood pressure and vascular compliance in 29 healthy individuals (normotensives and hypertensives) treated for one week: Miller[106] used 2.1 g/d Arg administered in two divided doses in a sustained release preparation to find that approximately 65% of hypertensive patients responded favorably with an average reduction of -4/-3.7 for the group as a whole that included normotensives and hypertensives. **Among patients who were "borderline or hypertensive" the average BP reduction was -11/-4.9 mm Hg.** Vascular elasticity assessed by digital pulse wave analysis showed a significant increase in large artery compliance (mean 23% improvement). Given the low dose, the short duration, and the low cost and absence of adverse effects, these results are worthy of clinical consideration and additional study. Consistent with many studies in clinical nutrition, the intervention provided an alterative, homeostatic effect in that—in contrast to the effects of pharmaceutical drugs—the effects are benign and rather minimal in healthy-normotensive persons and are clinically significant and therapeutic in patients with the index disease.

- o Randomized placebo-controlled trial: Effect of L-arginine on blood pressure in pregnancy-induced hypertension (n = 123): Inclusion criteria for this trial included maternal age range 16-45 years, diagnosis of gestational hypertension without proteinuria (patients normotensive until the 20th week), and gestational age ranging between 24 and 36 weeks. Subjects were allocated to receive either Arg 20 g/500 mL intravenously or placebo treatment through an i.v. line. Treatment or placebo was administered in the morning from 8-10 a.m. and was repeated for four consecutive days. The final analysis was performed on 62 women in the Arg group and 61 in the placebo group. "RESULTS: Maternal clinical features such as age, height, weight, and gestational age at inclusion were similar between groups. Both systolic and diastolic blood pressures were reduced by treatment, the effect of L-arginine being significantly higher than that of the placebo (systolic values F = 8.59, p < 0.005; diastolic values F = 3.36; p < 0.001). ... CONCLUSIONS: In conclusion, these data support the use of L-Arg as an antihypertensive agent for gestational hypertension especially in view of the other beneficial effects nitric oxide donors display in pregnancy. Further, L-Arg seems well tolerated since in this sample none of the patients reported adverse effects requiring study interruption."[107] According to Figure 4 of the article, BP reductions were approximately -5/-8 mm Hg.

- o Double-blind placebo-controlled clinical trial: Long-term N-acetylcysteine and L-arginine administration reduces endothelial activation and systolic blood pressure in hypertensive

---

[106] Miller AL. The effects of sustained-release-L-arginine formulation on blood pressure and vascular compliance in 29 healthy individuals. *Altern Med Rev*. 2006 Mar;11(1):23-9 http://www.thorne.com/altmedrev/.fulltext/11/1/23.pdf
[107] Neri I, Jasonni VM, Gori GF, Blasi I, Facchinetti F. Effect of L-arginine on blood pressure in pregnancy-induced hypertension: a randomized placebo-controlled trial. *J Matern Fetal Neonatal Med*. 2006 May;19(5):277-81

patients with type 2 diabetes: This double-blind trial included 24 male patients with type-2 DM and HTN divided into two groups of 12 patients that randomly received either placebo or NAC 1,200 mg/d and ARG 1,200 mg/d orally for 6 months. "RESULTS—The NAC + ARG treatment caused a reduction of both systolic and diastolic mean arterial blood pressure, total cholesterol, LDL cholesterol, oxidized LDL, high-sensitive C-reactive protein, intracellular adhesion molecule, vascular cell adhesion molecule, nitrotyrosine, fibrinogen, and plasminogen activator inhibitor-1, and an improvement of the intima-media thickness during endothelial postischemic vasodilation. HDL cholesterol increased. No changes in other parameters studied were observed. CONCLUSIONS—NAC + ARG administration seems to be a potential well-tolerated antiatherogenic therapy because it improves endothelial function in hypertensive patients with type 2 diabetes by improving NO bioavailability via reduction of oxidative stress and increase of NO production. Our study's results give prominence to its potential use in primary and secondary cardiovascular prevention in these patients.[108] The BP change in the treatment group was -5/-5 mm Hg; the results of this study are remarkable considering the low dose of Arg employed and the manifold biochemical benefits attained.

- Review: L-arginine and cardiovascular system: "The majority of experimental and clinical studies clearly show a beneficial effect of L-arginine on endothelium in conditions associated with its hypofunction and thus with reduced NO synthesis. Some clinical studies involving healthy volunteers or patients suffering from hypertension and diabetes indicate that it may also regulate vascular hemostasis."[109] The full text of this article goes on to itemize several clinical trials (at variable level of detail), the majority of these articles related to HTN will be summarized here:
    - Placebo controlled trial of 30 g (thirty grams) Arg infused intravenously over 30 minutes to healthy volunteers: Diastolic BP was "markedly reduced" more than was systolic BP; another study conducted in women found similar results.
    - Consumption of an Arg-enriched diet by healthy volunteers: BP reduction.
    - Oral administration of 21g daily to healthy young men for 3 days: No correlation of Arg with blood pressure.
    - Oral administration of 20g daily to healthy men for 28 days: No reduction in BP.
    - Oral administration of 9g daily to healthy subjects for 6 months: No reduction in BP; however, "long-term administration of this amino acid had a favorable effect on endothelium, improving its function and reducing concentration of endothelin." (Endothelins are peptides that constrict blood vessels and contribute to HTN.)
    - Intravenous Arg given at a dose of 500 mg/kg in patients with primary and secondary hypertension: "Considerable reduction both in systolic and diastolic pressure in all the cases."
    - Intravenous Arg given at a dose of 30g over 60 minutes in patients with treated/untreated HTN: Previously untreated HTN patients had the best clinical

---

[108] Martina V, Masha A, Gigliardi VR, et al. Long-term N-acetylcysteine and L-arginine administration reduces endothelial activation and systolic blood pressure in hypertensive patients with type 2 diabetes. *Diabetes Care*. 2008 May;31(5):940-4 http://care.diabetesjournals.org/content/31/5/940.long
[109] Cylwik D, Mogielnicki A, Buczko W. L-arginine and cardiovascular system. *Pharmacol Rep*. 2005 Jan-Feb;57(1):14-22 http://www.if-pan.krakow.pl/pjp/pdf/2005/1_14.pdf

response, followed by ACEi-treated patients, and a slight BP reduction in normal volunteers.
- <u>Oral Arg 5.6 or 12.6 g/day for 6 weeks in patients with heart failure</u>: Reduction in arterial blood pressure.
- <u>Oral Arg 21 g for 3 days to young men with coronary artery disease</u>: No changes in blood pressure despite improvement in brachial artery dilation.
- <u>Intravenous bolus of 3g Arg to healthy subjects and patients with insulin-independent diabetes, hypercholesterolemia and primary hypertension</u>: Best response was seen in young healthy patients (response inverse to age), then hypertensives, and lastly in patients with hypercholesterolemia and DM.
- <u>Oral Arg 21 g/d for 4 weeks in young patients with hypercholesterolemia</u>: Improved endothelium-dependent dilatation.
- <u>Intravenous infusion of Arg 30 g for 60 minutes in patients with limb ischemia</u>: "Marked reduction in diastolic and systolic pressure and an increased blood flow in the femoral artery."

- **Chiropractic spinal manipulative therapy**: Spinal manipulative therapy has proven safe and effective for musculoskeletal spinal pain as well as some extra-spinal disorders, notably asthma. Chiropractic manipulation differs from the types of manipulation provided by other professions (e.g., osteopathic, naturopathic) and thus research substantiating the effectiveness of chiropractic manipulation may not be applicable to different manipulative approaches.
    - <u>Double-blind, placebo-controlled pilot study of chiropractic manipulation for treatment of hypertension: Atlas vertebra realignment and achievement of arterial pressure goal in hypertensive patients (n=50)</u>: The authors introduce this study by writing, "Anatomical abnormalities of the cervical spine at the level of the Atlas vertebra are associated with relative ischemia of the brainstem circulation and increased blood pressure (BP). Manual correction of this mal-alignment has been associated with reduced arterial pressure." The authors used a double-blind, placebo-controlled design at a single center among 50 drug naïve (n=26) or washed out (n=24) patients with Stage 1 hypertension; patients were randomized to receive a National Upper Cervical Chiropractic (NUCCA) procedure or a sham procedure. Significant findings included the following, "At week 8, there were differences in systolic BP (-17 mm Hg, NUCCA versus -3 mm Hg, placebo) and diastolic BP (-10 mm Hg, NUCCA versus -2 mm Hg). … No adverse effects were recorded. We conclude that restoration of Atlas alignment is associated with marked and sustained reductions in BP similar to the use of two-drug combination therapy.."[110]
    - <u>Case report: Chiropractic management of a hypertensive patient</u>: In this single illustrative case report, the clinician authors describe their experience with a 38-year-old male previously diagnosed with and medicated for chronic essential HTN; the patient's presenting complaints were HTN, drug-related side effects, and low back pain. Chiropractic treatment emphasized specific contact, short lever arm spinal adjustments as the primary mode of chiropractic care. The authors noted, "**During the course of chiropractic treatment, the patient's need for hypertensive medication was reduced.**

---

[110] Bakris G, Dickholtz M Sr, Meyer PM, Kravitz G, Avery E, Miller M, Brown J, Woodfield C, Bell B. Atlas vertebra realignment and achievement of arterial pressure goal in hypertensive patients: a pilot study. *J Hum Hypertens*. 2007 May;21(5):347-52

The patient's medical physician gradually withdrew the medication over 2 months." Appreciating the BP-normalizing benefits of chiropractic manipulation and how these benefits may lead to complications in patients whose physiologic homeostasis is restored, the authors caution that "specific contact short lever arm spinal adjustments may cause a hypotensive effect in a medicated hypertensive patient that may lead to complications (e.g., hypotension). Since a medicated hypertensive patient's blood pressure may fall below normal while he or she is undergoing chiropractic care, it is advised that the blood pressure be closely monitored and medications adjusted, if necessary, by the patient's medical physician."[111]

- <u>Randomized, controlled trial (active treatment, placebo treatment, or no treatment): Effects of chiropractic treatment on blood pressure and anxiety</u>: This study (n=21) differs from the previously cited article "Atlas vertebra realignment and achievement of arterial pressure goal in hypertensive patients"[112] in that ❶ the thoracic spine (T1-T5) rather than the upper cervical spine was the area of treatment, ❷ the treatment used a mechanical chiropractic adjusting device rather than manual manipulation, and ❸ the study included assessment for anxiety as well as for changes in BP, rather than BP alone. The authors concluded, "**Results indicated that systolic and diastolic blood pressure decreased significantly in the active treatment condition**, whereas no significant changes occurred in the placebo and control conditions. State anxiety significantly decreased in the active and control conditions. **Results provide support for the hypothesis that blood pressure is reduced following chiropractic treatment**."[113]

- <u>Pilot study to determine the feasibility of a practice-based randomized controlled clinical trial with three parallel groups: Chiropractic adjustments and brief massage treatment at sites of subluxation in subjects with essential hypertension</u>: Treatment groups in this study consisted of ❶ chiropractic manipulation, ❷ brief soft tissue massage, or ❸ nontreatment control group. The patient group consisted of 23 subjects, 24-50 years of age, with systolic or diastolic primary HTN. In the active chiropractic treatment group, the intervention consisted of 2 months of full-spine chiropractic care using Gonstead technique, described as specific-contact, short-lever-arm adjustments delivered at motion segments exhibiting signs of subluxation. The massage group received brief effleurage at localized regions of the spine believed to be exhibiting signs of subluxation. The nontreatment control group rested alone for a period of approximately 5 minutes in a treatment room. In both the chiropractic and massage therapy groups, all subjects were classified as either overweight or obese; in the control group, only 2 subjects were overweight—these baseline differences in the study groups are important as they suggest that more patients in the chiropractic treatment group probably had HTN as a component of the metabolic syndrome rather than HTN due specifically and solely to a musculoskeletal lesion. The authors report that at the end of the study period, the BP change was -6.3 mm Hg in the chiropractic group, -1.0 mm Hg in the massage group, and -7.2 mm Hg in the relaxation group. The authors of this pilot feasibility study noted several methodological shortcomings and logistical complications of their study, most

---

[111] Plaugher G, Bachman TR. Chiropractic management of a hypertensive patient. *J Manipulative Physiol Ther*. 1993 Oct;16(8):544-9
[112] Bakris G, Dickholtz M Sr, Meyer PM, Kravitz G, Avery E, Miller M, Brown J, Woodfield C, Bell B. Atlas vertebra realignment and achievement of arterial pressure goal in hypertensive patients: a pilot study. *J Hum Hypertens*. 2007 May;21(5):347-52
[113] Yates RG, Lamping DL, Abram NL, Wright C. Effects of chiropractic treatment on blood pressure and anxiety: a randomized, controlled trial. *J Manipulative Physiol Ther*. 1988 Dec;11(6):484-8

notably the limited subject pool of patients who have hypertensive disease but who are not taking medications for its control. A larger study group would have allowed improved randomization and thus equilibration of baseline patient characteristics such as body mass index.[114]

- o <u>Review: Spinal manipulation and the efficacy of conservative therapeusis for the treatment of hypertension</u>: These authors review relevant chiropractic and osteopathic literature of the day (published in 1986) and conclude that manipulative therapy has a rational basis in the treatment of HTN based on the potential for spinal manipulation to promote restoration of homeostasis via reducing excess sympathetic tone and effecting a relative increase in parasympathetic tone. Spinal regions that are emphasized are ❶ the upper cervical spine (occiput-atlas) which correlates anatomically with the superior cervical sympathetic ganglia, ❷ the upper thoracic spine (T1-T6, especially T2-T3) which correlates with the thoracic sympathetic ganglia, and ❸ the lower thoracic spine (T11-T12) which correlates with sympathetic innervation via the renal ganglia/plexus that services the kidney. Clinicians should recall that sympathetic activation of the kidney increases production of renin, angiotensin-2, and aldosterone to effect systemic vasoconstriction and retention of sodium and water to increase blood volume and blood pressure. Treatment should involve manipulation of spinal segments, soft tissue massage, mobilization of the ribs, and the implementation of dietary, nutritional, exercise/lifestyle, sleep pattern, and psychoemotional interventions. The authors conclude that alleviating HTN via resolution of musculoskeletal dysfunction and restoration of homeostasis is a more logical and ethical approach than the suppression of HTN with the use of drugs that commonly have iatrogenic consequences.[115]

- **Vitamin C (ascorbic acid) 3 g/d or bowel tolerance**: Since ascorbic acid is biochemically synthesized from glucose, these molecules remain structurally similar; not surprisingly therefore, an excess of glucose (i.e., as in hyperglycemia) reduces cellular uptake of ascorbic acid, leading to a relative "cellular scurvy" even in the absence of the classic presentation of scurvy. "In neutrophils from different volunteers, glucose inhibited uptake and accumulation of ascorbic acid by both transport activities 3-9-fold. ... Glucose-induced inhibition of both ascorbic acid transport activities occurred in neutrophils of all donors tested and was fully reversible."[116]
  - o <u>Clinical trial: Vitamin C for refractory hypertension in elderly patients</u>: Treatment with ascorbic acid 600 mg/d for 6 months was evaluated for effects on blood pressure and levels of C-reactive protein, 8-isoprostane, and malondialdehyde-modified low-density lipoproteins among 12 elderly patients (average age 78.3y) and 12 adult patients (average age 54.6y) with refractory hypertension. **Chronic treatment with ascorbic acid markedly reduced systolic blood pressure and pulse pressure in ambulatory blood pressure monitoring in the elderly group from 154.9 to 134.8 mmHg** ($p < 0.001$) and from 79.1 to 63.4; respectively, which was accompanied by an increase in the serum levels of ascorbic

---

[114] Plaugher G, Long CR, Alcantara J, Silveus AD, Wood H, Lotun K, Menke JM, Meeker WC, Rowe SH. Practice-based randomized controlled-comparison clinical trial of chiropractic adjustments and brief massage treatment at sites of subluxation in subjects with essential hypertension: pilot study. *J Manipulative Physiol Ther*. 2002 May;25(4):221-39
[115] Crawford JP, Hickson GS, Wiles MR. The management of hypertensive disease: a review of spinal manipulation and the efficacy of conservative therapeusis. *J Manipulative Physiol Ther* 1986 Mar ;9(1):27-32
[116] Washko P, Levine M. Inhibition of ascorbic acid transport in human neutrophils by glucose. *J Biol Chem*. 1992 Nov 25;267(33):23568-74

acid and decreases in the levels of C-reactive protein, 8-isoprostane, and malondialdehyde-modified low-density lipoproteins. In contrast, ascorbic acid did not affect blood pressure in the adult group. These results suggest that ascorbic acid is useful for controlling blood pressure in elderly patients with refractory hypertension."[117]

Clinicians should appreciate that elevated systolic blood pressure is an important predictor of cardiovascular mortality in elderly patients, and that its ascorbate-induced reduction by -20 mmHg is highly clinically significant.

> **Clinical Pearl**
> Hypertension is always a manifestation of imbalance, underlying dysfunction, or disease.
>
> The astute clinician addresses the cause(s) of the problem directly.
>
> Except in the rare cases of an underlying disease process, HTN is almost always multifactorial—*not idiopathic*.

- **Urinary alkalinization**: In non-pathologic states, the pattern of dietary intake is the single most important determinant of systemic/urine acid-base balance.[118] The two main classes of acids of physiologic importance are 1) carbonic acid—formed when carbon dioxide ($CO_2$) from metabolism of carbohydrates and fatty acids combines with water ($H_2O$) to form carbonic acid ($H_2CO_3$), and 2) noncarbonic acids—these are primarily generated from the oxidation of sulfur-containing amino acids which results in the formation of sulfuric acid ($H_2SO_4$); avoidance of the former is mostly achieved via respiration (i.e., removal of $CO_2$) while elimination of the latter requires bicarbonate and renal excretion.[119] Average urine pH among societies consuming a Paleo-Mediterranean diet and obtaining daily physical exercise is 7.5-9; clearly this very alkaline state reflects a diet high in fruits and vegetables, and provides physiologic benefits including increased excretion of xenobiotics[120] and renal retention of potassium, magnesium, and calcium. For example, among New Guinean hunter-gatherer tribal groups living in the *primitive feral condition*, "urine pH of adults was usually between 7.5 and 9.0 because of potassium bicarbonate and carbonate excretion."[121] Excess urine alkalinity can predispose to urinary tract infections; thus some clinicians may be more comfortable with a urine pH goal of approximately 7.5-8.0.
  - Clinical trial: Neutralization of Western diet inhibits bone resorption independently of K intake and reduces cortisol secretion in humans: Acid-base neutralization by substituting equimolar amounts of sodium bicarbonate and potassium bicarbonate for NaCl and KCl "induced a significant cumulative calcium retention (10.7 +/- 0.4 mmol) and significantly reduced the urinary excretion of deoxypyridinoline, pyridinoline, and n-telopeptide. Mean daily plasma cortisol decreased from 264 +/- 45 to 232 +/- 43 nmol/l (P = 0.032), … An acidogenic Western diet results in mild metabolic acidosis in association with a state of cortisol excess, altered divalent ion metabolism, and increased bone resorptive indices. Acidosis-induced increases in cortisol secretion and plasma concentration may play a role in mild acidosis-induced alterations in bone metabolism and possibly in osteoporosis

---

[117] Sato K, Dohi Y, Kojima M, Miyagawa K, Takase H, Katada E, Suzuki S. Effects of ascorbic acid on ambulatory blood pressure in elderly patients with refractory hypertension. *Arzneimittelforschung*. 2006;56(7):535-40

[118] "Nutrition has long been known to strongly influence acid-base balance. Recently, we have shown that it is possible to appropriately estimate the renal net acid excretion (NAE) of healthy subjects from the composition of their diets." Remer T. Influence of nutrition on acid-base balance--metabolic aspects. *Eur J Nutr*. 2001 Oct;40(5):214-20

[119] Rennke HG, Denker BM. Renal Physiology: The Essentials. Second Edition. Philadelphia: Lippincott Williams and Wilkins; 2007, 129

[120] "Urine alkalinization is a treatment regimen that increases poison elimination by the administration of intravenous sodium bicarbonate to produce urine with a pH > or = 7.5." Proudfoot AT, Krenzelok EP, Vale JA. Position Paper on urine alkalinization. *J Toxicol Clin Toxicol*. 2004;42(1):1-26

[121] Sebastian A, Frassetto LA, Sellmeyer DE, Merriam RL, Morris RC Jr. Estimation of the net acid load of the diet of ancestral preagricultural Homo sapiens and their hominid ancestors. *Am J Clin Nutr*. 2002 Dec;76(6):1308-16

associated with an acidogenic Western diet."[122] Clinicians should appreciate that long-term reductions in cortisol along with renal retention of calcium would be expected to have a favorable effect on blood pressure.

- o <u>Review: Diet, evolution and aging--the pathophysiologic effects of the post-agricultural inversion of the potassium-to-sodium and base-to-chloride ratios in the human diet</u>: This excellent review article discusses the changes in mineral intake (i.e., less potassium complicated by more sodium) and the shift from a plant-based alkalinizing diet to a pseudo-food acidifying diet and the physiological ramifications of these dietary changes. Note their conclusion in the following quote which states that any level of acidosis may be unacceptable and that (conversely) a state of alkalinization is the normal and ideal human condition: "We argue that any level of acidosis may be unacceptable from an evolutionarily perspective, and indeed, that **a low-grade metabolic alkalosis may be the optimal acid-base state for humans.**"[123]

- **Mind-Body Approaches including Qigong, controlled breathing, transcendental meditation, and acupuncture**: Traditional therapeutics and lifestyle activities such as Qigong, controlled breathing, meditation, and acupuncture can effect statistically and clinically significant reductions in BP among hypertensive patients. Mechanisms of action include induction of beneficial neurohormonal responses (e.g., increased dehydroepiandrosterone and melatonin levels following meditation) as well as induction of a relaxed state. Avoidance of physiological stressors can play a role in blood pressure control and should be implemented on an as-appropriate basis. Sympathetic neural activity via beta-adrenergic receptors in the kidney stimulates release of renin, which is a peptidase enzyme that converts angiotensinogen to angiotensin-1 and thereby expedites the formation of angiotensin-2 in the lungs; angiotensin-2 is a vasoconstrictor and stimulates aldosterone production which increases sodium resorption and thus water retention.[124]; Thus, the net effect of sympathetic nervous activation is increased volume within a constricted vasculature, thus causing HTN. Data on therapeutic interventions in the following four subsections are derived from the review by Nahas.[125]

  - o <u>Qigong: A Chinese medicine form of movement, breathing, and meditation</u>: As a part of traditional Chinese medicine (TCM), Qigong incorporates movement, breathing, and meditation. Two systematic reviews involving hundreds of patients (n = > 900 to > 1,200 subjects) have examined the role of Qigong in the treatment of hypertension. Despite some methodological shortcomings, evidence shows that Qigong can reduce BP among hypertensives by -12 to -17 mm Hg systolic and -8.5 to -10 mm Hg diastolic. Thus, the BP-lowering results obtained by Qigong are comparable to drug treatment of HTN.
  - o <u>Controlled breathing</u>: Most studies (4 of 5) using slow controlled breathing have shown an antihypertensive benefit presumably mediated through increased parasympathetic

---

[122] Maurer M, Riesen W, Muser J, Hulter HN, Krapf R. Neutralization of Western diet inhibits bone resorption independently of K intake and reduces cortisol secretion in humans. *Am J Physiol Renal Physiol*. 2003 Jan;284(1):F32-40
[123] Frassetto L, Morris RC Jr, Sellmeyer DE, Todd K, Sebastian A. Diet, evolution and aging--the pathophysiologic effects of the post-agricultural inversion of the potassium-to-sodium and base-to-chloride ratios in the human diet. *Eur J Nutr*. 2001 Oct;40(5):200-13
[124] Benowitz NL. "Antihypertensive Agents." In Katzung BG (editor). <u>Basic and Clinical Pharmacology. Tenth Edition</u>. New York: McGraw Hill Medical; 2007, 161
[125] Nahas R. Complementary and alternative medicine approaches to blood pressure reduction: An evidence-based review. *Can Fam Physician*. 2008 Nov;54(11):1529-33 http://www.cfp.ca/cgi/content/full/54/11/1529

and reduced sympathetic activity; as expected, diabetics with autonomic dysfunction tend to receive less benefit.
- o Transcendental meditation: Twice-daily sessions of sitting quietly while repeating a specific mantra can effect a BP-lowering effect of approximately -4.7/-3.2 mm Hg.
- o Acupuncture: Acupuncture is difficult to study in a placebo-controlled manner due to the physical, individualized, and experiential nature of the treatment. Antihypertensive benefits of acupuncture have ranged from no different from the so-called placebo to reductions of -6 to -14 mm Hg for systolic BP and -3 to -7 mm Hg for diastolic BP.

- **Whey peptides, casokinins, and lactokinins**: Yet another benefit of whey protein consumption is the salutary effect on blood pressure, probably mediated by whey protein's anti-stress, anti-oxidant/pro-glutathione, and ACE-inhibiting properties. Very interestingly, the anti-hypertensive effects of milk peptides may depend on their specific hydrolysation by lactic acid producing bacteria in the intestines; thus, clinical anti-hypertensive benefit of milk/whey peptides may require establishment of eubiosis, eradication of intestinal dysbiosis, and/or co-supplementation with probiotics. (For extensive reviews on the clinical consequences of dysbiosis and the [re]establishment of eubiosis, see monographs[126] and book chapters[127] by Vasquez).
  - o Review: Lactokinins are whey protein-derived ACE inhibitory peptides: Whey protein contains lactokinins, peptides that function as ACE-inhibitors. "Peptides derived from the major whey proteins, i.e. alpha-lactalbumin (alpha-la) and beta-lactoglobulin (beta-lg) in addition to bovine serum albumin (BSA), inhibit ACE. ... While they do not have the inhibitory potency of synthetic drugs commonly used in the treatment of hypertension, these naturally occurring peptides may represent nutraceutical/functional food ingredients for the prevention/treatment of high blood pressure."[128]
  - o Review: Milk protein-derived peptide inhibitors of angiotensin-I-converting enzyme: "Numerous casein and whey protein-derived angiotensin-I-converting enzyme (ACE) inhibitory peptides/hydrolysates have been identified. **Clinical trials in hypertensive animals and humans show that these peptides/hydrolysates can bring about a significant reduction in hypertension.** These peptides/hydrolysates may be classified as functional food ingredients and nutraceuticals due to their ability to provide health benefits i.e. as functional food ingredients in reducing the risk of developing a disease and as nutraceuticals in the prevention/treatment of disease."[129]
  - o Review: Hypotensive peptides from milk proteins: "**Milk proteins, both caseins and whey proteins, are a rich source of ACE inhibitory peptides.** Several studies in spontaneously hypertensive rats show that these casokinins and lactokinins can significantly reduce blood pressure. Furthermore, a limited number of human studies have associated milk protein-derived peptides with statistically significant hypotensive effects (i.e., lower systolic and diastolic pressures)."[130]
- **Nattokinase**: Nattokinase is an enzyme extracted and purified from a Japanese food called Natto, a cheese-like food made from fermented soybeans.

---

[126] **Vasquez A**. Reducing Pain and Inflammation Naturally - Part 6: Nutritional and Botanical Treatments Against "Silent Infections" and Gastrointestinal Dysbiosis, Commonly Overlooked Causes of Neuromusculoskeletal Inflammation and Chronic Health Problems. *Nutritional Perspectives* 2006; 29 (January): 5-21
[127] Chapter Four in: **Vasquez A**. Integrative Rheumatology. IBMRC 2006, 2007. http://optimalhealthresearch.com/rheumatology.html
[128] FitzGerald RJ, Meisel H. Lactokinins: whey protein-derived ACE inhibitory peptides. *Nahrung*. 1999 Jun;43(3):165-7
[129] FitzGerald RJ, Meisel H. Milk protein-derived peptide inhibitors of angiotensin-I-converting enzyme. *Br J Nutr*. 2000 Nov;84 Suppl 1:S33-
[130] FitzGerald RJ, Murray BA, Walsh DJ. Hypotensive peptides from milk proteins. *J Nutr*. 2004 Apr;134(4):980S-8S

- o <u>Randomized, controlled trial: Effects of nattokinase on blood pressure</u>: 86 participants with pre-hypertension or stage-1 hypertension received nattokinase (2,000 FU/capsule) or a placebo capsule for 8 weeks. **Net changes in systolic and diastolic blood pressure were -5.55 mmHg and -2.84 mmHg, respectively, after the 8-week intervention.** Renin activity levels dropped by -1.17 ng/mL/h for the nattokinase group compared with the control group. The authors concluded, "nattokinase supplementation resulted in a reduction in SBP and DBP. These findings suggest that increased intake of nattokinase may play an important role in preventing and treating hypertension."[131]
- **Cocoa & Dark Chocolate (*Theobroma cacao*)**: Cacao has been cultivated for thousands of years in South and Central America; currently most production comes from Africa as well as various other countries such as Belize. The word chocolate came into English from Spanish and entered Spanish either from the Aztecs ("chocolatl" or "chicolatl") or the Maya ("chokol"). Among its numerous constituents, alkaloids such as theobromine and phenethylamine and various antioxidants such as epicatechin and procyanidins have received the most attention. Dark chocolate *without added sugar* and *without the addition of excess fat or cow's milk* provides antioxidant, cardioprotective, neuroprotective, and anticancer benefits. **People who regularly consume higher levels of cocoa (suggested range 10-30 grams up to 100 grams daily) have lower BP and a -50% relative reduction in cardiovascular and all-cause mortality**; regarding the mechanism of action for the BP-lowering effect of chocolate: **flavonoids in cacao upregulate nitric oxide synthase in endothelial cells, and thus chocolate improves endothelial function**.[132] The cocoa content should be at least 65% and preferably 85%-90%. In December 2009, MD Anderson Cancer Center endorsed dark chocolate for its probable cancer-preventive benefits.[133]
  - o <u>Systematic review and meta-analysis: Benefits of cocoa products on blood pressure</u>: For this systematic review, the authors performed a meta-analysis of randomized controlled trials assessing the antihypertensive effects of flavanol-rich cocoa products. They found that among 10 randomized controlled trials with a total of 297 individuals (either healthy normotensive adults or patients with prehypertension/stage 1 hypertension), **systolic BP dropped -4.5 mm Hg while diastolic BP dropped -2.5 mm Hg following cocoa consumption** for durations of 2-18 weeks. The authors concluded that "The meta-analysis confirms the BP-lowering capacity of flavanol-rich cocoa products...."[134] Rather than rendering the typical cautionary note ("…questions such as the most appropriate dose and the long-term side effect profile warrant further investigation before cocoa products can be recommended as a treatment option in hypertension."), the authors might have been more wise to suggest increased consumption of chocolate for its antihypertensive and cardioprotective benefits and its greater safety profile compared to pharmaceutical drugs.

---

[131] Kim JY, Gum SN, Paik JK, Lim HH, Kim KC, Ogasawara K, Inoue K, Park S, Jang Y, Lee JH. Effects of nattokinase on blood pressure: a randomized, controlled trial. *Hypertens Res*. 2008 Aug;31(8):1583-8
[132] Nahas R. Complementary and alternative medicine approaches to blood pressure reduction: An evidence-based review. *Can Fam Physician*. 2008 Nov;54(11):1529-33 http://www.cfp.ca/cgi/content/full/54/11/1529
[133] "In addition to being delicious, moderate amounts of dark chocolate may play a role in cancer prevention. ... To get those cancer prevention benefits, the chocolate should contain at least 65% cocoa. Winters R. Focused on Health - December 2009. http://www.mdanderson.org/publications/focused-on-health/issues/2009-december/share-the-health.html Accessed January 15, 2010
[134] Desch S, Schmidt J, Kobler D, Sonnabend M, Eitel I, Sareban M, Rahimi K, Schuler G, Thiele H. Effect of cocoa products on blood pressure: systematic review and meta-analysis. *Am J Hypertens*. 2010 Jan;23(1):97-103

- Randomized controlled trial: Effects of habitual cocoa intake on blood pressure and bioactive nitric oxide: The authors of this clinical trial review previously published research and note that regular intake of cocoa-containing foods is linked to lower cardiovascular mortality and that short-term interventions show that **high doses of cocoa can improve endothelial function and reduce BP due to the action of the cocoa polyphenols**. Their clinical trial design was a randomized, controlled, investigator-blinded, parallel-group trial involving 44 adults aged 56 through 73 years (24 women, 20 men) with untreated upper-range prehypertension or stage 1 hypertension without comorbidity; the treatment was 6.3 g (30 kcal) per day of dark chocolate containing 30 mg of polyphenols or a placebo of polyphenol-free white chocolate. Main outcome measures were ❶ BP, ❷ plasma markers of vasodilative nitric oxide (S-nitrosoglutathione), ❸ oxidative stress (8-isoprostane), and ❹ bioavailability of cocoa polyphenols. "RESULTS: From baseline to 18 weeks, **dark chocolate reduced mean systolic BP by -2.9 mm Hg and diastolic BP by -1.9 mm Hg** without changes in body weight, plasma levels of lipids, glucose, and 8-isoprostane. **Hypertension prevalence declined from 86% to 68%**. The BP decrease was accompanied by a sustained increase of S-nitrosoglutathione by 0.23 nmol/L, and a dark chocolate dose resulted in the appearance of cocoa phenols in plasma. White chocolate intake caused no changes in BP or plasma biomarkers. CONCLUSIONS: Data in this relatively small sample of otherwise healthy individuals with above-optimal BP indicate that **inclusion of small amounts of polyphenol-rich dark chocolate as part of a usual diet efficiently reduced BP and improved formation of vasodilative nitric oxide**."[135]

- Randomized controlled single-blind crossover trial: Benefits of acute dark chocolate and cocoa ingestion on endothelial function: The purpose of this clinical trial (n = 45, BMI = 30, age = 53y) was to assess the acute effects of solid dark chocolate and liquid cocoa intake on endothelial function and blood pressure in overweight adults. First, subjects were randomly assigned to consume a **solid dark chocolate bar (containing 22 g cocoa powder)** or a cocoa-free placebo bar (containing 0 g cocoa powder). In the second part of the trial, subjects were randomly assigned to consume **sugar-free cocoa** (containing 22 g cocoa powder), **sugared cocoa** (containing 22 g cocoa powder), or a **placebo** (containing 0 g cocoa powder). "RESULTS: **Solid dark chocolate and liquid cocoa** ingestion improved endothelial function (measured as flow-mediated dilatation) compared with placebo (**dark chocolate: 4.3** compared with -1.8; **sugar-free** and sugared cocoa: **5.7** and 2.0 compared with -1.5). **Blood pressure decreased after the ingestion of dark chocolate and sugar-free cocoa** compared with *placebo* (**dark chocolate: systolic, -3.2 mm Hg** compared with 2.7 mm Hg; and **diastolic -1.4 mm Hg** compared with 2.7 mm Hg; **sugar-free cocoa: systolic, -2.1 mm Hg** compared with 3.2 mm Hg; and **diastolic: -1.2** mm Hg compared with 2.8 mm Hg. **Endothelial function improved significantly more with sugar-free than with regular cocoa** (5.7 % compared with 2.0%). CONCLUSIONS: The acute ingestion of both solid dark chocolate and liquid cocoa improved endothelial function and lowered blood pressure in overweight adults. Sugar content may attenuate

---

[135] Taubert D, Roesen R, Lehmann C, Jung N, Schömig E. Effects of low habitual cocoa intake on blood pressure and bioactive nitric oxide: a randomized controlled trial. *JAMA*. 2007 Jul 4;298(1):49-60

these effects, and sugar-free preparations may augment them.."[136] The practical application of this research is important to communicate to patients: to obtain the cardioprotective benefits of chocolate, the chocolate must be consumed without added sugar, i.e., it must be **dark chocolate**, *not* sugar-sweetened milk chocolate.

- **Approaching an integrative model for the understanding of essential hypertension**: This diagram provides a reasonable representation of several of the key factors that generate and perpetuate the common clinical syndromes of overweight-obesity, hypertension, insulin resistance and diabetes mellitus type-2. Clinicians can use this single page for patient education so that patients will approach a more complete understanding of their condition and how the integration of various interventions such as dietary improvement, exercise, nutritional supplementation, and spinal manipulation can work together to provide additive and synergistic health benefits.

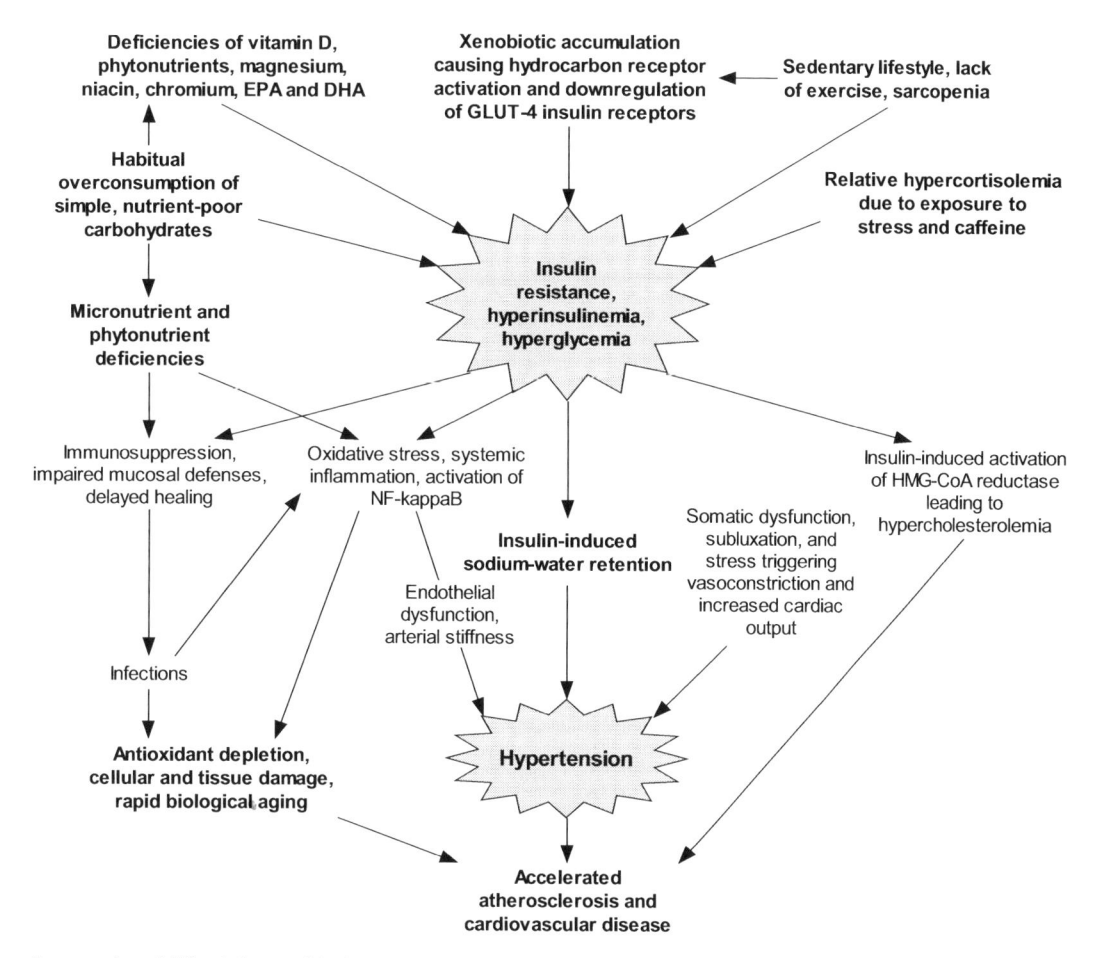

**A sample of lifestyle and interconnected mechanisms contributing to the hyperinsulinemia-hypertension syndrome commonly known as "idiopathic hypertension" and "type-2 diabetes"**

---

[136] Faridi Z, Njike VY, Dutta S, Ali A, Katz DL. Acute dark chocolate and cocoa ingestion and endothelial function: a randomized controlled crossover trial. *Am J Clin Nutr*. 2008 Jul;88(1):58-63 http://www.ajcn.org/cgi/content/full/88/1/58

- **Drug treatments for chronic HTN**: From a practical standpoint, the many drugs used for the suppression of HTN can be placed in one of five categories; the mnemonic offered in the *Saint-Frances Guide*[137] is "A.B.C.D.E." which stands for ❶ ACEi's/ARB's, ❷ beta-blockers, ❸ CCB, ❹ diuretics, and ❺ everything else (e.g., central alpha-agonists, alpha-blockers, vasodilators). For uncomplicated HTN, the initial treatment is a diuretic, generally hydrochlorothiazide (HCTZ), since the thiazide diuretics have the best cost-effectiveness of various drug classes; as noted by Howland and Mycek[138], "Current treatment recommendations are to **initiate therapy with a thiazide diuretic unless there are compelling reasons to employ other drug classes**. ... Recent data suggest that diuretics are superior to beta-blockers in older adults." For complicated HTN (resistant to treatment or with concomitant illness), a different first-line or additive second drug is chosen from a different class based on patient characteristics, as outlined below. While clinicians might choose a higher initial dose based on HTN severity or the doctor's experience and preference, as a general rule the most reasonable course is to start with a single drug at a low dose in order to minimize risk for adverse effects and to readily determine the offending agent in the event of an expected or idiosyncratic side effect. In the outline below, patient profiles are matched to drug classes; when specific drugs are listed, they are chosen based on general frequency of use with preference for those administered once daily due to improved compliance. If drug treatment is well tolerated but insufficient to achieve BP goal, then *treatment compliance is verified* before increasing the dose and eventually adding a second drug from a different class. For the patient-centered and drug-centered tables below, primary sources of information are Lippincott's Illustrated Reviews: Pharmacology, Third Edition[139] for pharmacology and The 5-Minute Clinical Consult, 18th Edition[140] for more clinical information and doses; Ebell's review and clinical worksheet ("Hypertension Encounter Guide") published in "Initial evaluation of hypertension" in *American Family Physician* (March 2004)[141] was also used as a

---

**Suggested Practical HTN Drug Protocol**
(Always ask about drug allergies/intolerances)

1. **Thiazide: Hydrochlorothiazide 12.5-25 mg/d** initially for most patients, not with renal insufficiency. For patients with DM or proteinuria, start with ACEi. Add **spironolactone 25-50 mg/d** if hypokalemia develops.
2. **ACEi: Lisinopril 10-40 mg/d**, give the first dose in the office to monitor for hypotensive syncope or angioedema. If cough or angioedema develop, switch to ARB, particularly **losartan 25-100 mg/d** due to modest uricosuric effect. ACEi and ARB are contraindicated in pregnancy.
3. **CCB: Amlodipine 2.5-10 mg/d**, particularly for patients with migraine, COPD, asthma.
4. **BB: Metoprolol 50-100 mg/d** (up to bid), especially with angina or MI; not with bradycardia, insulin-requiring DM, depression, or sexual dysfunction.
5. **Loop diuretic: Furosemide 20-320 mg/d** if patient has severe volume overload; effective with renal insufficiency.

Ebell MH. Initial evaluation of hypertension. *Am Fam Physician*. 2004 Mar 15;69:1485-7
http://www.aafp.org/afp/2004/0315/p1485.html
Domino FJ (editor in chief). The 5-Minute Clinical Consult. 2010. 18th Edition. Philadel.; WoltersKluwer: 2009, 656-7

---

[137] Bent S, Gensler LS, Frances C. Saint-Frances Guide: Clinical Clerkship in Outpatient Medicine. Second Edition. Philadelphia; Wolters Kluwer: 2008, 90
[138] Howland RD, Mycek MJ. Lippincott's Illustrated Reviews: Pharmacology, Third Edition. Baltimore: Lippincott Williams and Wilkins; 2006, 213-226
[139] Howland RD, Mycek MJ. Lippincott's Illustrated Reviews: Pharmacology, Third Edition. Baltimore: Lippincott Williams and Wilkins; 2006, 213-226
[140] Domino FJ (editor in chief). The 5-Minute Clinical Consult. 2010. 18th Edition. Philadelphia; Wolters Kluwer: 2009, 656-7
[141] Ebell MH. Initial evaluation of hypertension. *Am Fam Physician*. 2004 Mar 15;69(6):1485-7 http://www.aafp.org/afp/2004/0315/p1485.html

very practical point-of-care guide. The tables that follow were written by Alex Vasquez and reviewed by Robert Richard DO[142] in Jan 2010.

| Patient profile | Notes |
|---|---|
| **Uncomplicated** | Thiazide diuretics (especially **HCTZ**) are first choice (can worsen gout and dyslipidemia); BB have historically been a common second choice, but recently atenolol has fallen out of favor[143] and with the increasing prevalence of DM which indicates ACEi and ARB treatment, these medications may become the preferred second line; the ARB **losartan** would seem particularly favorable in patients with metabolic syndrome and type-2 DM due to its uricosuric effect. |
| **Diabetes mellitus** | ACEi's are renoprotective (but not used with renovascular disease), ARB's are second choice; beta-blockers are generally avoided in insulin-requiring DM due to blunting of protective responses to hypoglycemia. |
| **Renal disease** | ACEi's are renoprotective (but not used with renovascular disease), ARB's are second choice. Nondihydroperidine CCB reduce intrarenal filtration pressure thus reducing proteinuria. Thiazides require renal function and are generally not useful if creatinine is >2 mg/dl. |
| **African American** | African-Americans tend to respond better to diuretics and CCB than to BB or ACEi[144] |
| **Asthma and COPD** | Use a CCB. Generally avoid beta-blockers with any airway disease, B1-selective metoprolol might be considered |
| **Angina** | BB and CCB improve outcomes independent of BP-lowering; when BB and CCB are combined, the CCB should be a dihydropyridine (i.e., from the class of "-pyridines" or "-pines"). (Do not combine a BB with a negative inotropic non-dihydropyridine CCB so as to avoid inducing heart block.) |
| **Erectile dysfunction** | Avoid beta-blockers; thiazides may exacerbate. Consider concomitant administration of arginine and/or a phosphodiesterase-5 inhibitor; also consider treatment for excess estrogen in men with a serum estradiol greater than 30 picogram/mL (for details see the anti-estrogen protocol outlined in chapter 4 of *Integrative Rheumatology*[145]). |
| **Systolic HTN** | Dihydropyridine CCB ("-pyridines" or "-pines") are preferred |
| **CAD or prior MI** | BB are top choice if not contraindicated by problematic asthma, COPD, or DM |
| **Pregnancy** | Use methyldopa, hydralazine, magnesium; pregnancy contraindicates ACEi and ARB due to teratogenic effects |
| **CHF, atrial fibrillation** | BB are particularly useful for diastolic CHF to slow heart rate and allow greater filling time: Carvedilol is BB of choice in this situation. Monitor for signs of excessive cardiosuppression such as edema, SOB, rales, bradycardia. Carvedilol is a non-selective beta blocker/alpha-1 blocker indicated in the treatment of mild to moderate CHF. Do not use BB or CCB with bradycardia; generally do not use verapamil (negative inotrope CCB) with CHF. |
| **Bradycardia** | Do not use BB or CCB with bradycardia |
| **Edema** | Sodium and water restriction and use of loop diuretic (e.g., furosemide/Lasix) is common treatment |

---

[142] Robert Richard DO is Medical Director of the John Peter Smith Polytechnic Clinic and Chair of Community Medicine at Texas College of Osteopathic Medicine. Dr Richard's review of these tables does not imply his endorsement of their content nor of the content of this document as a whole. Furthermore, Dr Richard's review does not imply endorsement by JPS Health Network or Texas College of Osteopathic Medicine.
[143] Domino FJ (editor in chief). The 5-Minute Clinical Consult. 2010. 18th Edition. Philadelphia; Wolters Kluwer: 2009, 656-7
[144] Howland RD, Mycek MJ. Lippincott's Illustrated Reviews: Pharmacology, Third Edition. Baltimore: Lippincott Williams and Wilkins; 2006, 213-226
[145] **Vasquez A**. Integrative Rheumatology. IBMRC 2006, 2007 and all future editions. http://optimalhealthresearch.com/rheumatology.html

| *Drug class and description* | *Representative drugs and description* |
|---|---|
| **ACEi**: Blocking formation of angiotensin-2 reduces peripheral vascular resistance and aldosterone secretion; vasodilation is effected by reduced breakdown of bradykinin; sympathetic tone may be reduced.<br><br>For best safety, the initial dose of an ACEi can be given in the office under supervision due to risks for first-dose syncope and life-threatening angioedema; this advised practice is rarely followed. | • <u>Unique benefits of class</u>: ACE inhibitors provide renoprotection, hence their routine use in patients with DM, with or without HTN. Thiazide, BB, and ACEi can be safely used together. As summarized by Domino (ed)[146], "ACE inhibitors should be used in patients with diabetes, proteinuria, atrial fibrillation, or CHF but not in pregnancy."<br>• <u>Unique adverse effects and contraindications</u>: Not used with **renal artery stenosis** (causes ARF) or **pregnancy** (teratogenic); may cause **cough (10%) and angioedema** due to reduced breakdown of bradykinin. Reduced aldosterone secretion promotes hypotension and **hyperkalemia—potassium levels should be monitored** *especially in diabetic patients*; **coadministration of ACEi and spironolactone is generally contraindicated** due to risk for hyperkalemia.<br>• <u>Representative drugs of class (dose range)</u>: **Lisinopril 10-40 mg/d** |
| **ARB**: ARBs block reception of angiotensin-2 and thus reduce vasoconstriction and aldosterone secretion; risk-benefit profile is similar to ACEi except that bradykinin-mediated benefits (vasodilation) and risks (cough, angioedema) are not seen. | • <u>Unique benefits of class</u>: Hypotensive and renoprotective without the risks of cough and angioedema.<br>• <u>Unique adverse effects and contraindications</u>: Fetotoxicity contraindicates ARB use in pregnancy.<br>• <u>Representative drugs of class (dose range)</u>: **Losartan 25-100 mg/d**; among the ARBs, this drug provides the additional benefit of reducing uric acid levels |
| **BB**: Primary mechanism of action via B1 receptors is reduction in cardiac output; also reduce sympathetic tone and thus renin secretion.<br><br>Major adverse effects include bradycardia, fatigue, sexual dysfunction, exacerbation of asthma and COPD, and rebound hypertension. | • <u>Unique benefits of class</u>: Thiazide, BB, and ACEi can be safely used together. BB considered more effective in Caucasians than Africans, more effective in young than elderly. BB are particularly used in HTN patients who also have **supraventricular tachyarrhythmia, previous MI, angina, and migraine**.<br>• <u>Unique adverse effects and contraindications</u>: Do not use BB or CCB with **bradycardia** due to potential for inducing **heart block or hypotension**. Nonselective BB such as propranolol which target B1 (heart) and B2 (lungs) have potential to **exacerbate asthma and COPD**. Patients with PVD may have a worsening of limb ischemia secondary to reduced perfusion. **Hypotension, fatigue, depression, sexual dysfunction,** and **rebound hypertension** are common adverse BB effects; lowering of HDL and elevation of TRIGs has also been noted. Sudden discontinuation of BB can result in **rebound hypertension** (presumably due to upregulation of beta-adrenergic receptors under prolonged suppression).<br>• <u>Representative drugs of class (dose range)</u>: **Metoprolol in extended release (Toprol-XL) 50-100 mg/d** (up to bid), especially with angina or MI; not with bradycardia, insulin-requiring DM, depression, or sexual dysfunction. Of note, **atenolol** is no longer considered first-line treatment due to recent evidence of inefficacy in preventing HTN complications.[147] |

---

[146] Domino FJ (editor in chief). <u>The 5-Minute Clinical Consult. 2010. 18th Edition</u>. Philadelphia; Wolters Kluwer: 2009, 656
[147] Domino FJ (editor in chief). <u>The 5-Minute Clinical Consult. 2010. 18th Edition</u>. Philadelphia; Wolters Kluwer: 2009, 656-7

| Drug description (cont'd) | Representative drugs and description |
|---|---|
| **CCB—dihydropyridine**: The "-pyridines" block calcium entry into vascular smooth muscle and thus cause relative arterial dilation.<br><br>*Memory tool*: Remember that *pyridines* sounds like *pines* and that these drugs work on the *vascular tree* to lower blood pressure via systemic arterial dilation. | ▪ *Unique benefits of class*: Generally safe in HTN patients with asthma, DM, angina, and PVD.<br>▪ *Unique adverse effects and contraindications*: Do not use BB or non-dihydropyridine CCB with bradycardia. Constipation (10%, especially with nifedipine), headache, fatigue.<br>▪ *Representative drugs of class (dose range)*: **Amlodipine 2.5-10 mg/d**<br><br>Not detailed here are the non-dihydropyridine class of CCB (i.e., including diltiazem/Cardizem and Verapamil) which are not used for HTN but rather are used for their cardioselective effects. *Memory tool*: Remember that the *non*-dihydropyridine CCBs are cardiosuppressive via a *negative* inotropic effect. |
| **Diuretic—general information**: A key mechanism of action of most diuretics is enhanced excretion of sodium. Excess sodium (Na) promotes water retention and subsequent volume expansion, while also contributing to vasoconstriction and arterial stiffness via enhanced adrenergic reactivity and via promotion of intracellular hypercalcinosis (possibly due to enhanced sodium-calcium exchange).[148] | ▪ *Unique benefits of class*: Generally effective for all forms of HTN.<br>▪ *Unique adverse effects and contraindications*: Hypotension, hyponatremia; increased losses of water-soluble nutrients such as thiamine and minerals such as magnesium and potassium are seen especially with diuretics of the loop class, namely furosemide/Lasix.<br>▪ *Representative drugs of class (dose range)*: Listed in subclasses below.<br><br>*Clinical pearl*: Loop diuretics such as furosemide/Lasix are commonly used in the treatment of heart failure in elderly patients, but the depletion of thiamine, magnesium, potassium, and calcium can actually exacerbate heart failure[149] and contribute to co-morbidity such as depression and dementia. |
| **Diuretic—thiazide**: Drug of choice for initial treatment of HTN. Sulfa sensitivity does not necessarily contraindicate thiazide use, even though thiazides are sulfa derivatives; use with caution. | ▪ *Unique benefits of class*: Thiazide, BB, and ACEi can be safely used together. Particularly beneficial in elderly (as long as renal function is intact) and Africans. Promotion of calcium retention may benefit osteoporosis and reduce calcium nephrolithiasis.<br>▪ *Unique adverse effects and contraindications*: Not useful in patients with renal insufficiency (creatinine clearance < 50 mL/min).<br>   o Thiazide diuretics can worsen **hyperuricemia** (70% of patients) and **gout** due to competition for renal excretion (organic acids).<br>   o **Hypokalemia (70%)** —potassium levels should be monitored in patients predisposed to cardiac arrhythmia and those treated with digitalis. Coadministration with ACEi/lisinopril helps negate the tendency toward hypokalemia.<br>   o **Hyperglycemia (10%)**<br>   o **Dyslipidemia**<br>   o **Hypomagnesemia**<br>   o Promotion of calcium retention can promote **hypercalcemia**, even with the addition of modest doses of vitamin D (e.g., 2,000 IU/d)<br>     (author's clinical experience, also mentioned in citation #150)<br>▪ *Representative drugs of class (dose range)*: **Hydrochlorothiazide 12.5-25 mg/d** initially for most patients |

---

[148] Benowitz NL. "Antihypertensive Agents." In Katzung BG (editor). Basic and Clinical Pharmacology. Tenth Edition. New York: McGraw Hill Medical; 2007, 163
[149] Felípez L, Sentongo TA. Drug-induced nutrient deficiencies. *Pediatr Clin North Am*. 2009 Oct;56(5):1211-24
[150] **Vasquez A**, Manso G, Cannell J. The clinical importance of vitamin D (cholecalciferol): a paradigm shift with implications for all healthcare providers. *Altern Ther Health Med*. 2004 Sep-Oct;10(5):28-36 http://optimalhealthresearch.com/cholecalciferol.html

| *Drug description (cont'd)* | *Representative drugs and description* |
|---|---|
| **Diuretic—loop:** | - *Unique benefits of class*: Fast action even in patients with renal insufficiency.<br>- *Unique adverse effects and contraindications*: Chronic use promotes depletion of potassium, magnesium, and thiamine.<br>- *Representative drugs of class (dose range)*: **Furosemide 20-320 mg/d**, commonly used PRN for outpatients; dose must be step-wise increased to find patient-specific threshold dose and frequency for individual patient, works for 6 hours, avoid nighttime use to avoid nocturia; higher doses not better than threshold dose. |
| **Diuretic—potassium sparing:** Weak diuretics; spironolactone is the prototype and also has anti-androgen action and is therefore used in hirsutism. | - *Unique benefits of class*: Spironolactone is commonly used with HCTZ; beneficially diminishes cardiac remodeling seen in CHF. Spironolactone reduces incidence of spontaneous bacterial peritonitis (SBP) in patients with cirrhosis.<br>- *Unique adverse effects and contraindications*: Spironolactone has antiandrogen effects, can promote ED and gynecomastia; can precipitate hyperkalemia and hypermagnesemia.<br>- *Representative drugs of class (dose range)*: **Spironolactone 25-50** mg/d in patients with hypokalemia, cirrhosis, or hirsutism. |
| **Alpha-1-blocker**: Reduce BP via relaxation of venous and arterial smooth muscle; sodium-water retention, hypotension and **reflex tachycardia are common**. First-dose syncope is common with prazosin. | - *Unique benefits of class*: Can be used when other drugs have not been effective; can benefit men with prostatic hyperplasia.<br>- *Unique adverse effects and contraindications*: Sodium-water retention, hypotension, syncope, and reflex tachycardia are common; tachycardia can be prevented with BB.<br>- *Representative drugs of class*: **Prazosin 1-10 mg twice daily**: first dose syncope is common. **Doxazosin 4 mg**: chronic doxazosin use is associated with an increased risk for CHF. |
| **Alpha-2 agonists**: Centrally acting drugs reduce sympathetic output via feedback inhibition. Rebound hypertension with clonidine withdrawal mandates tapering discontinuation. | - *Unique benefits of class*: Safe for use in renal disease; generally used with diuretic.<br>- *Unique adverse effects and contraindications*: Generally used with a diuretic to counteract the sodium-water retention. Sedation and dry nose may occur. Rebound hypertension mandates *tapering* discontinuation. **Alpha-2 agonists are best avoided due to high risk of rebound HTN following noncompliance or skipped dose(s).** |
| **Vasodilators**: Direct-acting smooth muscle relaxants. **Warning**: Vasodilators cause reflex tachycardia that can precipitate MI and CHF. | - *Unique benefits of class*: **These are last-resort medications** for resistant HTN, especially in African-Americans.<br>- *Unique adverse effects and contraindications*: Sodium-water retention can be avoided with BB and diuretic. BB can be used to avoid vasodilator-induced tachycardia.<br>- *Representative drugs of class*: **Hydralazine 25-150 mg twice daily**: Monotherapy is only used in the treatment of pregnancy-induced HTN; side effects include headache and drug-induced systemic lupus erythematosus (SLE). |

Abbreviations: **25-OH-D** = serum 25-hydroxy-vitamin D, **ACEi** = angiotensin converting enzyme inhibitor, **alpha-blocker** = alpha-adrenergic antagonist, **ARB** = angiotensin-2 receptor blocker/antagonist, **ARF** = acute renal failure, **BB** = beta blocker or beta-adrenergic antagonist, **CAD** = coronary artery disease, **CCB** = calcium channel blocker/antagonist, **CHF** = congestive heart failure, **CRF** = chronic renal insufficiency, **CVD** = cardiovascular disease, **DM** = diabetes mellitus, **ECG** or **EKG** = electrocardiogram, **HDL** = high density lipoprotein cholesterol, **HTN** = hypertension, **MI** = myocardial infarction, **PVD** = peripheral vascular disease, **TRIGs** = serum triglycerides, **UA** = urinalysis, **US** = ultrasound

# Intracellular Hypercalcinosis: A Functional Nutritional Disorder with Implications Ranging from Myofascial Trigger Points to Affective Disorders, Hypertension, and Cancer

## Alex Vasquez, D.C., N.D.

This article was originally published in *Naturopathy Digest*
http://www.naturopathydigest.com/archives/2006/sep/vasquez.php

**Introduction**:
Let's explore the possibility that elevated levels of calcium *within the cell* (intracellular hypercalcinosis) might predispose toward a wide range of clinical problems including migraine, hypertension, myofascial trigger points, inflammation, and cancer. Further, let's review the data showing that several commonly employed nutritional interventions can be used synergistically to counteract and correct this problem. By the time readers complete this article, they will have 1) an understanding of this problem, 2) a protocol for how to correct this problem, and 3) be able to explain the biochemical rationale for using these nutritional protocols in patients who might otherwise be treated with drugs in general and calcium-channel-blocking drugs in particular.

Although prescription drugs are often used by medical doctors in a "willy-nilly manner" (according to Harvard Medical School Professor Dr. Jerry Avorn[151]), let's assume for a moment that legitimate reasons exist for the widespread use of drugs that block calcium channels in cell membranes—the "calcium-channel-blocking drugs." Although it is counterintuitive to promote health by interfering with the body's natural function, calcium-channel-blocking drugs are routinely used in pharmaceutical medicine for a broad range of problems including hypertension, heart rhythm disturbances, bipolar disorder, and anxiety/panic disorders. Widespread medical use of calcium-channel-blocking drugs appears to validate the supposition that excess intracellular calcium is an important contributor to these and perhaps other problems. Therefore, if intracellular hypercalcinosis is the problem, then any safe and cost-effective treatment that can correct this problem should be met with the same widespread acceptance given to calcium-channel-blocking drugs, which are universally accepted and utilized in the allopathic "conventional medicine" society.

At the very least, we can generally state that all phenomena that contribute to calcium deficiency result in an increase in intracellular calcium levels (the "calcium paradox") due to the effect of parathyroid hormone, which specifically promotes calcium uptake in cells while mobilizing calcium from bone. Additionally, a few other nutritional influences (such as fatty acid imbalances) modulate cellular calcium balance, and these will be discussed in the section on clinical interventions.

**The Problem of Excess Intracellular Calcium**:
Although the current author is the first to coin the phrase "intracellular hypercalcinosis"[152], several other authors have pointed to the problem of the "calcium paradox" and the means by which *body-wide calcium deficiency* can result in *intracellular calcium overload*, which triggers a cascade of events leading to adverse health effects. Most notably, the work of Takuo Fujita[153,154] stands out in its clarity

---

[151] America The Medicated. http://www.cbsnews.com/stories/2005/04/21/health/main689997.shtml
[152] http://optimalhealthresearch.com/archives/intracellular-hypercalcinosis
[153] Fujita T. Calcium paradox: consequences of calcium deficiency manifested by a wide variety of diseases. *J Bone Miner Metab*. 2000;18(4):234-6

and specificity in linking intracellular hypercalcinosis with disorders such as hypertension, arteriosclerosis, diabetes mellitus, neurodegenerative diseases, malignancy, and degenerative joint disease.

Mechanisms by which intracellular hypercalcinosis contributes to disease have been defined, at least partially. However, we must remember that nutritional disorders never occur in isolation, and that the effects of intracellular hypercalcinosis observed clinically are overlaid with manifestations of the primary nutritional/metabolic disorder. Stated differently, contrary to what the pharmaceutical paradigm's monotherapeutic use of calcium-channel-blocking drugs would imply, intracellular hypercalcinosis never occurs by itself. For example, if intracellular hypercalcinosis is contributed to by vitamin D3 deficiency, then some of the observed clinical complications of that condition are due to and yet independent from the excess intracellular calcium since the primary problem (vitamin D3 deficiency) causes adverse effects and deficiency symptoms that are independent of its effect on intracellular calcium levels. To better understand the specific effects of excess intracellular calcium, a brief review of a few specific biochemical/physiologic mechanisms by which intracellular hypercalcinosis can contribute to disease is warranted. We must start by realizing that calcium is much more than a "bone nutrient" and that it functions as an electrolyte, intracellular messenger, and regulator of cell replication and metabolism. Let's talk about four pathways by which increased intracellular calcium promotes disease:

1. <u>*Adverse effects on membrane receptors and intracellular transduction*</u>: The concentration of extracellular calcium exceeds the concentration of intracellular calcium by a ratio of 10,000 to one. When intracellular calcium levels rise even slightly, receptors and messaging systems in the cell membrane fail to function optimally. Thereby, increased intracellular calcium can predispose to insulin resistance (via interference with insulin receptors) and can promote neurodegeneration by amplifying the intracellular cascade of effects that follows activation of the brain's NMDA-receptors (excitoneurotoxicity). More specifically, we must note that the recently discovered "calcium-sensing receptor" (CaR, a G protein-coupled plasma membrane receptor) senses minute alterations in serum calcium levels and then ultimately translates these variations into changes in cellular function, notably alterations in cell replication (think cancer) and eicosanoid production (think inflammation).[155,156] Given that CaR are found in a wide range of cell types, including those found in bone, the kidneys, and immune system, we can see a pathway by which alterations in calcium balance could be implicated in a wide range of diseases. CaR-mediated alterations in cell function are likely to be complicated by disorders of vitamin D3 nutrition and metabolism (that commonly complicate disorders of calcium homeostasis), which affect an even wider range of cell types including those of the breast, prostate, ovary, lung, skin, lymph nodes, colon, pancreas, adrenal medulla, brain (pituitary, cerebellum, and cerebral cortex), aortic endothelium, and immune system, including monocytes, transformed B-cells, and activated T-cells. This is an example of the complexity involved in understanding nutrition in general and the effects of nutritional deficiency (always multifaceted) in particular.

---

[154] Fujita T, Palmieri GM. Calcium paradox disease: calcium deficiency prompting secondary hyperparathyroidism and cellular calcium overload. *J Bone Miner Metab*. 2000;18(3):109-25
[155] Peterlik M, Cross HS. Vitamin D and calcium deficits predispose for multiple chronic diseases. *Eur J Clin Invest*. 2005 May;35(5):290-304
[156] Heaney RP. Long-latency deficiency disease: insights from calcium and vitamin D. *Am J Clin Nutr*. 2003 Nov;78(5):912-9

2. *Mitochondrial failure and cell death*: According to the most recent edition of the classic text Robbins Pathologic Basis of Disease (pages 15-16), increased intracellular calcium is a major cause of cell death. When calcium levels are increased within the cell, one adverse effect is the inhibition of mitochondrial function. Since calcium is pumped out of the cell in an energy-dependent process, and because dysfunctional mitochondria pour calcium into the intracellular space, calcium-induced mitochondrial failure results in an additional increase in intracellular calcium. Further complicating this problem is the fact that the cell membrane becomes increasingly permeable to calcium as calcium levels increase. Elevated intracellular calcium levels activate enzymes such as ATPase, phospholipase, proteases, and endonucleases that synergistically promote cell death.

3. *Pro-inflammatory effects of intracellular calcium*: The recent finding that intracellular calcium activates NF-kappaB[157] has obvious implications given the pivotal role of NF-kappaB in the promotion of systemic inflammation and diseases such as rheumatoid arthritis.[158] Thus, increased intracellular calcium appears to promote inflammation. This may explain in part how vitamin D3 supplementation (which lowers intracellular calcium levels) exerts its clinically impressive anti-inflammatory and immunomodulatory benefits.[159]

4. *Enhanced production of lipid peroxides*: Fujita notes that lipid peroxides lead to an increase in cell membrane permeability to calcium, which results in increased intracellular calcium; this activates metabolic pathways that increase oxidative stress, thus leading to a vicious cycle stimulated by the production of additional lipid peroxides. Thus, intracellular hypercalcinosis promotes oxidative stress, which becomes self-perpetuating by this and other mechanisms. Of course, we all know by now that increased production of free radicals contributes to the development of many health problems, such as cancer, cardiovascular disease, arthritis, autoimmunity, diabetes, and other forms of rapid biological aging.

5. *Myofascial trigger points, chronic muscle spasm, and increased vascular tone (hypertension)*: The release of calcium from the sarcoplasmic reticulum triggers muscle contraction and plays a role in hypertension (hence the use of calcium-channel-blocking drugs in the treatment of hypertension), chronic muscle spasm (especially when complicated by magnesium deficiency[160]), and the perpetuation of myofascial trigger points.[161] Reducing the levels of cytosolic and sarcoplasmic calcium promotes muscle relaxation.

---

[157] "Furthermore, a calcium chelator, BAPTA-AM, attenuated the NF-kappaB activation… CONCLUSIONS: Induction of NF-kappaB within 30 min by TNF-alpha- and IL-1beta was mediated through intracellular calcium but not ROS." Chang JW, Kim CS, Kim SB, Park SK, Park JS, Lee SK. Proinflammatory cytokine-induced NF-kappaB activation in human mesangial cells is mediated through intracellular calcium but not ROS: effects of silymarin. *Nephron Exp Nephrol.* 2006;103:e156-65

[158] Tak PP, Firestein GS. NF-kappaB: a key role in inflammatory diseases. *J Clin Invest.* 2001 Jan;107(1):7-11. See also: **Vasquez A**. Reducing pain and inflammation naturally - Part 4: Nutritional and Botanical Inhibition of NF-kappaB, the Major Intracellular Amplifier of the Inflammatory Cascade. A Practical Clinical Strategy Exemplifying Anti-Inflammatory Nutrigenomics. *Nutritional Perspectives* 2005;July: 5-12 http://optimalhealthresearch.com/part4

[159] Timms PM, Mannan N, Hitman GA, et al. Circulating MMP9, vitamin D and variation in the TIMP-1 response with VDR genotype: mechanisms for inflammatory damage in chronic disorders? *QJM.* 2002 Dec;95(12):787-96. See also: **Vasquez A**, Manso G, Cannell J. The clinical importance of vitamin D (cholecalciferol): a paradigm shift with implications for all healthcare providers. *Altern Ther Health Med.* 2004 Sep-Oct;10(5):28-36 http://optimalhealthresearch.com/monograph04

[160] **Vasquez A**. Integrative Orthopedics. www.OptimalHealthResearch.com/orthopedics.html

[161] Simons DG. Cardiology and myofascial trigger points: Janet G. Travell's contribution. *Tex Heart Inst J.* 2003;30(1):3-7

**Nutritional Interventions to Ameliorate Intracellular Hypercalcinosis**:
Now that we've reviewed the data implicating intracellular hypercalcinosis as a legitimate contributor to a wide range of clinical disorders and diseases, let's explore some nutritional solutions.

1. *Correction of vitamin D deficiency*: Vitamin D deficiency causes calcium deficiency which increases parathyroid hormone production resulting in increased intracellular calcium levels. Vitamin D deficiency is common (40-80% of most populations) and can be established via history and more objectively by measurement of serum 25-hydroxyl-vitamin D. Replacement doses are in the range of 1,000 IU per day for infants, 2,000 IU per day for children, and 4,000 IU per day for adults.[162] Vitamin D2 (ergocalciferol) should be avoided, and vitamin D3 (cholecalciferol) should be used, preferably in emulsified form to facilitate absorption, especially in older patients and those with impaired digestion and absorption.[163]

2. *Reduction in dietary arachidonic acid intake*: Arachidonic acid promotes intracellular calcium uptake, as demonstrated in a recent study using human erythrocytes.[164] Rich sources of arachidonic acid include beef, liver, pork, lamb, and cow's milk.

3. *Increase intake of eicosapentaenoic acid (EPA)*: EPA reduces intracellular calcium levels in experimental models[165] and anticancer, antihypertensive, and anti-inflammatory effects of EPA are seen clinically. One to three grams per day is reasonable for adults.

4. *Urinary alkalinization*: Diet-induced chronic metabolic acidosis[166] promotes loss of calcium in urine[167] and thus indirectly contributes to calcium deficiency and the resultant rise in parathyroid hormone and intracellular calcium levels. An alkalinizing plant-based Paleo-Mediterranean diet should be the foundational treatment for numerous reasons[168]; however some patients may need to supplement with vegetable culture, potassium citrate, potassium bicarbonate, and/or sodium bicarbonate either chronically or on an "as needed" basis.

5. *Ensuring adequate intake of calcium*: A healthy diet can supply upwards toward 1,000 mg of calcium per day, and some people may choose to supplement with an additional 500 to 1,500 mg daily. Calcium supplementation should be used with magnesium, vitamin D and other components of the supplemented Paleo-Mediterranean diet.[169]

6. *Avoiding other dietary and lifestyle factors that promote calcium loss in urine*: Caffeine, sugar, alcohol/ethanol, and psychoemotional stress all increase calcium loss in urine and thus contribute to secondary hyperparathyroidism and intracellular hypercalcinosis.

---

[162] **Vasquez A**, Manso G, Cannell J. The clinical importance of vitamin D (cholecalciferol): a paradigm shift with implications for all healthcare providers. Altern Ther Health Med. 2004 Sep-Oct;10(5):28-36 http://optimalhealthresearch.com/monograph04

[163] **Vasquez A**. Subphysiologic Doses of Vitamin D are Subtherapeutic: Comment on the Study by The Record Trial Group. *The Lancet* 2005 Published on-line May 6   http://optimalhealthresearch.com/lancet

[164] "The Ca(2+) influx rate varied from 0.5 to 3 nM Ca(2+)/s in the presence of AA and from 0.9 to 1.7 nM Ca(2+)/s with EPA." Soldati L, Lombardi C, Adamo D, Terranegra A, Bianchin C, Bianchi G, Vezzoli G. Arachidonic acid increases intracellular calcium in erythrocytes. *Biochem Biophys Res Commun*. 2002 May 10;293(3):974-8

[165] "This is a consequence of the ability of EPA to release Ca2+ from intracellular stores while inhibiting their refilling via capacitative Ca2+ influx that results in partial emptying of intracellular Ca2+ stores and thereby activation of protein kinase R." Palakurthi SS, Fluckiger R, Aktas H, Changolkar AK, Shahsafaei A, Harneit S, Kilic E, Halperin JA. Inhibition of translation initiation mediates the anticancer effect of the n-3 polyunsaturated fatty acid eicosapentaenoic acid. *Cancer Res*. 2000 Jun 1;60(11):2919-25

[166] Maurer M, Riesen W, Muser J, Hulter HN, Krapf R. Neutralization of Western diet inhibits bone resorption independently of K intake and reduces cortisol secretion in humans. *Am J Physiol Renal Physiol*. 2003 Jan;284(1):F32-40

[167] Sellmeyer DE, Schloetter M, Sebastian A. Potassium citrate prevents increased urine calcium excretion and bone resorption induced by a high sodium chloride diet. *J Clin Endocrinol Metab*. 2002 May;87(5):2008-12

[168] **Vasquez A**.  A Five-Part Nutritional Protocol that Produces Consistently Positive Results. *Nutritional Wellness* 2005 September http://optimalhealthresearch.com/protocol

[169] **Vasquez A**.  Integrative Rheumatology.  http://www.optimalhealthresearch.com/rheumatology.html

**Conclusions**:
In this brief article, I have introduced and reviewed important concepts related to diet-induced alterations in cellular calcium balance. Notice that this discussion of calcium has transcended the usual conversation of simple "deficiency" and "excess." What I've done here is review data showing that we can indirectly modulate certain aspects of intracellular nutrition to promote optimal biochemical balance within the cell in order to optimize health and prevent and correct disease and dysfunction. Next time someone tells you that there is no scientific basis for interventional nutrition, sit them down and give them a lecture on causes and treatments for intracellular hypercalcinosis. Tell them it is only the tip of the iceberg, and that they'd be wise to take interventional nutrition seriously. Just because we buy groceries and nutritional supplements without a prescription (for now), this does not mean that these choices are not powerful or lacking in scientific merit. Amazing results can be achieved with diet modification and nutritional/botanical supplementation.

## Nutritional Treatments for Hypertension

*Alex Vasquez, D.C., N.D.*

This article was originally published in *Naturopathy Digest*
http://www.naturopathydigest.com/archives/2006/nov/vasquez.php

**Introduction**:
Clinical problems associated with hypertension can be divided into two categories dependent upon the severity and duration of the elevated blood pressure. Mild elevations in blood pressure that are sustained over a period of many years and decades increases the risk of atherosclerosis, stroke, myocardial infarction, heart failure, and renal failure. Acute elevations in blood pressure, even if sustained for a relatively short time, can cause hypertensive encephalopathy, stroke, retinal hemorrhage, acute myocardial infarction, and acute left ventricular failure with pulmonary edema. Many different etiologies exist for hypertension, including but not limited to metabolic syndrome, hypothyroidism, renal failure, and adverse drug effects; the scope of this article is limited to uncomplicated prehypertension and Stage One Hypertension. Obviously, the goals of therapy are to bring the blood pressure down into the normal range and to prevent end-organ damage, especially to heart, brain, eyes, and kidneys.

Guidelines for the assessment and therefore management of hypertension change periodically based on new consensus and new research data. "Prehypertension" or early hypertension begins at 120 systolic over 80 diastolic, while "Stage One hypertension" is in the range of 140/90 - 160/100. Patients beyond Stage One Hypertension or those with a complex clinical presentation should generally be co-managed pharmaceutically (at least initially); a table describing hypertensive categories is provided below (Table 1). Doctors who choose to manage hypertension for their patients must include proper history, physical examination, laboratory assessment (e.g., chemistry/metabolic panel, urinalysis, thyroid and cardiovascular panels), and the treatment plan must include frequent follow-up (e.g., every 2-4 weeks) until the problem is resolved. If effectiveness cannot be obtained, sustained, or documented then the patient should receive both verbal and written referral to another physician, particularly an internist or cardiologist.

**Table 1: Hypertension categorization***

| | |
|---|---|
| Prehypertension: | >120/80 |
| Stage One: | 140/90 - 160/100 |
| Stage Two: | 160/100 - 210/120 without symptoms and without end-organ damage (i.e., no renal damage, headache, or edema). Clinicians should generally refer or co-manage these patients. |
| Urgent: | SBP ≥ 220 or DBP 125 - 129, or Stage 2 with symptoms or end-organ damage. Immediate referral for drug treatment is appropriate. |
| Emergency: | >220/130 is an emergency: 911 or ER |

* Additional considerations that affect treatment and management: Insulin resistance / pre-diabetes / metabolic syndrome: dyslipidemia / high cholesterol, obesity, inactivity, personal and family medical history, other chief complaints and clinical and laboratory findings.

**Nutritional treatments for hypertension**:

Nutritional treatments for hypertension include the following considerations, which can generally be used in combination (rather than in isolation, as studied in the research). These will be listed and discussed in order of general effectiveness (see Table 2).

1. Short-term supervised fasting: Short-term inpatient supervised fasting appears to be the most effective treatment for chronic hypertension that has ever been documented. Working closely with his multidisciplinary team, **pioneering chiropractic physician Alan Goldhamer DC** documented reductions in hypertension of 60/17 in patients with severe hypertension and reductions of 37/13 in patients with moderate hypertension.[170,171,172] Generally the program begins with 4-7 days of a raw vegetarian diet followed by 1-2 weeks of fasting and concluded with reintroduction of a vegetarian and health-promoting diet. Laboratory tests and professional supervision help ensure patient safety.

2. Healthy diet and exercise: Health-promoting diets such as either Paleo- and Mediterranean-style diets can lower blood pressure by as much as 17/13 according to some reports. Please see my previous articles in this magazine for description of the "supplemented Paleo-Mediterranean Diet."[173]

3. CoQ10: Coenzyme Q-10 in doses of 100-225 mg/day can lower blood pressure quite effectively, as documented in several clinical studies, some of which showed that CoQ-10 is more effective and safer than the use of antihypertensive drugs.[174,175,176] Reductions in blood

---

[170] Goldhamer A, et al. Medically supervised water-only fasting in the treatment of hypertension. *J Manipulative Physiol Ther* 2001 Jun;24(5):335-9
[171] Goldhamer AC, et al. Medically supervised water-only fasting in the treatment of borderline hypertension. *J Altern Complement Med*. 2002 Oct;8(5):643-50
[172] Goldhamer AC. Initial cost of care results in medically supervised water-only fasting for treating high blood pressure and diabetes. *J Altern Complement Med*. 2002 Dec;8(6):696-7
[173] **Vasquez A**. A Five-Part Nutritional Protocol that Produces Consistently Positive Results. *Nutritional Wellness* 2005 Sept. http://nutritionalwellness.com/archives/2005/sep/09_vasquez.php and http://optimalhealthresearch.com/protocol
[174] "RESULTS: The mean reduction in systolic blood pressure of the CoQ-treated group was 17.8 +/- 7.3 mm Hg (mean +/- SEM). None of the patients exhibited orthostatic blood pressure changes. CONCLUSIONS: Our results suggest CoQ may be safely offered to hypertensive patients as an alternative treatment option." Burke BE, Neuenschwander R, Olson RD. Randomized, double-blind, placebo-controlled trial of coenzyme Q10 in isolated systolic hypertension. *South Med J*. 2001 Nov;94(11):1112-7
[175] "These findings indicate that treatment with coenzyme Q10 decreases blood pressure possibly by decreasing oxidative stress and insulin response in patients with known hypertension receiving conventional antihypertensive drugs." Singh RB, Niaz MA, Rastogi SS, Shukla PK, Thakur AS. Effect of hydrosoluble coenzyme Q10 on blood pressures and insulin resistance in hypertensive patients with coronary artery disease. *J Hum Hypertens*. 1999 Mar;13(3):203-8
[176] "...51% of patients came completely off of between one and three antihypertensive drugs at an average of 4.4 months after starting CoQ10." Langsjoen P, Langsjoen P, Willis R, Folkers K. Treatment of essential hypertension with coenzyme Q10. *Mol Aspects Med*. 1994;15 Suppl:S265-72

pressure are generally in the range of 17/12 and are dose-dependent. A patient who does not respond to 100 mg per day may respond very well to 200 mg per day. Since it is a fat-soluble nutrient, CoQ-10 should be administered with dietary fat and/or consumed in a "pre-emulsified" form to enhance absorption which is a prerequisite for clinical effectiveness. Several trials have been reported showing enhanced absorption of CoQ-10 when administered in pre-emulsified form. CoQ-10 is very safe, and drug interactions are rare; caution should be used in patients taking coumadin.

4. <u>Sodium restriction</u>: Clinical responsiveness to low-sodium diets ranges from minimal to a maximal reduction in the range of 22/14 - 16/9.[177] Contraindications to low-sodium diet are uncommon (e.g., hyponatremia); low-sodium diets should generally be a component of all anti-hypertensive treatment plans.

5. <u>Vitamin D and calcium</u>: Vitamin D3 (cholecalciferol) and calcium supplementation can reduce blood pressure in hypertensive patients by approximately 13/7.[178] As I have discussed in extensive detail elsewhere, a reasonable dose of vitamin D3 for adults is in the range of 2,000 - 4,000 IU per day, and doctors new to vitamin D therapy should read my clinical monograph published in 2004 and available on-line.[179] The most important drug interaction with vitamin D is seen with hydrochlorothiazide, a commonly-used antihypertensive diuretic that promotes hypercalcemia; vitamin D therapy in patients taking hydrochlorothiazide must be implemented slowly, with professional supervision, and with weekly laboratory monitoring of serum calcium. Vitamin D probably corrects hypertension via several mechanisms, including but not limited to increased absorption of magnesium and reduction in intracellular calcium, as I described previously in this magazine.[180] Since vitamin D absorption decreases with age and in patients with intestinal disease (including dysbiosis[181]), absorption of fat-soluble vitamin D3 is enhanced when administered in pre-emulsified form.[182]

6. <u>Prescription drugs</u>: Use of the nutritional treatments described in this article can complement or replace antihypertensive drug therapy in many patients. When used singly, prescription antihypertensive drugs average a reduction in blood pressure of approximately 12/6. Initial reductions of 20/10 require combination therapy, according to a review article published in American Family Physician in 2003.[183]

7. <u>Exercise</u>: Moderate exercise can reduce blood pressure by approximately 7/7 in the short term. Longer-term exercise, particularly along with diet improvements and weight loss, can

---

[177] "The average fall in blood pressure from the highest to the lowest sodium intake was 16/9 mm Hg." MacGregor GA, Markandu ND, Sagnella GA, Singer DR, Cappuccio FP. Double-blind study of three sodium intakes and long-term effects of sodium restriction in essential hypertension. *Lancet*. 1989 Nov 25;2(8674):1244-7

[178] "A short-term supplementation with vitamin D(3) and calcium is more effective in reducing SBP than calcium alone. Inadequate vitamin D(3) and calcium intake could play a contributory role in the pathogenesis and progression of hypertension and cardiovascular disease in elderly women." Pfeifer M, Begerow B, Minne HW, Nachtigall D, Hansen C. Effects of a short-term vitamin D(3) and calcium supplementation on blood pressure and parathyroid hormone levels in elderly women. *J Clin Endocrinol Metab*. 2001 Apr;86(4):1633-7

[179] **Vasquez A**, Manso G, Cannell J. The clinical importance of vitamin D (cholecalciferol): a paradigm shift with implications for all healthcare providers. *Altern Ther Health Med*. 2004 Sep-Oct;10(5):28-36 http://optimalhealthresearch.com/monograph04

[180] **Vasquez A**. Intracellular Hypercalcinosis. A Functional Nutritional Disorder With Implications Ranging From Myofascial Trigger Points to Affective Disorders, Hypertension and Cancer. Naturopathy *Digest* 2006, September http://www.naturopathydigest.com/archives/2006/sep/vasquez.php

[181] **Vasquez A**. Reducing Pain and Inflammation Naturally. Part 6: Nutritional and Botanical Treatments Against "Silent Infections" and Gastrointestinal Dysbiosis, Commonly Overlooked Causes of Neuromusculoskeletal Inflammation and Chronic Health Problems. *Nutritional Perspectives* 2006; January. http://optimalhealthresearch.com/dysbiosis

[182] **Vasquez A**. Subphysiologic Doses of Vitamin D are Subtherapeutic: Comment on the Study by The Record Trial Group. *Lancet* 2005 published online May 6 http://optimalhealthresearch.com/lancet

[183] Magill MK, Gunning K, Saffel-Shrier S, Gay C. New developments in the management of hypertension. *Am Fam Physician*. 2003 Sep 1;68(5):853-8 http://www.aafp.org/afp/20030901/853.html

result in synergistic and curative benefits. Patients who have been sedentary for years and those with probable or documented cardiovascular disease should be evaluated by a physician and ECG before beginning an exercise program.

8. <u>Fish oil</u>: Fish oil supplementation had been shown to reduce blood pressure by approximately 3/2. For reasons that I have detailed elsewhere[184], fish oil should be co-administered with a source of GLA such as borage oil in order to maximize effectiveness and minimize subtle biochemical adverse effects. Importantly, fish oil is safer, less expensive, and more effective than "statin" antihypercholesterolemic drug treatment for reducing total and cardiovascular mortality.

9. <u>Food allergy elimination</u>: According to a clinical study of migraineurs published in *The Lancet*, identification and avoidance of food allergens can normalize blood pressure in hypertensive migraine patients.[185] The anti-hypertensive response to food allergy avoidance can be seen clinically even in patients who do not have migraine or other manifestations of allergy, but the more allergic symptoms that are seen and the more complete the response to allergy elimination, the more likely is a reduction in blood pressure.

**Table 2: General effectiveness of therapies for chronic essential hypertension**

1. <u>Short-term supervised fasting:</u>   -60/-17 for severe HTN and -37/-13 for moderate HTN*
2. <u>Healthy diet and exercise:</u>   -17/-13
3. <u>CoQ10 100-225 mg/day:</u>   -17/-12
4. <u>Sodium restriction:</u>   22/14 - 16/-9
5. <u>Vitamin D and calcium:</u>   -13/-7
6. <u>Prescription drugs:</u>   -12/-6   * Reductions of 20/10 require combination therapy
7. <u>Exercise:</u>   -7/-7
8. <u>Fish oil:</u>   -3/-2
9. <u>Food allergy elimination:</u>   <u>variable response</u> ranging from insignificant to curative

**Conclusions**:

Many nutritional treatments for hypertension are documented in the research literature, and several of these treatments appear safer and more cost-effective than pharmaceutical antihypertensive drugs. Furthermore, the synergistic use of the nutritional and lifestyle interventions described above—e.g., supplemented Paleo-Mediterranean diet along with exercise, fish oil, vitamin D, CoQ-10, and sodium restriction-results in clinical benefits that far exceed the results published in the single-intervention clinical trials that have documented the effectiveness of the individual components. The major drug interaction that one must look out for is the combination of vitamin D with hydrochlorothiazide. Switching from pharmaceutical drugs to nutrients for the management of hypertension requires diligent follow-up, informed consent, and documentation of beneficial clinical response and should be undertaken only by skilled and experienced clinicians.

---

[184] **Vasquez A**. Reducing Pain and Inflammation Naturally. Part 2: New Insights into Fatty Acid Supplementation and Its Effect on Eicosanoid Production and Genetic Expression. *Nutritional Perspectives* 2005; January: 5-16 http://optimalhealthresearch.com/part2.html
[185] Grant EC. Food allergies and migraine. *Lancet*. 1979 May 5;1(8123):966-9

# Twilight of the Idiopathic Era and The Dawn of New Possibilities in Health and Healthcare

*Alex Vasquez, D.C., N.D.*

This article was originally published in *Naturopathy Digest*
http://www.naturopathydigest.com/archives/2006/mar/idiopathic.php

Among the perplexing paradoxes that exist in healthcare is coexistence of our adoration of allopathy for its "scientific method" along with the description of most chronic diseases as "idiopathic." If the allopathic use of the scientific method were so adroit, then why are so many conditions described as having "no known cause"? Is it that the scientific method is inadequate, or that the allopathic lens is incapable of bringing disease causation into focus? Perhaps a third option exists: could it be that some groups—namely the allopaths and the pharmaceutical companies—benefit by convincing us that most diseases have "no known cause" and that therefore the best doctors and patients can hope for is additive and endless pharmaceuticalization of all health problems? When the cause of our health problems is "unknown", we are disempowered, and we must depend on "experts" to help us. When the cause of our problems is known, we are empowered to take effective action. Certainly, some groups have financial and political interests in keeping us confused and disempowered.

## The End of the Idiopathic Era
A stark contrast exists between primary research literature and the "facts" that are selectively reported in medical textbooks and which are used to buttress "conventional wisdom" and the resulting status quo. While I have been aware of this contrast for many years, the divergency was impressed upon me with renewed vigor during the preparation of a recent article[186] and the completion of my recent textbook on *Integrative Rheumatology*.[187] Arthritis in general and autoimmune and rheumatic diseases in particular are frequently described as "idiopathic" and as having "no known cause" by most mainstream medical books like *The Merck Manual* and *Current Medical Diagnosis and Treatment*. These contentions are inconsistent with the abundant and diverse research showing that—rather than being *idiopathic*—most chronic musculoskeletal disorders are *multifactorial*. When a disease is codified as idiopathic, doctors lose their incentive to look for and treat the *causes* of the disease (because the causes have not been identified), and patients are convinced to give up their hope of ever being cured—they chose the second best option: lifelong medicalization.

## Idiopathic, or Multifactorial?
Let's look at psoriasis and rheumatoid arthritis as two *idiopathic* examples. If one looks into a regular medical textbook, one sees that these conditions have no known cause and therefore the lifelong prescription of anti-inflammatory medications is presumptively justified. On the

---

[186] **Vasquez A.** Reducing Pain and Inflammation Naturally. Part 6: Nutritional and Botanical Treatments Against "Silent Infections" and Gastrointestinal Dysbiosis, Commonly Overlooked Causes of Neuromusculoskeletal Inflammation and Chronic Health Problems. *Nutritional Perspectives* 2006; January http://www.optimalhealthresearch.com/part6
[187] **Vasquez A.** *Integrative Rheumatology. The Art of Creating Wellness While Effectively Managing Acute and Chronic Musculoskeletal Disorders. Volume One: Autoimmune Diseases.* 2006 http://www.optimalhealthresearch.com/rheumatology.html

contrary, if one spends a few days in the local medical library, one can find articles that point to the causes of these diseases and then illuminate the path by which doctors and patients can arrive at permanent cure. Most patients can be cured of psoriasis, and a large percentage of rheumatoid arthritis patients can avoid the complications and medicalization associated with their disease, particularly if *the causes* of their condition are treated early. We now know that most autoimmune diseases are caused by and/or perpetuated by chronic infections, food allergies, a proinflammatory lifestyle, hormonal imbalances, and exposure to chemicals and metals that cause immune dysfunction. When the cause(s) of the disease is treated, the disease is cured. When the disease is cured, lifelong medicalization becomes unnecessary, the patient is free to fully resume his/her life, and doctors are liberated from their roles as drug representatives and can resume their proper positions as healers.

Asserting an empowered stance toward disease prevention and treatment carries implications beyond those for the doctor and the patient. These implications also point to new ways of living and stewarding the world. When we look at a disease like Parkinson's disease and then determine that it is *idiopathic*, then nothing happens to change or shape our view of the world, our place in it, and the interconnected natures of health and disease. Everyone agrees that that clinical manifestations of Parkinson's disease result from the death of dopaminergic neurons. From the allopathic perspective, the disease is *idiopathic*, while from an integrative naturopathic perspective, we see Parkinson's disease as a multifaceted disorder associated with defective mitochondrial function, impaired xenobiotic detoxification, and occupational and/or recreational exposure to toxicants, particularly pesticides. These associations align to create a new model for the illness based on exposure to neurotoxicants such as pesticides,[188] which are ineffectively detoxified[189] and then accumulate in the brain[190] and induce mitochondrial dysfunction[191] and resultant oxidative stress,[192] which leads to death of dopaminergic neurons. Therefore, from the perspective of both prevention and treatment, the clinical approach to Parkinson's disease would include pesticide avoidance and optimization of detoxification to prevent the neuronal accumulation of neurotoxic mitochondrial poisons. The plan must also include optimization of nutritional status, antioxidant capacity, and mitochondrial function.[193] Further, if our goal is to reduce the societal prevalence of Parkinson's disease, then we must begin living in better harmony with nature and thinking of ways to reduce our use of pesticides and herbicides, the very chemicals that are consistently shown to cause premature neuronal death.

### The Dawn of New Possibilities in Health and Healthcare
The time is past when credible physicians can assert that most diseases are "of unknown origin." The truth is that we already have access to the information we need to help our patients. The truth is that we can often offer our patients the *probability of cure* rather than *lifelong and endless prescriptions for symptom-modifying drugs*. These truths imply that healthcare and our systems of

---

[188] Ritz B, Yu F. Parkinson's disease mortality and pesticide exposure in California 1984-1994. Int J Epidemiol. 2000 Apr;29(2):323-9.
[189] Menegon A, Board PG, Blackburn AC, Mellick GD, Le Couteur DG. Parkinson's disease, pesticides, and glutathione transferase polymorphisms. Lancet. 1998;352(9137):1344-6.
[190] Kamel F, Hoppin JA. Related Articles, Association of pesticide exposure with neurologic dysfunction and disease. Environ Health Perspect. 2004;112(9):950-8.
[191] Parker WD Jr, Swerdlow RH. Mitochondrial dysfunction in idiopathic Parkinson disease. Am J Hum Genet. 1998;62(4):758-62.
[192] Davey GP, Peuchen S, Clark JB. Energy thresholds in brain mitochondria. Potential involvement in neurodegeneration. J Biol Chem. 1998;273(21):12753-7.
[193] Kidd PM. Parkinson's disease as multifactorial oxidative neurodegeneration: implications for integrative management. Altern Med Rev. 2000 Dec;5(6):502-29.

healthcare delivery must change, because the pharmaceutical and medical icons that stand before us were built upon feet and legs of clay and interspersed lead. We stand at the dawn of a new era in healthcare—one in which patients with chronic diseases in general and autoimmune diseases in particular—have a real opportunity to regain their health.

## Thinking Outside the (Pill) Box: Is the "Battle Against Hypertension and Diabetes" Truly Meant to be "Won" for Patients…or for the Drug Companies?

The Most Profitable "Wars" are the ones that are Fought Indefinitely and which Require Reliance on Private Industry: As with most modern sociopolitical fights, wars, and missions, a keen observer (or any high-school student who read George Orwell's classic novel *1984*) might question whether the current "**Mission**: To **Combat** High Blood Pressure in America"[194] is actually meant to ever be won. The US National Heart, Lung, and Blood Institute (NHLBI) invokes the language of battle, e.g., "to **mobilize** all Americans in the **fight against high blood pressure** and reduce the more than 1 million heart attacks, strokes, and kidney failure cases that it causes each year. The CDC and the NHLBI have **joined forces** to **disseminate** these materials…"[195] Ironically, the NHLBI's document entitled "Physician Fact Sheet: What Every Physician Should Know" (http://hp2010.nhlbihin.net/mission/partner/physcian_factsheet.pdf) contains zero practical information on diet, exercise, or nutritional supplementation. Likewise, the document under the heading "Real Possibilities for America's Health Care Providers"[196] provides nothing that a clinician or patient could use to authentically correct the common causes of HTN; it provides near-meaningless mention of "diet and exercise" accompanied by a photo of people sitting at a table with food and encourages that doctors "Support Adherence to Treatment" accompanied by a photo of a woman taking pills.

"Common Objectives" …with Drug Companies: For more than a decade, the American Heart Association has been "advised" by their "Pharmaceutical Roundtable" (PRT) comprised of monolithic drug companies which must each pay a least $1 million per year for each 3-year term of membership.[197] According to the American Heart Association's website in a document updated August 2009[198], "The American Heart Association Pharmaceutical Roundtable (PRT) is a strategic coalition of 10 leading pharmaceutical companies and association volunteers and staff. It allows our association and members of the **pharmaceutical industry** to identify and pursue **common objectives** to improve cardiovascular health in the United States through research, patient education, and public and professional programs."

---

[194] National Heart, Lung, and Blood Institute (NHLBI). The Mission: To Combat High Blood Pressure in America http://hp2010.nhlbihin.net/mission/ Accessed December 22, 2009
[195] Centers for Disease Control and Prevention. State Heart Disease and Stroke Prevention Program Addresses High Blood Pressure. http://www.cdc.gov/dhdsp/library/fs_state_hbp.htm Accessed December 22, 2009
[196] National Heart, Lung, and Blood Institute (NHLBI). http://www.nhlbi.nih.gov/health/prof/heart/hbp/mp/mp_health.htm Accessed December 22, 2009
[197] "Each industry participant of the PRT will sign a separate agreement with AHA that will be binding only between the AHA and that individual industry member. The agreements will commit each industry member to contribute $1,000,000 per year for three years." Letter dated March 20, 1998 from Joel I. Klein (Assistant Attorney General), US Department of Justice Antitrust Division. http://www.justice.gov/atr/public/busreview/1608.htm Accessed December 23, 2009
[198] http://www.americanheart.org/presenter.jhtml?identifier=2366 Accessed December 23, 2009

Current (or recent) members of the American Heart Association Pharmaceutical Roundtable include:

1. AstraZeneca L.P.
2. Eli Lilly and Company
3. Bristol-Myers Squibb Company
4. GlaxoSmithKline
5. Merck/Schering-Plough Pharmaceuticals
6. Merck Pharmaceuticals
7. Novartis Pharmaceuticals Corporation
8. Pfizer, Inc.
9. Sanofi-Aventis
10. Takeda Pharmaceuticals

Promoting Unhealthy Eating: Proatherosclerotic Recipes Endorsed by the US National Heart, Lung, and Blood Institute (NHLBI): The following is a partial list of atherosclerosis-promoting recipes listed under the title "Stay Young at Heart: Cooking the Heart-Healthy Way"[199] advocated on the website of the NHLBI in December 2009. Notice the lack of nutrient density, the emphasis on simple carbohydrates, the frequent use of baking with oil to create the effect of frying, the lack of raw foods, and the scarcity of phytonutrients:

- "Stir-fried beef" with boiled potatoes and white rice
- "Beef stroganoff" with 6 cups of cooked macaroni pasta
- "Crispy oven-fried chicken" cooked in cornflakes and buttermilk
- "Classic macaroni and cheese"
- "Candied yams" with brown sugar, margarine, white flour, and orange juice
- "Oven French fries" (white potatoes oven-fried in vegetable oil)
- "White rice" cooked with vegetable oil and salt
- "Sunshine (white) rice" cooked with vegetable oil, orange juice, and lemon juice
- "Homestyle biscuits" made from white flour, salt, and sugar
- "Banana-nut bread" made from mashed ripe bananas, low-fat buttermilk, packed brown sugar, margarine, all-purpose white flour, egg and salt.
- "Apricot-orange bread" made from dried apricots, margarine, white sugar, egg, white flour, dry milk powder, salt and orange juice
- "Apple coffee cake" made with peeled apples (please note that >90% of the antioxidants contained in apples are in the peel—thus when the peel is removed, virtually all that remains is antioxidant-poor carbohydrate), one cup of sugar, one cup of dark raisins, one-quarter cup vegetable oil, 1 egg, and two-and-a-half cups of sifted all-purpose white flour
- "Frosted cake" with 2 1/4 cups cake flour, 4 tablespoons margarine, 1 1/4 cups sugar, 4 eggs, low fat cream cheese, and 2 cups sifted confectioners sugar!!
- "Topical fruit compote" with sugar
- "Peach cobbler" with sugar, white flour, margarine, canned peaches "packed in juice", peach nectar, and cornstarch
- "Rice pudding" with white rice, 3 cups of skim milk, and 2/3 cup sugar

The list goes on to include many other proatherosclerotic and prodiabetic meals. Any reasonable person might ask why US National Heart, Lung, and Blood Institute would promote a diet plan that is ensured to contribute to the pandemics of hypertension, obesity, and diabetes mellitus.

---

[199] US National Heart, Lung, and Blood Institute (NHLBI). Stay Young at Heart: Cooking the Heart-Healthy Way. http://www.nhlbi.nih.gov/health/public/heart/other/syah/index.htm Accessed December 23, 2009

# Wellness Promotion: Re-Establishing the Foundation for Health

<u>Topics:</u>
- **Re-establishing the Foundation for Health**
    - **Healthcare, Health, and Wellness**
    - **Daily living**
        - Lifestyle habits
        - Motivation: background and clinical applications
        - Exceptional living: the key to exceptional results
        - Recognize and affirm individual uniqueness
        - Individuation & conscious living: alternatives to common paradigms
        - Quality and quantity of sleep: concepts and clinical applications
        - Exercise, obesity, BMI, and proinflammatory activity of adipose tissue
    - **Diet is a powerful tool for the prevention and treatment of disease**
        - Make "whole foods" the foundation of the diet
        - Increase consumption of fruits and vegetables
        - Phytochemicals: food-derived anti-inflammatory nutrients
        - Eat the right amount of protein
        - Benefits of complex carbohydrates
        - Reducing consumption of sugars: exceptions for supercompensation
        - Avoiding artificial sweeteners, colors, and other additives
        - Reducing or eliminating caffeine
        - To the extent possible, eat "organic" foods
        - Recognize the importance of avoiding food allergens
        - Supplement your healthy diet with vitamins, minerals, and fatty acids
        - Putting it all together: *the supplemented Paleo-Mediterranean diet*
    - **Advanced concepts in nutrition**
        - "Biochemical Individuality" and "Orthomolecular Medicine"
        - Nutrigenomics: Nutritional Genomics
        - General guidelines for the safe use of nutritional supplements
    - **Emotional, mental, and social health**
        - Stress management and authentic living
        - Stress always has a biochemical/physiologic component
        - The body functions as a whole
        - Healing past experiences
        - Autonomization, intradependence, emotional literacy, corrective experience
    - **Environmental health**
        - Environmental exposures and the importance of detoxification
        - Avoid unnecessary chemical medications and medical procedures
        - Intestinal health, bowel function, and introduction to dysbiosis
- **Natural holistic healthcare contrasted to standard medical treatment**
- **Opposite influences of health promotion vs. disease promotion**
- **Select Previously Published Essays**
    - Five-Part Nutritional Wellness Protocol That Produces Consistently Positive Results
    - Implementing the Five-Part Nutritional Wellness Protocol for the Treatment of Various Health Problems
    - Common Oversights and Shortcomings in the Study and Implementation of Nutritional Supplementation

> **Lifestyle Support**
> This section details the lifestyle modifications that can support a wellness-promoting antihypertensive cardioprotective health program.

# Introduction Wellness Promotion

The *Foundation for Health* refers to the lifestyle and nutrition **basics** that need to be attended to in order for a person to have a chance at being truly healthy. Without a basic, healthy foundation, *survival* is possible, but *long-term health*—let alone *wellness*—is not possible. Indeed, **many so-called "diseases" may be effectively treated with comprehensive lifestyle improvements** and *without disease-specific treatments.* The research literature on the management of chronic illnesses is replete with documentation supporting the effectiveness of non-drug non-surgical healthcare; yet these natural treatments continue to be labeled as "unscientific" and "unproven" and are cast aside in favor of "medical" treatments simply because the latter conform to the financially-leveraged nationally-televised medical paradigm[1,2] of patient passivity, medicalization, surgery, and superfluous technological sophistication.[3] One of the most thoroughly documented conditions responsive to lifestyle interventions is heart disease. The work of Dr. Dean Ornish[4,5] has shown that coronary atherosclerosis can be reversed with intensive lifestyle intervention; previous to his pioneering research, patients were forced to submit to expensive/hazardous drugs and invasive surgery as their only treatment options. **Atherosclerosis, hypertension, and hypercholesterolemia are virtually unknown in societies that follow healthy diets and lifestyles[6], yet each of these is a multibillion-dollar medical business in industrialized nations.**[7] The safest and most effective treatments for chronic hypertension ever documented—short-term fasting[8,9,10], supplemented protein-sparing caloric restriction for obese and type-2 diabetic hypertensives[11,12,13], and nutritional supplementation as

> **Common sense is "unconventional"**
> "How did we get to a place in medicine," Ornish asked, "where it's considered radical to ask people to stop smoking, meditate, walk, and eat a healthy diet, and conventional to cut people open and blow balloons up in their arteries and put radioactive stents in there?"
>
> Dean Ornish, MD. Ornish: Heart-healthy diet also aids prostate. *Houston Chronicle* July 5, 2002. Houston section, page 3.
> http://www.chron.com/CDA/archives/archive.mpl?id=2002_3560710

---

[1] "...many ads may be targeted specifically at women and older viewers. Our findings suggest that Americans who watch average amounts of television may be exposed to more than 30 hours of direct-to-consumer drug advertisements each year, far surpassing their exposure to other forms of health communication." Brownfield ED, Bernhardt JM, Phan JL, Williams MV, Parker RM. Direct-to-consumer drug advertisements on network television: an exploration of quantity, frequency, and placement. *J Health Commun.* 2004 Nov-Dec;9(6):491-7

[2] Kaphingst KA, DeJong W, Rudd RE, Daltroy LH. A content analysis of direct-to-consumer television prescription drug advertisements. *J Health Commun.* 2004 Nov-Dec;9(6):515-2

[3] "...despite lush advertisements from companies with obvious vested interests, and authoritative testimonials from biased investigators who presumably believe in their own work to the point of straining credulity and denying common sense... (translate: economic improvement, not biological superiority)." Stevens CW, Glatstein E. Beware the Medical-Industrial Complex. *Oncologist* 1996;1(4):IV-V http://theoncologist.alphamedpress.org/cgi/reprint/1/4/190-iv.pdf on July 4, 2004

[4] "More regression of coronary atherosclerosis occurred after 5 years... In contrast, in the control group, coronary atherosclerosis continued to progress and more than twice as many cardiac events occurred." Ornish D, et al. Intensive lifestyle changes for reversal of coronary heart disease. *JAMA.* 1998 Dec 16;280(23):2001-7

[5] Ornish D. *Dr. Dean Ornish's Program for Reversing Heart Disease: The Only System Scientifically Proven to Reverse Heart Disease Without Drugs or Surgery*. Ballentine; 1990

[6] O'Keefe JH, Cordain L, Harris, WH, Moe RM, Vogel R. Optimal low-density lipoprotein is 50 to 70 mg/dl. Lower is better and physiologically normal. *J Am Coll Cardiol* 2004;43: 2142-6

[7] "The economic impact of hypertension is enormous, representing $US23.74 billion in the US ...and hypertension represents one of the 3 leading causes of visits to primary healthcare centres." Pardell H, et al. Pharmacoeconomic considerations in the management of hypertension. *Drugs*. 2000;59 Suppl 2:13-20; discussion 39-40

[8] Goldhamer A, et al. Medically supervised water-only fasting in the treatment of hypertension. *J Manipulative Physiol Ther* 2001 Jun;24(5):335-9

[9] Goldhamer AC, et al. Medically supervised water-only fasting in the treatment of borderline hypertension. *J Altern Complement Med.* 2002 Oct;8(5):643-50

[10] Goldhamer AC. Initial cost of care results in medically supervised water-only fasting for treating high blood pressure and diabetes. *J Altern Complement Med.* 2002 Dec;8(6):696-7

[11] Vertes V, Genuth SM, Hazelton IM. Supplemented fasting as a large-scale outpatient program. *JAMA.* 1977 Nov 14;238(20):2151-3

[12] Bauman WA, Schwartz E, Rose HG, Eisenstein HN, Johnson DW. Early and long-term effects of acute caloric deprivation in obese diabetic patients. *Am J Med.* 1988 Jul;85(1):38-46

[13] "Average weight loss was 63.9 kg... Concomitant with weight reduction, there were significant decrements in blood pressure... This study demonstrates that massively obese persons can achieve marked weight reduction, even normalization of weight, without hospitalization, surgery, or pharmacologic

# Wellness Promotion: Re-Establishing the Foundation for Health

with coenzyme Q-10[14,15,16] and vitamin D3[17]—are unknown to and underutilized by most allopathic cardiologists and are not offered to most hypertensive patients who must then resort to dependence upon chemical drugs, which—according to one study—are inaccurately prescribed 40% of the time.[18] Meanwhile, the nation's only doctorate-level healthcare providers with graduate-level training in diet therapy and clinical nutrition—*the chiropractic and naturopathic physicians*—are excluded from full participation in the national healthcare system despite clear evidence that such integration has the potential to address the nation's healthcare crisis with effectiveness, safety, and major cost savings.[19,20,21,22]

Preventive research by Orme-Johnson and Herron[23] utilizing a "multicomponent prevention program" that included 1) twice-daily meditation, 2) daily yoga, 3) herbal dietary supplements, and 4) "recommendations for diet and daily routine" documented that total medical expenses were reduced by 59% over 4 years and by 63% over 11 years compared to outcomes obtained by patients relegated to standard allopathic medical treatment. Hospital admission rates were reduced 11.4-fold for cardiovascular disease, 3.3-fold for cancer, and 6.7-fold for mental health and substance abuse. Based on these and other illustrative examples described later in this text, we might reasonably conclude that American healthcare would be more effective, more affordable, and safer if **chiropractic and naturopathic physicians** were fully integrated into the healthcare system rather than being politically excluded (e.g., restrictive licensure laws[24]) or functionally excluded (e.g., discriminatory CPT codes and HMO policies[25]) by a system of drug- and surgery-based healthcare that financially depletes the people[26], business[27], and communities

---

intervention." Kempner W, Newborg BC, Peschel RL, Skyler JS. Treatment of massive obesity with rice/reduction diet program. An analysis of 106 patients with at least a 45-kg weight loss. *Arch Intern Med*. 1975 Dec;135(12):1575-84

[14] "RESULTS: The mean reduction in systolic blood pressure of the CoQ-treated group was 17.8 +/- 7.3 mm Hg (mean +/- SEM). None of the patients exhibited orthostatic blood pressure changes. CONCLUSIONS: Our results suggest CoQ may be safely offered to hypertensive patients as an alternative treatment option." Burke BE, Neuenschwander R, Olson RD. Randomized, double-blind, placebo-controlled trial of coenzyme Q10 in isolated systolic hypertension. *South Med J*. 2001 Nov;94(11):1112-7

[15] "These findings indicate that treatment with coenzyme Q10 decreases blood pressure possibly by decreasing oxidative stress and insulin response in patients with known hypertension receiving conventional antihypertensive drugs." Singh RB, Niaz MA, Rastogi SS, Shukla PK, Thakur AS. Effect of hydrosoluble coenzyme Q10 on blood pressures and insulin resistance in hypertensive patients with coronary artery disease. *J Hum Hypertens*. 1999 Mar;13(3):203-8

[16] "...51% of patients came completely off of between one and three antihypertensive drugs at an average of 4.4 months after starting CoQ10." Langsjoen P, Langsjoen P, Willis R, Folkers K. Treatment of essential hypertension with coenzyme Q10. *Mol Aspects Med*. 1994;15 Suppl:S265-72

[17] "..supplementation with vitamin D(3) and calcium resulted in...a decrease in systolic blood pressure (SBP) of 9.3% (P = 0.02), and a decrease in heart rate of 5.4% (P = 0.02)... Inadequate vitamin D(3) and calcium intake could play a contributory role in the pathogenesis and progression of hypertension and cardiovascular disease in elderly women." Pfeifer M, Begerow B, Minne HW, Nachtigall D, Hansen C. Effects of a short-term vitamin D(3) and calcium supplementation on blood pressure and parathyroid hormone levels in elderly women. *J Clin Endocrinol Metab*. 2001 Apr;86(4):1633-7

[18] "We identified 815,316 prescriptions (40%) for which an alternative regimen appeared more appropriate according to evidence-based recommendations. Such changes would have reduced the costs to payers in 2001 by 11.6 million dollars (nearly a quarter of program spending on antihypertensive medications), as well as being more clinically appropriate overall." Fischer MA, Avorn J. Economic implications of evidence-based prescribing for hypertension: can better care cost less? *JAMA* 2004 Apr 21;291(15):1850-6

[19] "Systematic access to managed chiropractic care not only may prove to be clinically beneficial but also may reduce overall health care costs." Legoretta A, Metz D, Nelson C, Ray S, Chernicoff H, DiNubile N. Comparative Analysis of Individuals With and Without Chiropractic Coverage. *Archives of Internal Medicine* 2004; 164: 1985-1992

[20] Orme-Johnson DW, Herron RE. An innovative approach to reducing medical care utilization and expenditures. *Am J Manag Care*. 1997 Jan;3(1):135-44 http://www.ajmc.com/Article.cfm?Menu=1&ID=2154

[21] Goldhamer A, et al. Medically supervised water-only fasting in the treatment of hypertension. *J Manipulative Physiol Ther* 2001 Jun;24(5):335-9

[22] Herron R, Schneider RH, Mandarino JV, Alexander CN, Walton KG. Cost-effective hypertension management: Comparison of drug therapies with an alternative program. *American Journal of Managed Care* 1996; 2(4): 427-437 http://www.ajmc.com/article.cfm?ID=2345

[23] Orme-Johnson DW, Herron RE. An innovative approach to reducing medical care utilization and expenditures. *Am J Manag Care* 1997 Jan;3:135-44

[24] **Getzendanner S. Permanent injunction order against AMA. *JAMA*. 1988 Jan 1;259(1):81-2** http://optimalhealthresearch.com/archives/wilk-ama-judgement.pdf

[25] "The Solla plaintiffs argued that each HMO defendant is "by itself a combination in restraint of trade, and that there is no concerted action requirement for an illegal combination."" Solla Case DISMISSED! *Dynamic Chiropractic*; August 24, 1998, Volume 16, Issue 18 http://www.chiroweb.com/archives/16/18/22.html on July 12, 2004

[26] "A national study released today reports 20 million American families — or one in seven families — faced hardships paying medical bills last year, which forced many to choose between getting medical attention or paying rent or buying food..." Freeman, Liz. 'Working poor' struggle to afford health

of our nation[28,29] while failing to deliver consistently competent healthcare[30,31,32] and cost-effective nationwide health improvements[33] that are proportional to the continuous increase in spending.[34]

***Patients*** *are* ***people with health problems*, and they have their health problems because some event** (e.g., injury or other trauma) **or group of events and processes** (chronic stress, dysbiosis, chemical exposure, metabolic disease) **has disrupted their physiology to such an extent that they are functionally compromised and have developed symptoms** (pain, fatigue, depression, anxiety), **signs** (inflammation from conditions such as arthritis, lupus, bursitis, colitis), **or loss of organ function** (diabetes, weakness). In pursuit of relief from their ailment(s), they come to doctors for advice and treatment. However, the advice that they get varies tremendously in safety, effectiveness, and method of delivery depending upon the paradigm of the provider and the sociopolitical context in which the patient has come to view reality and healthcare options.

Since patients have been indoctrinated into the passive medical model of disease treatment[35,36], which relies on abdication and passivity rather than empowerment and personal responsibility, they generally come to doctors for the wrong answer to the wrong question. The question that people generally ask is, "What can *you* do to solve *my problem*?" This question implies that the doctor does the work, the patient does nothing other than implementing a rather minor interventional plan, and that the problem is rather simple, linear, and one-dimensional. Patients have been taught to think this way by the dominant medical-drug system[37] that can function most profitably if patients are convinced that they are powerless to effect significant self-directed improvements in their health status and if they are convinced that low-cost simple natural

---

care. Naples Daily News. Published in Naples, Florida and online at http://www.naplesnews.com/npdn/news/article/0,2071,NPDN_14940_3000546,00.html Accessed July 28, 2004

[27] "The USA's 5.8 million small companies… Health care costs are rising about 15% this year for those with fewer than 200 workers vs. 13.5% for those with 500 or more… But many small employers cite increases of 20% or more. That's made insurance the No. 1 small business problem…" Jim Hopkins. Health care tops taxes as small business cost drain. USA TODAY. http://www.usatoday.com/news/health/2003-04-20-small-business-costs_x.htm. Accessed July 28, 2004

[28] "In 1994, we spent $1 trillion on health care in the US, or, more accurately, we spent most of this astounding sum on disease treatment. …Corporations now spend an incredible 48% of their after-tax profits on health care, …." Pizzorno JE. Total Wellness. Rocklin: Prima; 1996 page 7

[29] "Though the U.S. has slightly fewer doctors per capita than the typical developed nation, we have almost twice as many MRI machines and perform vastly more angioplasties. …at least 31 percent of all the incremental income we'll earn between 1999 and 2010 will go to health care." Pat Regnier, *Money Magazine*. Healthcare myth: We spend too much. October 13, 2003: 11:29 AM EDT http://money.cnn.com/2003/10/08/pf/health_myths_1/ Accessed Monday, July 12, 2004

[30] "Although they spend more on health care than patients in any other industrialized nation, Americans receive the right treatment less than 60 percent of the time, resulting in unnecessary pain, expense and even death…" Ceci Connolly. U.S. Patients Spend More but Don't Get More, Study Finds: Even in Advantaged Areas, Americans Often Receive Inadequate Health Care. Washington Post, May 5, 2004; Page A15. On-line at http://www.washingtonpost.com/ac2/wp-dyn/A1875-2004May4 accessed on July 28, 2004

[31] "Participants received 54.9 percent (95 percent confidence interval, 54.3 to 55.5) of recommended care…CONCLUSIONS: **The deficits we have identified in adherence to recommended processes for basic care pose serious threats to the health of the American public**." McGlynn EA, Asch SM, Adams J, Keesey J, Hicks J, DeCristofaro A, Kerr EA. The quality of health care delivered to adults in the United States. *N Engl J Med*. 2003 Jun 26;348(26):2635-45

[32] "CONCLUSIONS: There is a substantial amount of injury to patients from medical management, and many injuries are the result of substandard care." Brennan TA, Leape LL, Laird NM, Hebert L, Localio AR, Lawthers AG, Newhouse JP, Weiler PC, Hiatt HH. Incidence of adverse events and negligence in hospitalized patients: results of the Harvard Medical Practice Study I. 1991. *Qual Saf Health Care*. 2004;13(2):145-51; discussion 151-2

[33] "Basically, you die earlier and spend more time disabled if you're an American rather than a member of most other advanced countries." Christopher Murray MD PhD, Director of World Health Organization's Global Program on Evidence for Health Policy http://www.who.int/inf-pr-2000/en/pr2000-life.html Accessed July 12, 2004

[34] "The results of the study demonstrate that, over the past four decades, the United States has been spending more and accomplishing less when compared with other industrialized nations." Shi L. Health care spending, delivery, and outcome in developed countries: a cross-national comparison. *Am J Med Qual* 1997;12(2):83-93

[35] "…many ads may be targeted specifically at women and older viewers. Our findings suggest that Americans who watch average amounts of television may be exposed to more than 30 hours of direct-to-consumer drug advertisements each year, far surpassing their exposure to other forms of health communication." Brownfield ED, Bernhardt JM, Phan JL, Williams MV, Parker RM. Direct-to-consumer drug advertisements on network television: an exploration of quantity, frequency, and placement. *J Health Commun*. 2004 Nov-Dec;9(6):491-7

[36] Kaphingst KA, DeJong W, Rudd RE, Daltroy LH. A content analysis of direct-to-consumer television prescription drug advertisements. *J Health Commun*. 2004 Nov-Dec;9(6):515-2

[37] Mintzes B, Barer ML, Kravitz RL, Kazanjian A, Bassett K, Lexchin J, Evans RG, Pan R, Marion SA. Influence of direct to consumer pharmaceutical advertising and patients' requests on prescribing decisions: two site cross sectional survey. *BMJ*. 2002 Feb 2; 324(7332): 278-9

treatments are "**unscientific**" (which implies that they do not follow logic), "**unconventional**" (which implies that they are radical and unpredictable), and "**alternative**" (which implies that they are of secondary quality, presumably behind drugs and surgery). The answer that patients have been conditioned to accept is, *"Take this drug, and it will solve your problem. You don't have to do anything else."* Patients like this answer because, when the focus remains on an external treatment, the implication is that they are exonerated from personal responsibility for their health problems even though their lifestyle and dietary choices may have caused the problem in the first place. Patients and doctors are creatures of habit in both thought and action; getting them to appreciate and implement lifestyle change for the prevention and treatment of disease is a major challenge—yet it offers our best opportunity for improving health outcomes on an individual basis as well as on a national level.

Patients ask for care in different ways depending on the specifics of their current health. They want a doctor to "give me a treatment" that will "relieve my pain," "lower my cholesterol" or "help me feel better." Most patients have no concept of wellness and the health possibilities that are available to them and the level of self-reliance, self-direction, and self-development that are necessary for them to attain optimal functioning in all aspects of their lives—physical, emotional, spiritual, and social. For practical reasons, we have to start from where they are, take care of the major problems and then move them toward optimal health after they are stabilized and have re-attained normal health. However the latter statement implies that *the promotion and attainment of optimal health* and *the treatment of problems* are distinct, while often they are connected and interdependent. Many times in clinical practice, for a patient to attain sufficient improvement with their primary complaint, we must look *beyond the problem* to the environment, diet, lifestyle, attitudes, beliefs, activities, habits, and emotional landscape (intrapersonal and interpersonal) that set the stage for the problem to have developed in the first place.

Healthcare is delivered along a continuum that ranges from reductionistic to holistic, from micromanagement to macromanagement, from "solving problems" to "healing lives." The latter is generally inclusive of the former, but ending at the "accomplishment" of problem-solving never attains the larger goal of healing of an entire person. For practical purposes as clinicians, we have to begin with a problem-oriented model of healthcare and ensure that major, life-threatening problems are addressed before moving on to more subtle—yet still highly important—problems such as poor lifestyle habits and self-defeating behavior. If a patient comes to you with back pain, and you overlook their *cauda equina syndrome* for the sake of dealing with their *unrecognized childhood issues* and *poor diet*, you are more likely to find yourself out of a career than praised for your holistic approach, no matter how good your intentions. Even the best holistic physicians with the broadest perspectives and most comprehensive wellness-promoting goals must utilize effective micromanagement strategies for acute and life-threatening problems. Thus, with **recognition of the importance of** *simultaneous* **problem management** *and* **wellness promotion**, we begin this chapter that provides minimal and elemental building blocks for the restoration of health and the attainment of optimal wellness.

*Notes*:

# Re-Establishing the Foundation for Health

> "The work of the naturopathic physician is to elicit healing by helping patients to create or recreate conditions for health to exist within them.
> **Health will occur where the conditions for health exist.**
> **Disease is the product of conditions which allow for it."** *Jared Zeff, N.D.*[38]

One of the most important concepts within the philosophy and practice of naturopathic medicine is that of "re-establishing the foundation for health." This means that instead of first looking to a specific treatment or "magic bullet" to solve a health problem, we first look at the environment in which the problem arose to determine if the patient's environment has initiated or perpetuated the problem. The term *environment* as used here means much more than the patient's immediate surroundings at home and work; it is used as a term to include all modifiable factors that may have an effect on the patient's health, such as lifestyle, diet, exercise, supplementation, chronic and situational stress, exposure to toxicants and microbes, nutritionally-modifiable genetic factors[39], emotions, feelings, and unconscious assumptions[40], and many other considerations.

> "Virtually all human diseases result from the interaction of genetic susceptibility factors and modifiable environmental factors, broadly defined to include infectious, chemical, physical, nutritional, and behavioral factors." *Centers for Disease Control and Prevention*[41]

"Optimal health" does not *and never will* come in a pill or tonic—the human body and the interactions that we each have between our genes, outlooks, environments, and lifestyles are far too complex to ever be addressed wholly and completely by a simplistic paradigm or single treatment. Even a superficial observation of the complexity of human physiology and the complexity of our environments (including noise, toxins such as benzene from pollution, chemicals such as formaldehyde from building materials, work stress and multitasking, radiation exposure, microwaves) shows that **our modern lifestyles subject the human body to many more "stressors" than ever before in the history of human existence.** Each of these stressors depletes our psychic and physiologic reserves, such that daily replenishment and protection are necessary.

Research in nutrition and physiology is revealing the mechanisms by which "simple" lifestyle practices and dietary interventions exert their powerful benefits. For example, whole foods such as fruits and vegetables contain over 8,000 phytochemicals with different physiologic effects[42], and simple practices such as meditation and massage can significantly alter hormone and neurotransmitter levels.[43,44] On the surface, a simple practice such as consumption of fruits and

---

[38] Zeff JL. The process of healing: a unifying theory of naturopathic medicine. *Journal of Naturopathic Medicine* 1997; 7: 122-5
[39] Kaput J, Rodriguez LR. Nutritional genomics: the next frontier in the postgenomic era. *Physiol Genomics* 16: 166–177 http://physiolgenomics.physiology.org/cgi/content/full/16/2/166
[40] Miller A. The truth will set you free: overcoming emotional blindness and finding your true adult self. New York: Basic Books; 2001
[41] Gene-Environment Interaction Fact Sheet by the Centers for Disease Control and Prevention, August 2000
[42] "We propose that the additive and synergistic effects of phytochemicals in fruit and vegetables are responsible for their potent antioxidant and anticancer activities, and that the benefit of a diet rich in fruit and vegetables is attributed to the complex mixture of phytochemicals present in whole foods." Liu RH. Health benefits of fruit and vegetables are from additive and synergistic combinations of phytochemicals. *Am J Clin Nutr*. 2003 Sep;78(3 Suppl):517S-520S
[43] "The significant decrease of the catecholamine metabolite VMA (vanillic-mandelic acid) in meditators, that is associated with a reciprocal increase of 5-HIAA supports as a feedback necessity the "rest and fulfillment response" versus "fight and flight"." Bujatti M, Riederer P. Serotonin, noradrenaline, dopamine metabolites in transcendental meditation-technique. *J Neural Transm*. 1976;39(3):257-67

vegetables and a multivitamin/multimineral supplement may seem to be a way to provide merely "good nutrition"; however the clinical effects can include antidepressant[45] and anti-inflammatory benefits[46], by enhancing the efficiency of biochemical reactions[47] and by reducing excess activity of NF-kappaB[48], respectively. The power of interventional nutrition utilizing high-doses and/or synergistic formulations of nutraceuticals and phytonutraceuticals becomes much more clinically apparent when patients first (re)establish a healthy foundation of diet and lifestyle practices upon which these additive treatments can be added; I estimate that the effectiveness of treatments for complex illness such as inflammatory diseases and cancer is *at least* doubled when patients implement these lifestyle changes in addition to specific natural treatments rather than relying on natural treatments alone without a healthy supportive lifestyle. In other words, "*foundation for health* + natural treatments" is much more effective than "**un**healthy *lifestyle* + natural treatments." This explains, in part, the discrepancy between the relatively lackluster response seen in single intervention clinical trials* compared to the better results that we attain clinically when using a holistic approach characterized by multicomponent treatment plans. The biochemical and "scientific" reasons for this positive/negative synergism will become clear during the course of this chapter in particular and this textbook in general.

*Single intervention clinical trials (i.e., clinical trials that utilize only one treatment) are the "gold standard" in allopathic drug-based research because their goal is to quantify and qualify the nature of positive and negative responses. However, this approach loses much of its luster in clinical settings where neither patients nor lifestyles and treatment plans can be standardized due to the unique constitution, lifestyle, history, and treatment plan of each patient. Single intervention clinical trials have a place in the researching of all treatments, including natural interventions. However, clinicians—especially recent graduates—must pry themselves away from this research tool when it comes to treating individual patients in clinical practice, where **single interventions are the antithesis of holistic treatment**.

## *Daily Living*

Life occurs on a moment-to-moment and daily basis. Choices that we make in relationships, occupations, exercise, and diet have profound and powerful influence over the course of our lives—particularly our health and happiness. Despite the previous and ongoing obfuscation of health

> Realize that the choices that are made on a daily basis greatly influence whether or not we will be healthy in the future. Doctors and patients should choose a healthy diet, appropriate supplementation, healthy relationships, and physical activity rather than junk foods, toxic relationships, and physical inactivity.

---

[44] "By the end of the study, the massage therapy group, as compared to the relaxation group, reported experiencing less pain, depression, anxiety and improved sleep. They also showed improved trunk and pain flexion performance, and their serotonin and dopamine levels were higher." Hernandez-Reif M, Field T, Krasnegor J, Theakston H. Lower back pain is reduced and range of motion increased after massage therapy. *Int J Neurosci* 2001;106(3-4):131-45
[45] Benton D, Haller J, Fordy J. Vitamin supplementation for 1 year improves mood. *Neuropsychobiology*. 1995;32(2):98-105
[46] Church TS, Earnest CP, Wood KA, Kampert JB. Reduction of C-reactive protein levels through use of a multivitamin. *Am J Med*. 2003 Dec 15;115(9):702-7
[47] Ames BN, Elson-Schwab I, Silver EA. High-dose vitamin therapy stimulates variant enzymes with decreased coenzyme binding affinity (increased K(m)): relevance to genetic disease and polymorphisms. *Am J Clin Nutr*. 2002 Apr;75(4):616-58 http://www.ajcn.org/cgi/content/full/75/4/616
[48] **Vasquez A**. Reducing pain and inflammation naturally - part 4: nutritional and botanical inhibition of NF-kappaB, the major intracellular amplifier of the inflammatory cascade. A practical clinical strategy exemplifying anti-inflammatory nutrigenomics. *Nutritional Perspectives*, July 2005:5-12. www.OptimalHealthResearch.com/part4

information by allopathic groups[49,50,51,52,53] and the pharmaceutical industry[54,55], enough valid information and common sense is available to doctors and the public such that **ignorance is no longer a viable excuse for deferring responsibility for lifestyle-induced disease and misery**.[56] Eating too much sugar and fat while not eating enough fruits and vegetables is making a choice to have an increased probability of developing diabetes, cancer, heart disease, arthritis, and obesity. Exercising regularly, eating a healthy diet, and supplementing the diet with high-quality nutrients and botanicals is making the choice to greatly reduce your risk of health problems[57,58] and to nurture your life and your body so that you can make the most of your life experience and enjoy your life, your hobbies, life purpose(s), and time with friends and family.

When we were children, we looked to other people to provide for us and to "take care of us." **As adults, we have to assume responsibility for the course of our own lives, to make decisions based on long-term considerations rather than instant gratification and selective ignorance.** Of course, this does not mean that we have to abandon enjoyment; but it does mean that we can make decisions based on priorities, and if health is a priority then it follows that we should take steps to attain and maintain it. For people who have chosen to make their health a priority, sugar- and fat-laden food begins to lose its appeal, and exploring new adventures in healthy cooking becomes an activity that can be transformed into an art—one that is particularly amenable to building relationships and connections with other people. **The improved sense of wellbeing and improved physical and intellectual performance obtained from consumption of a health-promoting Paleo-Mediterranean diet (described later) supercedes any short-term gratification from the disease-promoting diet commonly referred to as the Standard American Diet (SAD).** When people want to be healthy, exercising and spending enjoyable time outdoors becomes more fun than the inactivity and passivity of watching television. When we consider that the average American watches 3-4 hours of television per day then it is no surprise that, with such inactive lifestyles, Americans show increasingly high rates of obesity, cancer, heart disease, and diabetes. Such an inactive lifestyle also affects our children: on average, each American child watches more than 23 hours of television per week[59]—a national habit that unquestionably contributes to the high levels of obesity and (social) illiteracy demonstrated by America's youth. Adults who watch average amounts of television are exposed to (indoctrinated by) more than 2.5 hours of direct-to-consumer drug advertisements each month—more than 30 hours of drug advertisements per year—far exceeding their exposure to other, potentially more authentic,

---

[49] Wolinsky H, Brune T. The Serpent on the Staff: The Unhealthy Politics of the American Medical Association. GP Putnam and Sons, New York, 1994
[50] Wilk CA. Medicine, Monopolies, and Malice: How the Medical Establishment Tried to Destroy Chiropractic. Garden City Park: Avery, 1996
[51] Carter JP. Racketeering in Medicine: The Suppression of Alternatives. Norfolk: Hampton Roads Pub; 1993
[52] National Alliance of Professional Psychology Providers. AMA Seeks To Control and Restrict Psychologist's Scope of Practice. http://www.nappp.org/scope.pdf Accessed November 25, 2006
[53] "In an effort to marshal the medical community's resources against the growing threat of expanding scope of practice for allied health professionals, the AMA has formed a national partnership to confront such initiatives nationwide… The committee will use $25,000..." Daly R, American Psychiatric Association. AMA Forms Coalition to Thwart Non-M.D. Practice Expansion. *Psychiatric News* 2006 March; 41: 17 http://pn.psychiatryonline.org/cgi/content/full/41/5/17-a?eaf Accessed November 25, 2006
[54] Angell M. The Truth About the Drug Companies: How They Deceive Us and What to Do About it. Random House; August 2004
[55] "**It begins on the first day of medical school… It starts slowly and insidiously, like an addiction, and can end up influencing the very nature of medical decision-making and practice… Attempts to influence the judgment of doctors by commercial interests serving the medical industrial complex are nothing if not thorough.**" Editorial. Drug-company influence on medical education in USA. *Lancet.* 2000 Sep 2;356(9232):781
[56] "Error is not blindness, error is cowardice. Every acquisition, every step forward in knowledge is the result of courage, of severity towards oneself, of cleanliness with respect to oneself." Nietzsche FW. Ecce Homo: How One Becomes What One Is. [Translator: Hollingdale RJ] Penguin Books:1979,34
[57] Orme-Johnson DW, Herron RE. An innovative approach to reducing medical care utilization and expenditures. *Am J Manag Care.* 1997;3(1):135-44
[58] **Vasquez A**. A Five-Part Nutritional Protocol that Produces Consistently Positive Results. *Nutritional Wellness* 2005Sept. http://nutritionalwellness.com/archives/2005/sep/09_vasquez.php and http://optimalhealthresearch.com/reprints/vasquez-nutritional-wellness-5-part-protocol-2005-sept.pdf
[59] "American children view over 23 hours of television per week. * Teenagers view an average of 21 to 22 hours of television per week. * By the time today's children reach age 70, they will have spent 7 to 10 years of their lives watching television." American Academy of Pediatrics http://www.aapca1.org/aapca1/tv.html accessed September 30, 2003

health-promoting information.[60] Not only does television siphon time and energy that could be used more productively, more socially, or more enjoyably, but at a cost of $540 to $900 per year ($45-75 per month), **cable television subtracts from the available resources (i.e., time, money, attention/focus) that could be directed toward health-promoting choices**. Cable television is only one of many examples of how everyday choices can have an impact on long-term health. **Encourage your patients to become mindful of their choices and the impact these choices have on long-term health and vitality.**

<u>Lifestyle habits</u>: Without the conscious decision that **health is a priority** and the realization that **optimal health has to be earned rather than taken for granted**, patients and doctors alike can fall into the belief that healthcare and health maintenance are *burdens* and *inconveniences* rather than opportunities for fulfillment and self-care. Taking an **empowered** and **pro-active** role in one's healthcare may include a coordinated program of diet changes (such as eating certain foods, while avoiding others), regular exercise, nutritional supplementation, stress reduction, and relationship improvement. Unhealthy habits such as eating junk foods, using tobacco, and watching too much television rob people of the time, energy, motivation, and financial resources that could otherwise be used to improve health and prevent unnecessary illness. As described later in this chapter, the choices that are made on a daily basis from this point forward are the most powerful predictors of future health and are generally more powerful than past habits or genetic inheritance. We can all greatly increase our probability of enjoying a future of high-energy health rather than painful illness by consistently choosing health-promoting options instead of foods, behaviors, and emotional states that promote illness.

While prevention of lung cancer and heart disease are important enough, smoking cessation has taken on new importance recently now that **the connection between tobacco smoking and the induction of autoimmunity—rheumatoid arthritis and systemic lupus erythematosus—is becoming increasingly well established**. Patients with any form of autoimmunity should not smoke tobacco and should minimize any exposure to second-hand smoke.[61]

*Notes*:

---

[60] "…many ads may be targeted specifically at women and older viewers. Our findings suggest that Americans who watch average amounts of television may be exposed to more than 30 hours of direct-to-consumer drug advertisements each year, far surpassing their exposure to other forms of health communication." Brownfield ED, Bernhardt JM, Phan JL, Williams MV, Parker RM. Direct-to-consumer drug advertisements on network television: an exploration of quantity, frequency, and placement. *J Health Commun*. 2004 Nov-Dec;9(6):491-7

[61] "Counseling against smoking should be mandatory in rheumatological practice both to patients and to their relatives. Studies on the mechanisms whereby smoking triggers rheumatoid arthritis and systemic lupus erythematosus may provide fundamental new knowledge about the cause and molecular pathogenesis of these diseases." Klareskog L, Padyukov L, Alfredsson L. Smoking as a trigger for inflammatory rheumatic diseases. *Curr Opin Rheumatol*. 2007 Jan;19(1):49-54

**One hour of time per day and/or about $2 - $8 per day:**

| Active self-care | Benefits | Distraction | Result |
|---|---|---|---|
| 1. Meditation<br>2. Yoga, stretching<br>3. Walking, jogging, biking, no-cost calisthenics<br>4. Martial arts, Tai Chi<br>5. Hot bath<br>6. Cooking new healthy meals<br>7. Herbal teas (especially green tea) provide anti-inflammatory, anticancer, and antioxidant benefits<br>8. Basic nutritional supplementation (less than $2 per day): 1) High-potency multivitamin and multimineral supplement, 2) Complete balanced, fatty acid supplementation, 3) 2,000 – 4,000 IU vitamin D per day for adults, 4) probiotics and/or synbiotics.<br><br>*At $2 per day for meditation, stretching, calisthenics, (etc.) and basic supplementation, the total comes to $730 per year.* | 1. Increased flexibility and joint mobility<br>2. Reduction in blood pressure<br>3. Reduced risk for cancer<br>4. Increased strength<br>5. Improved cognitive function<br>6. New and enjoyable meals<br>7. Relaxation<br>8. New life skills<br>9. Improved heart health<br>10. The opportunity to develop social skills and more friends and a better social support network<br>11. Reduced risk for Alzheimer's and Parkinson's diseases | 1. Cable television ($1.50 - $2.50 per day)<br>2. 1 pack of cigarettes per day ($3 per day)<br>3. Grande Café Latte ($3 per day)<br><br>*At $8 per day for cable television, designer coffee, and cigarettes, the total comes to approximately $3,000 per year.* | 1. Watching an hour of television may or may not contribute significantly to life and long-term goals. (Cable television costs between $600 and $800 per year.)<br>2. One pack of cigarettes per day at $2.88 per pack equals $1,051 per year for increased risk of cancer and heart disease.<br>3. Grande Café Latte at $3.05 per day costs $1,113 per year for 7-per-week and $793 per year for 5-per-week. |

## Wellness Promotion: Re-Establishing the Foundation for Health

**Motivation**: We all have a combination of reasons, feelings, inclinations, and unconscious influences that support and perpetuate our health behaviors[62,63]; getting in touch with those motivations can help us to better understand the healthy/functional (health-promoting) and unhealthy/dysfunctional (illness-promoting) aspects of our psyches. Uncovering and "upgrading" these motivations can help us and our patients to develop more authentic lives and improved health. Self-defeating behaviors, such as 1) a willingness to remain ignorant of factors which influence health, 2) a willingness to frequently consume disease-promoting processed and "fast foods", and 3) submission to confinement within the boundaries of one's insurance coverage (which often confines one to drugs and surgery as the only treatment options), reflect—*at best*—the willingness to settle for mediocrity and—*at worst*—an unconscious movement in the direction of illness and early death—masochism and suicide by lifestyle. Conversely, an unencumbered drive toward health will create the greatest opportunity for wellness. Since **actions originate from beliefs and goals**, we can surmise much about undisclosed beliefs and goals in others and ourselves simply by observing outward behavior. Effectively changing actions (such as diet and lifestyle choices) therefore must include not only behavior modification but also careful examination and reconsideration of largely unconscious goals and beliefs that motivate and underlie those behaviors. **When a fully empowered motivation toward health is matched with accurate informational insight, we have the *potential* for health-promoting change—*potential* which only becomes *manifest* after the habitual application of appropriate action.** Patients and doctors alike can benefit from considering the factors that incline them *toward* or *away* from behaviors that promote health or disease.

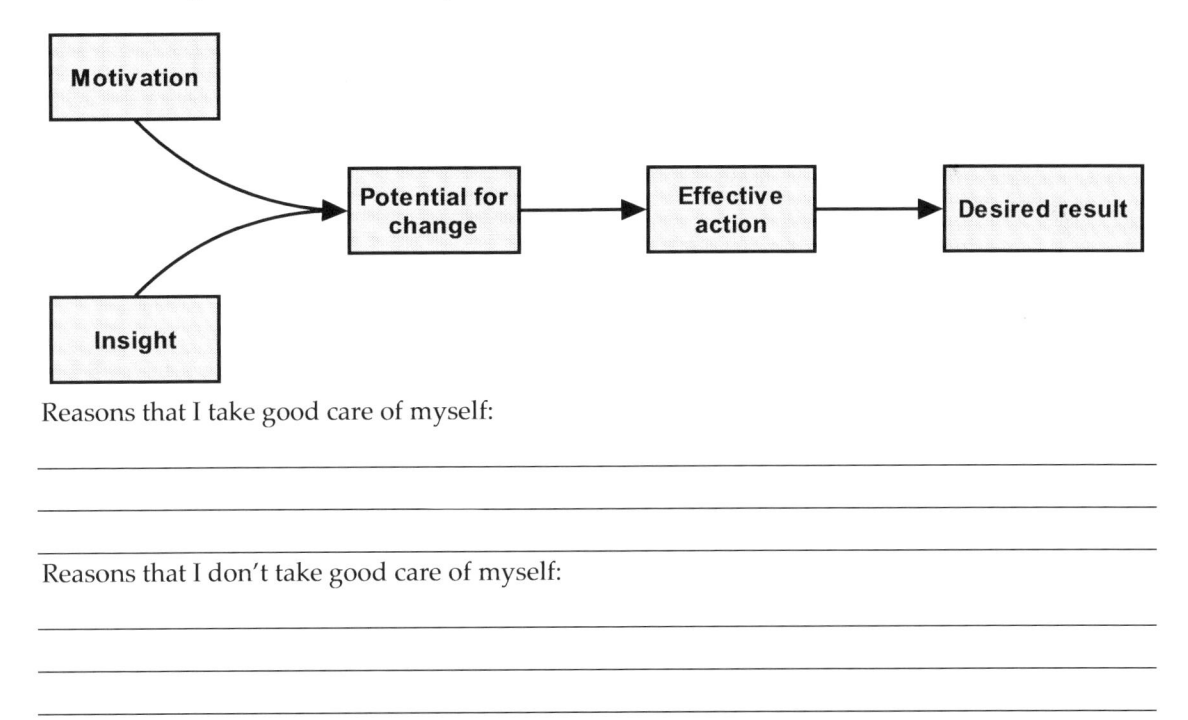

Motivation ⟶ ⎫
              ⎬ Potential for change → Effective action → Desired result
Insight    ⟶ ⎭

Reasons that I take good care of myself:
_____
_____

Reasons that I don't take good care of myself:
_____
_____
_____

---

[62] Bradshaw J. Healing the Shame that Binds You [Audio Cassette (April 1990) Health Communications Audio; ISBN: 1558740430]
[63] Miller A. The Drama of the Gifted Child: The Search for the True Self. Basic Books: 1981

**Motivation: moving from theory to practice**: Many recently-graduated doctors start with the erroneous assumption that all patients actually want to become healthier, and furthermore, that all the doctor has to do is "enlighten" them to the error of their ways and the patient will be dutifully compliant unto the attainment of his or her health-related goals. In reality, many people are indifferent about their health. Many people do not care if they are 30 lbs overweight or have hypertension or will die early as a result of their lifestyle; they often have to be encouraged to begin to *consider* making positive changes.

At our 2004 Functional Medicine Symposium, Dr. James Prochaska[64] elucidated the different stages of patient preparedness, and we note that each of these five levels of thought and action produces specific results and requires different types of support from the doctor. I have paraphrased, translated, and embellished Dr. Prochaska's lecture in the following table; for additional information and insights, obtain his lecture from the Institute for Functional Medicine or his book *Changing for Good*.[65]

**Level of preparedness and readiness for change**

| *Stage/level* | *Doctor's interventions and social support* |
|---|---|
| 1. **Pre-contemplation**: "I am not seriously thinking about making a change to be healthier." | <ul><li>Outreach</li><li>Retainment</li></ul> |
| 2. **Contemplation**: "I am thinking about making a change, but I am not ready for action." | <ul><li>Resolve resistance</li><li>Emphasize benefits</li><li>Address ambivalence</li></ul> |
| 3. **Preparation**: "I am getting ready to make a change, but I am not taking effective action yet." | <ul><li>Ensure adequate preparation</li><li>Prevent relapse following initial action</li></ul> |
| 4. **Action**: "I am beginning to make changes to become healthier." | <ul><li>Support (group support is best)</li><li>Encouragement</li><li>Reward system</li></ul> |
| 5. **Maintenance**: "I take action every day and on a consistent basis to reach my goals." | <ul><li>Continued provision for continuation of health changes: facilities, supplements, social support, affirmation</li></ul> |

Recognizing the different levels of patient preparedness and addressing individual patients with a customized approach not only for their *disease* but also for their *level of preparedness* for action can help doctors deliver more effective healthcare. Also, patients may have different levels of preparedness for different aspects of their treatment plans. He/she may be ready for **action** with regard to exercise, in **preparation** for dietary change, but in **precontemplation** for the use of supplements and botanicals.

---

[64] Prochaska JO. Changing for good: motivating diabetic patients. The Coming Storm: Reversing the Rising Pandemic of Diabetes and Metabolic Syndrome. The Eleventh International Symposium on Functional Medicine. May 13-15, 2004 in Vancouver, British Columbia, Canada. Pages 173-180. Presented by the Institute for Functional Medicine in Gig Harbor, Washington. www.FunctionalMedicine.org
[65] Prochaska, JO, Norcross, JC, and DiClemente, CC (1994). Changing for Good: A Revolutionary Six-Stage Program for Overcoming Bad Habits and Moving Your Life Positively Forward. NY, William Morrow and Company; 1994

Here is the secret to being exceptionally healthy: *You have to live in an exceptional way*. We cannot expect to achieve the goal of being vibrantly healthy or exceptionally happy if we live in the same way as everyone else, particularly when our fellow citizens are likely to be overweight, depressed, unhealthy, taking multiple pharmaceutical medications[66], and experiencing a state of progressively declining health.[67] *Healthy lifestyle* not only includes the basics of adequate sleep, healthy whole-foods diet, supportive relationships, and regular exercise, but it also includes preventive medicine and pro-active healthcare. **Despite the fact that we as a nation spend more on medical treatments than any other country in the world, Americans have the worst health outcomes of all the major industrialized countries.**[68,69,70] This is largely because *American medicine* is centered on a *disease-oriented model of medicine* which means that instead of having a healthcare system and social structure that proactively promotes health and prevents disease before it happens, our systems are *reactive*—treating disease *after* it occurs rather than emphasizing the prevention of disease *before* it occurs. It is also reductionistic: focusing on the small problem (micromanagement) rather than the big picture (macromanagement). The problem is compounded by the use of expensive pharmaceutical drugs which carry high rates of inefficacy (50-70%[71]) and which can exacerbate the diseases they are designed to treat or which result in adverse health effects that outweigh the purported benefits.[72,73,74,75,76,77,,78,79,80,81,82,83,84,85,86] **Every**

> **Americans have poor health outcomes compared to citizens of other industrialized nations**
>
> "Basically, you die earlier and spend more time disabled if you're an American rather than a member of most other advanced countries."
>
> Christopher Murray MD PhD, Director of World Health Organization's Global Program on Evidence for Health Policy. Press release on June 4, 2000.
> http://www.who.int/inf-pr-2000/en/pr2000-life.html

---

[66] "According to the latest available data, total health care costs reached $1.3 trillion in 2000. This represents a per capita health care expenditure of $4,637. The total prescription drug expenditure in 2000 was $121.8 billion, or approximately $430 per person." Presentation to the U.S. Senate Commerce Committee April 23, 2002 "Drug Pricing & Consumer Costs" Kathleen D. Jaeger, R.Ph., J.D. http://commerce.senate.gov/hearings/042302jaegar.pdf

[67] Zack MM, Moriarty DG, Stroup DF, Ford ES, Mokdad AH. Worsening trends in adult health-related quality of life and self-rated health-United States, 1993-2001. *Public Health Rep*. 2004 Sep-Oct;119(5):493-505 http://www.pubmedcentral.nih.gov/articlerender.fcgi?tool=pubmed&pubmedid=15313113

[68] "[America] also has the fewest hospital days per capita, the highest hospital expenditures per day, and substantially higher physician incomes than the other OECD countries. On the available outcome measures, the United States is generally in the bottom half, and its relative ranking has been declining since 1960." Anderson GF, Poullier JP. Health spending, access, and outcomes: trends in industrialized countries. *Health Aff* (Millwood) 1999 May-Jun;18(3):178-92 http://content.healthaffairs.org/cgi/reprint/18/3/178.pdf

[69] "However, on outcomes indicators such as life expectancy and infant mortality, the United States is frequently in the bottom quartile among the twenty-nine industrialized countries, and its relative ranking has been declining since 1960." Anderson GF. In search of value: an international comparison of cost, access, and outcomes. *Health Aff* 1997 Nov-Dec;16(6):163-71

[70] "Basically, you die earlier and spend more time disabled if you're an American rather than a member of most other advanced countries," says Christopher Murray, MD, PhD, Director of WHO's Global Program on Evidence for Health Policy. http://www.who.int/inf-pr-2000/en/pr2000-life.html

[71] "The vast majority of drugs - more than 90 percent - only work in 30 or 50 percent of the people." Allen Roses, M.D., worldwide vice-president of genetics at GlaxoSmithKline. http://commondreams.org/headlines03/1208-02.htm

[72] Whitaker R. **The case against antipsychotic drugs: a 50-year record of doing more harm than good**. *Med Hypotheses*. 2004;62(1):5-13

[73] Titier K, Canal M, Deridet E, Abouelfath A, Gromb S, Molimard M, Moore N. Determination of myocardium to plasma concentration ratios of five antipsychotic drugs: comparison with their ability to induce arrhythmia and sudden death in clinical practice. *Toxicol Appl Pharmacol*. 2004;199(1):52-60

[74] Ray WA, Meredith S, Thapa PB, Meador KG, Hall K, Murray KT. **Antipsychotics and the risk of sudden cardiac death**. *Arch Gen Psychiatry*. 2001;58(12):1161-7

[75] Straus SM, Bleumink GS, Dieleman JP, van der Lei J, 't Jong GW, Kingma JH, Sturkenboom MC, Stricker BH. **Antipsychotics and the risk of sudden cardiac death**. *Arch Intern Med*. 2004 Jun 28;164(12):1293-7

[76] Ray WA, Meredith S, Thapa PB, Hall K, Murray KT. **Cyclic antidepressants and the risk of sudden cardiac death**. *Clin Pharmacol Ther*. 2004;75(3):234-41

[77] Relling MV, Rubnitz JE, Rivera GK, Boyett JM, Hancock ML, Felix CA, Kun LE, Walter AW, Evans WE, Pui CH. High incidence of secondary brain tumours after radiotherapy and antimetabolites. *Lancet*. 1999 Jul 3;354(9172):34-9

[78] "The leukemia risk associated with partial-body radiotherapy for uterine corpus cancer was small; about 14 excess leukemia cases were due to radiation per 10,000 women followed for 10 years." Curtis RE, Boice JD Jr, Stovall M, Bernstein L, Holowaty E, Karjalainen S, Langmark F, Nasca PC, Schwartz AG, Schymura MJ, et al. Relationship of leukemia risk to radiation dose following cancer of the uterine corpus. *J Natl Cancer Inst*. 1994 Sep 7;86(17):1315-24

year "medication errors" kill over 7,000 people in America[87], and at least 180,000 Americans (493 patients per day) die due to "hospital errors."[88] Drug-related morbidity and mortality cost America more than $136 billion a year.[89]

Examples of allopathic iatrogenesis abound, and some of the more notable problems will be cited here:

- Many non-steroidal anti-inflammatory drugs for arthritis may actually exacerbate joint destruction.[90,91,92]
- A recent study evaluating arthroscopic knee surgery found it to be no more effective than placebo[93], yet it continues to be used "on at least 225,000 middle-age and older Americans each year at a cost of more than a billion dollars to Medicare, the Department of Veterans Affairs and private insurers."[94]
- The so-called "safer" new COX-2 inhibitors, which cost seven times the price of other analgesics with no improvement in efficacy over older medications[95], increase the risk for heart attack, stroke, other cardiovascular events including sudden unexplained death[96], and hypertension.[97]

---

[79] "Platinum-based treatment of ovarian cancer increases the risk of secondary leukemia." Travis LB, Holowaty EJ, Bergfeldt K, Lynch CF, Kohler BA, Wiklund T, Curtis RE, Hall P, Andersson M, Pukkala E, Sturgeon J, Stovall M. Risk of leukemia after platinum-based chemotherapy for ovarian cancer. *N Engl J Med*. 1999 Feb 4;340(5):351-7

[80] Zhang F, Chen Y, Pisha E, Shen L, Xiong Y, van Breemen RB, Bolton JL. **The major metabolite of equilin, 4-hydroxyequilin, autoxidizes to an o-quinone which isomerizes to the potent cytotoxin 4-hydroxyequilenin-o-quinone.** *Chem Res Toxicol*. 1999 Feb;12(2):204-13

[81] Pisha E, Lui X, Constantinou AI, Bolton JL. **Evidence that a metabolite of equine estrogens, 4-hydroxyequilenin, induces cellular transformation in vitro**. *Chem Res Toxicol*. 2001;14(1):82-90

[82] Zhang F, Swanson SM, van Breemen RB, Liu X, Yang Y, Gu C, Bolton JL. Equine estrogen metabolite 4-hydroxyequilenin induces DNA damage in the rat mammary tissues: formation of single-strand breaks, apurinic sites, stable adducts, and oxidized bases. *Chem Res Toxicol*. 2001;14(12):1654-9

[83] "At...concentrations comparable to those... in the synovial fluid of patients treated with the drug, several NSAIDs suppress proteoglycan synthesis... These NSAID-related effects on chondrocyte metabolism ... are much more profound in osteoarthritic cartilage than in normal cartilage, due to enhanced uptake of NSAIDs by the osteoarthritic cartilage." Brandt KD. Effects of nonsteroidal anti-inflammatory drugs on chondrocyte metabolism in vitro and in vivo. *Am J Med*. 1987 Nov 20; 83(5A): 29-34

[84] "The case of a young healthy man, who developed avascular necrosis of head of femur after prolonged administration of indomethacin, is reported here." Prathapkumar KR, Smith I, Attara GA. Indomethacin induced avascular necrosis of head of femur. *Postgrad Med J*. 2000 Sep; 76(899): 574-5

[85] "This highly significant association between **NSAID use and acetabular destruction** gives cause for concern, not least because of the difficulty in achieving satisfactory hip replacements in patients with severely damaged acetabula." Newman NM, Ling RS. Acetabular bone destruction related to non-steroidal anti-inflammatory drugs. *Lancet*. 1985 Jul 6; 2(8445): 11-4

[86] Vidal y Plana RR, Bizzarri D, Rovati AL. Articular cartilage pharmacology: I. In vitro studies on glucosamine and non steroidal antiinflammatory drugs. *Pharmacol Res Commun*. 1978 Jun;10(6):557-69

[87] "In 1983, 2876 people died from medication errors. ... By 1993, this number had risen to 7,391 - a 2.57-fold increase." Phillips DP, Christenfeld N, Glynn LM. Increase in US medication-error deaths between 1983 and 1993. *Lancet*. 1998 Feb 28;351(9103):643-4

[88] "Recent estimates suggest that each year more than 1 million patients are injured while in the hospital and approximately 180,000 die because of these injuries. Furthermore, drug-related morbidity and mortality are common and are estimated to cost more than $136 billion a year." Holland EG, Degruy FV. Drug-induced disorders. *Am Fam Physician*. 1997;56:1781-8, 1791-2

[89] "Recent estimates suggest that each year more than 1 million patients are injured while in the hospital and approximately 180,000 die because of these injuries. Furthermore, drug-related morbidity and mortality are common and are estimated to cost more than $136 billion a year." Holland EG, Degruy FV. Drug-induced disorders. *Am Fam Physician*. 1997;56:1781-8, 1791-2

[90] Dingle JT. The effects of NSAID on the matrix of human articular cartilages. *Z Rheumatol* 1999 Jun;58(3):125-9

[91] Hugenberg ST, Brandt KD, Cole CA. Effect of sodium salicylate, aspirin, and ibuprofen on enzymes required by the chondrocyte for synthesis of chondroitin sulfate. *J Rheumatol* 1993 Dec;20(12):2128-33

[92] Fujii K, et al. Effects of nonsteroidal antiinflammatory drugs on collagen biosynthesis of cultured chondrocytes. *Semin Arthritis Rheum* 1989;18(3 Suppl 1):16-8

[93] Moseley JB, O'Malley K, Petersen NJ, Menke TJ, Brody BA, Kuykendall DH, Hollingsworth JC, Ashton CM, Wray NP. A controlled trial of arthroscopic surgery for osteoarthritis of the knee. *N Engl J Med* 2002 Jul 11;347(2):81-8

[94] Gina Kolata. A Knee Surgery for Arthritis Is Called Sham. *The New York Times*, July 11, 2002

[95] "In these trials rofecoxib 12.5-25 mg/day was no more effective than the comparators (ibuprofen or diclofenac) used at maximal recommended doses." Rofecoxib: new preparation. A disappointing NSAID analgesic. *Prescrire Int* 2000 Dec;9(50):166-7, 169

[96] "The results from VIGOR showed that the relative risk of developing a confirmed adjudicated thrombotic cardiovascular event (myocardial infarction, unstable angina, cardiac thrombus, resuscitated cardiac arrest, sudden or unexplained death, ischemic stroke, and transient ischemic attacks) with rofecoxib treatment compared with naproxen was 2.38." Mukherjee D, Nissen SE, Topol EJ. Risk of cardiovascular events associated with selective COX-2 inhibitors. *JAMA* 2001; 286(8):954-9

[97] "Systolic blood pressure increased significantly in 17% of rofecoxib- compared with 11% of celecoxib-treated patients (P = 0.032) at any study time point." Whelton A, Fort JG, Puma JA, Normandin D, Bello AE, Verburg KM; SUCCESS VI Study Group.Cyclooxygenase-2--specific inhibitors and cardiorenal function: a randomized, controlled trial of celecoxib and rofecoxib in older hypertensive osteoarthritis patients. *Am J Ther* 2001 Mar-Apr;8(2):85-95

- Several antidepressant drugs *increase* the risk of suicide in children[98] as well as adults.[99]
- Long-term use of so-called antipsychotic medications is clinically unsatisfying[100] and may worsen long-term outcomes in a large percentage of patients.[101]
- Although adenoidectomy for the treatment of recurrent ear infections in children is no more effective than placebo[102], it is routinely performed at a cost of approximately $4,000 per procedure.[103] Naturopathic treatment is safer, more effective, and more cost-effective.[104]
- As a final example, some authors have argued that reliance upon mammography (e.g., diagnostic radiation) as a "cancer preventive" may be inefficacious and possibly unsafe[105,106] especially when emphasis on mammography supersedes emphasis on a cancer-preventing diet and lifestyle.[107]

> "The vast majority of drugs - more than 90 percent - only work in 30 or 50 percent of the people."
>
> Allen Roses, M.D., worldwide vice-president of genetics at GlaxoSmithKline
> http://commondreams.org/headlines03/1208-02.htm

Clearly, the most effective method for avoiding expensive and potentially dangerous medical procedures and drug treatments is for us as a nation and as individuals to shift our thinking from a *disease treatment* model of healthcare to a more logical program of aggressive *disease prevention* and *wellness promotion* via the use of safe natural treatments rather than heroic interventions.[108,109] Of course, this means that our concept and view of health and healthcare will have to change. As noted by Shi[110], "**Redesigning the system of health care delivery in the United States may be the only viable option to improve the quality of health care**." In the meantime, while we work for change on a national level, we are wise to change our personal habits and healthcare choices in favor of natural and preventive healthcare.

---

[98] "In addition, the pooled results showed that suicidal thoughts, suicide attempts and episodes of self-harm were more frequent among the paroxetine users (5.3% of 378 children) than among those in the placebo group (2.8% of 285 children)." Wooltorton E. Paroxetine (Paxil, Seroxat): increased risk of suicide in pediatric patients. *CMAJ*. 2003 Sep 2;169(5):446 http://www.cmaj.ca/cgi/content/full/169/5/446 on July 4, 2004

[99] "Similarly for fatal suicide, the RR among patients who were first prescribed an antidepressant within 1 to 9 days before their index date was 38.0... **The risk of suicidal behavior is increased in the first month after starting antidepressants**, especially during the first 1 to 9 days." Jick H, Kaye JA, Jick SS. Antidepressants and the risk of suicidal behaviors. *JAMA*. 2004 Jul 21;292(3):338-43

[100] "CONCLUSIONS: The majority of patients in each group discontinued their assigned treatment owing to inefficacy or intolerable side effects or for other reasons." Lieberman JA, Stroup TS, McEvoy JP, Swartz MS, Rosenheck RA, Perkins DO, Keefe RS, Davis SM, Davis CE, Lebowitz BD, Severe J, Hsiao JK; Clinical Antipsychotic Trials of Intervention Effectiveness (CATIE) Investigators. Effectiveness of antipsychotic drugs in patients with chronic schizophrenia. *N Engl J Med*. 2005 Sep 22;353(12):1209-23. Epub 2005 Sep 19

[101] "...standard of care in developed countries is to maintain schizophrenia patients on neuroleptics, this practice is not supported by the 50-year research record for the drugs. ...this paradigm of care worsens long-term outcomes, ... 40% of all schizophrenia patients would fare better if they were not so medicated." Whitaker R. The case against antipsychotic drugs: a 50-year study of doing more harm than good. *Med Hypotheses*. 2004;62(1):5-1

[102] "Adenoidectomy, as the first surgical treatment of children aged 10 to 24 months with recurrent acute otitis media, is not effective in preventing further episodes. It cannot be recommended as the primary method of prophylaxis." Koivunen P, Uhari M, Luotonen J, Kristo A, Raski R, Pokka T, Alho OP. Adenoidectomy versus chemoprophylaxis and placebo for recurrent acute otitis media in children aged under 2 years: randomised controlled trial. *BMJ*. 2004 Feb 28;328(7438):487

[103] See cost estimations at http://www.healthcentral.com/peds/top/003011.cfm#Cost: July 4, 2004

[104] Sarrell EM, Cohen HA, Kahan E. Naturopathic treatment for ear pain in children. *Pediatrics*. 2003 May;111(5 Pt 1):e574-9

[105] "INTERPRETATION: Screening for breast cancer with mammography is unjustified. If the Swedish trials are judged to be unbiased, the data show that for every 1000 women screened biennially throughout 12 years, one breast-cancer death is avoided whereas the total number of deaths is increased by six." Gotzsche PC, Olsen O. Is screening for breast cancer with mammography justifiable? *Lancet*. 2000 Jan 8;355(9198):129-34

[106] "...no large study has shown the effectiveness of breast cancer screening by either CBE or mammography for women whose risk of breast cancer is higher than the general population." *Patient Care Archive* January 15, 1998

[107] Sellman S. Breast cancer awareness: seeing deception is your only protection. *Alternative Medicine* November 2001, pages 68-74 See also: "...mammography improves early cancer detection and survival in post-menopausal women, no such benefit is demonstrable for younger women." "Mammograms increase the risk for developing breast cancer and raise the risk of spreading or metastasizing an existing growth," says Dr. Charles Simone, former clinical associate in immunology and pharmacology at NCI. Sellman S. Seeing Deception is your Only Protection: The Breast Cancer Awareness Month Story. Available at http://www.mercola.com/2000/oct/29/breast_cancer_awareness.htm on July 4, 2004

[108] "Systematic access to managed chiropractic care not only may prove to be clinically beneficial but also may reduce overall health care costs." Legorreta A, Metz D, Nelson C, Ray S, Chernicoff H, DiNubile N. Comparative Analysis of Individuals With and Without Chiropractic Coverage. *Archives of Internal Medicine* 2004; 164: 1985-1992

[109] Orme-Johnson DW, Herron RE. An innovative approach to reducing medical care utilization and expenditures. *Am J Manag Care*. 1997;3(1):135-44

[110] Shi L. Health care spending, delivery, and outcome in developed countries: a cross-national comparison. *Am J Med Qual* 1997;12(2):83-93

**Recognize and affirm that you are a unique individual with unique needs**: Your "personality" extends far beyond and far deeper than your sense of humor and your choice of clothing; you are also very unique on a physiologic and biochemical level as well. So-called *normal* and *apparently healthy* individuals vary greatly in their biochemical efficiency and nutritional needs. This is the concept of "biochemical individuality" which was first detailed in 1956 by the renowned scientist Roger J Williams from the University of Texas. In his historic work, Dr. Williams[111] reviews research that conclusively proves that among *apparently healthy* individuals, we can objectively determine great differences in physiology, organ efficiency, enzyme function, and nutritional needs. For example, variables that promote health include increased enzyme efficiency and efficient digestion and assimilation of nutrients, while internal factors that reduce health can include inadequate digestion, inefficient absorption, increased excretion of nutrients, impaired detoxification, nutritional deficiencies, poor enzyme function and "partial genetic blocks"—a term now understood to imply single nucleotide polymorphisms[112] and related enzyme defects, which result in **supradietary requirements for specific vitamins and minerals** for the prevention of disease and maintenance of health.[113] What this means for us as doctors and for our patients in practical terms is that in order for us to become as healthy as possible, we will almost certainly have to give attention to each person's unique abilities/disabilities in order to maximize the function of the various body systems and to optimize genetic expression.[114] This means that what works for your neighbor, spouse, or best friend in terms of exercise, diet and nutrition may not work for your unique physiology. Have the courage to affirm that, in order for you to attain your goal of better health, you will have to learn about how your body works and will have to learn to make changes in your lifestyle and daily routine which reflect and honor your body's way of working. This may mean modifying work, sleep, and exercise schedules, avoiding some foods and eating others, and customizing nutrient intake to meet the body's needs as they are *in the present*. The process of learning how a person's body works requires time, patience, and the process of trial and error—from patient and doctor—but achieving the goal of improved health and increased energy are well worth the effort.

*Notes*:

---

[111] Williams RJ. Biochemical Individuality : The Basis for the Genetotrophic Concept. Austin and London: University of Texas Press, 1956
[112] Ames BN. Cancer prevention and diet: help from single nucleotide polymorphisms. *Proc Natl Acad Sci U S A*. 1999 Oct 26;96(22):12216-8
[113] Ames BN, Elson-Schwab I, Silver EA. High-dose vitamin therapy stimulates variant enzymes with decreased coenzyme binding affinity (increased K(m)): relevance to genetic disease and polymorphisms. *Am J Clin Nutr*. 2002 Apr;75(4):616-58 http://www.ajcn.org/cgi/content/full/75/4/616
[114] "The combination of biochemical individuality and known functional utilities of allelic variants should converge to create a situation in which nutritional optima can be specified as part of comprehensive lifestyle prescriptions tailored to the needs of each person." Eckhardt RB. Genetic research and nutritional individuality. *J Nutr* 2001;131(2):336S-9S

**Individuation and the practice of conscious living**: Our visions of reality are influenced by religious institutions, large corporations, advertising networks[115], corporate-owned mass media[116], and what Professors Stevens and Glatstein called **"the medical-industrial complex."**[117] Some of the paradigms that are advocated are both *unhistorical* (having no historical precedent) and *antihistorical* (contrary to the available historical precedent, which includes sustainability). Some of these companies and organizations offer us a view of reality and vision of our individual potentials that is fashioned in such a way as to promote the financial and political interests of the company or organization. Conversely, the actualization of our true physical, emotional, intellectual, and spiritual potentials may require that we separate from or at least attain a conscious appreciation of the (pseudo)reality that we have been advised to follow.[118,119] Critiques of and reasonable alternatives to our current paradigms of school[120], work[121], and money[122] have been discussed elsewhere and are worthy of consideration. Becoming mindful of the paradigms and assumptions under which we live is the first step in true individuation, characterized by choosing (creating the best option: freedom) rather than deciding (selecting one of the offered options: the illusion of freedom). Different "layers of illusions" create our "working reality" which represents the way that we see things and the paradigm by which we *act in* and *interact with* the larger world. These layers come from our own families, schools, teachers, churches, companies, friends, parents, and ourselves—our previous interpretations and misinterpretations of ourselves and events. Becoming conscious of these illusions allows us the opportunity to discard those views that are inaccurate, dysfunctional, and harmful and to accept a truer reality based on what we experience, feel, and know to be real. Once we are freed from *unreality*, we can live true to ourselves in a way that is authentically responsible to our own needs *and* the needs of our communities so that we can simultaneously sustain our obligations to society[123,124] while being free to be unique individuals.[125]

*Notes*:

_____

_____

_____

_____

---

[115] "Patients' requests for medicines are a powerful driver of prescribing decisions. In most cases physicians prescribed requested medicines but were often ambivalent about the choice of treatment. If physicians prescribe requested drugs despite personal reservations, sales may increase but appropriateness of prescribing may suffer." Mintzes B, Barer ML, Kravitz RL, Kazanjian A, Bassett K, Lexchin J, Evans RG, Pan R, Marion SA. Influence of direct to consumer pharmaceutical advertising and patients' requests on prescribing decisions: two site cross sectional survey. *BMJ*. 2002 Feb 2; 324(7332): 278-9

[116] Manufacturing Consent: Noam Chomsky and the Media. Movie directed by Mark Achbar and Peter Wintonick. 1992. See www.imdb.com/title/tt0104810/and www.zeitgeistfilms.com

[117] "...despite lush advertisements from companies with obvious vested interests, and authoritative testimonials from biased investigators who presumably believe in their own work to the point of straining credulity and denying common sense... (translate: economic improvement, not biological superiority)." Stevens CW, Glatstein E. Beware the Medical-Industrial Complex. *Oncologist* 1996;1(4):IV-V http://theoncologist.alphamedpress.org/cgi/reprint/1/4/190-iv.pdf on July 4, 2004

[118] Breton D, Largent C. The Paradigm Conspiracy: Why Our Social Systems Violate Human Potential-And How We Can Change Them. Center City; Hazelden: 1996

[119] Pearce JC. Exploring the Crack in the Cosmic Egg: Split Minds and Meta-Realities. New York: Washington Square Press; 1974

[120] Gatto JT. Dumbing us down: the hidden curriculum of compulsory education. Gabriola Island, Canada; New Society Publishers: 2005

[121] "No one should ever work. In order to stop suffering, we have to stop working. That doesn't mean we have to stop doing things. It does mean creating a new way of life based on play..." Black B. The abolition of work and other essays. Port Townsend: Loompanics Unlimited; 1985, pages 17-33

[122] Dominguez JR. Transforming Your Relationship With Money. Sounds True; Book and Cassette edition: 2001 Audio tape.

[123] Bly R. The Sibling Society. Vintage Books USA; Reprint edition (June 1, 1997) ISBN: 0679781285 (Abridged audio edition (May 1, 1996), ASIN: 0679451609)

[124] Bly R. Where have all the parents gone? A talk on the Sibling Society. New York: Sound Horizons, 1996 Highly recommended.

[125] Rick Jarow. Creating the Work You Love: Courage, Commitment and Career; Inner Traditions Intl Ltd; 1995 [ISBN: 0892815426]

## Examples of commonly accepted paradigms and their reasonable alternatives

| Commonly advocated/accepted paradigms<br>↳ Implication and effect | Alternate paradigm<br>↳ Implication and effect |
|---|---|
| **It is OK to be irresponsible in daily choices and then blame health problems on bad luck, bad genes, or both.**<br>↳ Many people fail to take responsibility for their lives and thereby become victims of circumstances—negative circumstances that they themselves helped to create. | **Lifestyle, especially diet and nutrition, is the most powerful influence on health outcomes. Therefore, an educated patient is empowered to direct his/her health destiny.**<br>↳ Optimal health *per individual* is attained when people take responsibility for their lives, seek health information, and then incorporate this information into their daily lives in the form of healthy living: healthy lifestyle, healthy eating, healthy exercise, healthy supplementation, healthy relationships, and healthy occupational and social activities, including socio-political involvement to protect the environment and resist the privatization of life and the spoliation of the environment in which we live and upon which our lives and health depend.[126,127] |
| **In general, chemical medications are the answer to nearly all health problems.**<br>↳ The belief in medications as the primary treatment of disease creates a patient population that is apathetic, disempowered, and dependent upon the medical-pharmaceutical industry, which grows richer and more powerful despite so-called 'earnest' attempts at cost containment.[128] | **Many acute and chronic problems can be more effectively managed in terms of prevention, safety, efficacy, and cost-effectiveness when phytonutritional interventions are either used as primary therapy or, when necessary, used in conjunction with medications.**<br>↳ A reduction in disease prevalence via health-promoting diet and lifestyle along with integrative treatments offers the best opportunity for benefit to patients, doctors, and third-party payers.[129] |

---

[126] "**Your lack of interest in the past, your lack of involvement, your unwillingness to develop coherent strategies, your unwillingness to challenge authority - these have created a vacuum in decision-making, that has been filled by professional groups with close relationships with the chemical industries...**" Samuel Epstein MD, 1993. Professor of Occupational and Environmental Medicine at the School of Public Health, University of Illinois Medical Center Chicago. http://www.converge.org.nz/pirm/pestican.htm accessed September 11, 2004

[127] Kristin S. Schafer, Margaret Reeves, Skip Spitzer, Susan E. Kegley. Chemical Trespass: Pesticides in Our Bodies and Corporate Accountability. Pesticide Action Network North America. May 2004 Available at http://www.panna.org/campaigns/docsTrespass/chemicalTrespass2004.dv.html on August 1, 2004

[128] "In this paper I offer four hypotheses to help explain why use of pharmaceuticals has continued to grow even as managed care and other cost containment efforts have flourished." Berndt ER. The U.S. pharmaceutical industry: why major growth in times of cost containment? *Health Aff* (Millwood). 2001 Mar-Apr;20(2):100-14

[129] "Hospital admission rates in the control group were 11.4 times higher than those in the MVAH group for cardiovascular disease, 3.3 times higher for cancer, and 6.7 times higher for mental health and substance abuse. …MVAH patients older than age 45…had 88% fewer total patients days compared with control patients." Orme-Johnson DW, Herron RE. An innovative approach to reducing medical care utilization and expenditures. *Am J Manag Care*. 1997 Jan;3(1):135-44

## Examples of commonly accepted paradigms and their reasonable alternatives—*continued*

| *Commonly advocated/accepted paradigms*<br>↪ *Implication and effect* | *Alternate paradigm*<br>↪ *Implication and effect* |
|---|---|
| **Work ethic: a belief that "hard work" has moral value and makes a person "better."**<br>↪ Belief in the principle of "work ethic" encourages people to mindlessly engage in work for the sake of engaging in work without considering the implications of their actions or other alternatives that might produce a more beneficial outcome.[130] | **Work is the means rather than an end unto itself (except when the "work" is enjoyable, in which case it is no longer "work").**<br>↪ Occupations and professions can be designed for the enhancement of life (health, pleasure, relationships, the environment, care of the poor) rather than as an end to themselves at the expense of the individual, society, and the environment. |
| **It is "normal" for adults to give 10.5-12 hours per day 5 days per week to work.**<br>↪ In most corporate environments, employee's work at least 8.5 hours per day, with 1 additional hour spent in commuting[131] and another hour spent in preparation, transportation, and maintenance of work-related clothing, preparing work-related meals, maintaining the auto that is used for work-related tasks. With 10.5 hours given directly to work, 0.5-1 additional hours are needed for recuperation from work-related stress ("daily decompression"); thus the average amount of time given to work-related activities is much larger than commonly believed.[132] Because of the time and energies devoted to "work" the vast majority of people feel that they do not have sufficient time for themselves, their families and friends, their creativity, learning about the world, political involvement, and other more important aspects of life. "Not enough time" is the most common reason given by patients for not exercising. | **A paradigm of a 4-day workweek is just as valid and perhaps more so than one that advocates a 5-day workweek. A paradigm of a 6-hour workday is at least as valid as one of an 8-10 hour workday.**<br>↪ Many people in our culture are chronically overworked, undernourished, tired and suffer from an insufficiency of time to simply be in community, to rest, to be creative. It is no surprise that they then behave addictively (e.g., drugs, alcohol) and destructively (e.g., over-eating, alcohol, sugar, fat)—their behaviors are simply frustrated and maladaptive coping strategies to combat the stress caused by a damaging, unnatural paradigm from which they cannot escape.[133] Redesigning our societal structures and expectations in ways that conform to our natural humanity and biologic, nutritional, and emotional needs is more rational than forcing *en masse* all of humanity to contort and conform to an artificial posture and cadence of performance, productivity, professionalism, and other unnatural expectations. Less time dedicated to "work" and all that it entails leaves more time for 1) healthy cooking, 2) relaxed, conscious, and enjoyable eating, 3) exercise, 4) creativity and hobbies, 5) keeping informed of and involved with political change, and 6) participation in social relationships.[134] |

---

[130] "Conventional wisdom is the habitual, the unexamined life, absorbed into the culture and the fashion of the time, lost in the mad rush of accumulation, lulled to sleep by the easy lies of political hacks and newspaper scribblers, or by priests who wouldn't know a god if they met one." Nisker W. Crazy Wisdom. Berkeley; Ten Speed Press: 1990, page 7

[131] Monday, September 8, 2003 -- The average daily one-way commute to work in the United States takes just over 26 minutes, according to the Bureau of Transportation Statistics' Omnibus Household Survey. Omnibus Household Survey Shows Americans' Average Commuting Time is Just Over 26 Minutes. http://www.bts.gov/press_releases/2003/bts020_03/html/bts020_03.html on August 3, 2004

**Quality and quantity of sleep**: Anything less than 8 hours of solid sleep each and every night is insufficient for the vast majority of people, and many people feel their best with 9 hours of sleep. Not only is it important to get a sufficient *quantity* of sleep, but we need to ensure that the *quality* of the sleep receives appropriate attention, as well. Sleep should be mostly continuous, not "broken" or interrupted for extended periods of time. Some experts believe that people should be able to recall their dreams at night, as this may be a sign of proper neurotransmitter status, especially with regard to serotonin, which is affected by pyridoxine[135] as well as other factors. Going to bed at a regular hour (not later than 10 or 11 at night) helps to synchronize the daily schedule with the body's inherent hormonal rhythms and "physiological clock" which expects one to be in deep sleep by midnight and to be waking at approximately 8 o'clock in the morning. Recent research has shown that **sleep deprivation causes a systemic inflammatory response manifested objectively by increases in high-sensitivity C-reactive protein**.[136] Correspondingly, sleep apnea, a condition associated with repetitive sleep disturbances, is also associated with an elevation of CRP[137], and effective treatment of sleep apnea results in a normalization of CRP levels.[138] We could therefore conclude that **sleep deprivation creates a proinflammatory condition**. Furthermore, **sleep deprivation has been proven to impair intellectual functioning, emotional state, and immune function**, with abnormalities in immune status already evident the morning after sleep deprivation.[139] Wakefulness and exposure to light at night result in a suppression of melatonin production and may therefore contribute to cancer development since melatonin has anticancer actions that would be abrogated by its reduced production.[140,141] Limited evidence also suggests that melatonin production is

> **The Importance of Sleep**
> Regulation of sleep-wake cycles and the regular satisfaction of sleep needs are important for preservation of immune function, intellectual performance, emotional stability, and the internal regulation of the body's inflammatory tendency.

---

[132] Dominguez JR. Transforming Your Relationship With Money. Sounds True; Book and Cassette edition: 2001
[133] Breton D, Largent C. The Paradigm Conspiracy: Why Our Social Systems Violate Human Potential-And How We Can Change Them. Hazelden: 1998
[134] TAKE BACK YOUR TIME is a major U.S./Canadian initiative to challenge the epidemic of overwork, over-scheduling and time famine that now threatens our health, our families and relationships, our communities and our environment. http://www.simpleliving.net/timeday/ on August 3, 2004
[135] "…a significant difference in dream-salience scores (this is a composite score containing measures on vividness, bizarreness, emotionality, and color) between the 250-mg condition and placebo over the first three days of each treatment… An hypothesis is presented involving the role of B-6 in the conversion of tryptophan to serotonin." Ebben M, Lequerica A, Spielman A. Effects of pyridoxine on dreaming: a preliminary study. *Percept Mot Skills* 2002 Feb;94(1):135-40
[136] "CONCLUSIONS: Both acute total and short-term partial sleep deprivation resulted in elevated high-sensitivity CRP concentrations… We propose that sleep loss may be one of the ways that inflammatory processes are activated and contribute to the association of sleep complaints, short sleep duration, and cardiovascular morbidity observed in epidemiologic surveys." Meier-Ewert HK, Ridker PM, et al. Effect of sleep loss on C-reactive protein, an inflammatory marker of cardiovascular risk. *J Am Coll Cardiol*. 2004 Feb 18;43(4):678-83
[137] "OSA is associated with elevated levels of CRP, a marker of inflammation and of cardiovascular risk. The severity of OSA is proportional to the CRP level." Shamsuzzaman AS, Winnicki M, Lanfranchi P, Wolk R, Kara T, Accurso V, Somers VK. Elevated C-reactive protein in patients with obstructive sleep apnea. *Circulation*. 2002 May 28;105(21):2462-4
[138] "CONCLUSIONS: Levels of CRP and IL-6 and spontaneous production of IL-6 by monocytes are elevated in patients with OSAS but are decreased by nCPAP." Yokoe T, Minoguchi K, Matsuo H, Oda N, Minoguchi H, Yoshino G, Hirano T, Adachi M. Elevated levels of C-reactive protein and interleukin-6 in patients with obstructive sleep apnea syndrome are decreased by nasal continuous positive airway pressure. *Circulation*. 2003 Mar 4;107(8):1129-34 Available on-line at http://circ.ahajournals.org/cgi/reprint/107/8/1129.pdf on August 2, 2004
[139] "Taken together, SD induced a deterioration of both mood and ability to work, which was most prominent in the evening after SD, while the maximal alterations of the host defence system could be found twelve hours earlier, i.e., already in the morning following SD." Heiser P, Dickhaus B, Opper C, Hemmeter U, Remschmidt H, Wesemann W, Krieg JC, Schreiber W. Alterations of host defense system after sleep deprivation are followed by impaired mood and psychosocial functioning. *World J Biol Psychiatry* 2001 Apr;2(2):89-94
[140] "Observational studies support an association between night work and cancer risk. We hypothesise that the potential primary culprit for this observed association is the lack of melatonin, a cancer-protective agent whose production is severely diminished in people exposed to light at night." Schernhammer ES, Schulmeister K. Melatonin and cancer risk: does light at night compromise physiologic cancer protection by lowering serum melatonin levels? *Br J Cancer*. 2004 Mar 8;90(5):941-3
[141] "This is the first biological evidence for a potential link between constant light exposure and increased human breast oncogenesis involving MLT suppression and stimulation of tumor LA metabolism." Blask DE, Dauchy RT, Sauer LA, Krause JA, Brainard GC. Growth and fatty acid metabolism of human breast cancer (MCF-7) xenografts in nude rats: impact of constant light-induced nocturnal melatonin suppression. *Breast Cancer Res Treat*. 2003 Jun;79(3):313-20

altered in patients with the inflammatory conditions eczema[142] and psoriasis[143] and that this sleep-related hormone has anti-rheumatic/anti-autoimmune benefits that may be relevant for the suppression of inflammatory diseases such as multiple sclerosis[144] and sarcoidosis.[145]

---

### Helping patients improve quality and quantity of sleep

- Reduce intake of stimulants such as caffeine, tobacco, and aspartame. Some patients will need to reduce intake only in the evening, while others will need to reduce intake even in the morning in order to have improved quality and quantity of sleep later at night.
- Exercise early in the day (morning or early afternoon) to promote restful sleep at night.[146]
- Avoid aggressive or arousing physical activity in the evening to avoid increases in norepinephrine, epinephrine, and cortisol, which can discourage sleep.
- Dim lights at night to promote melatonin production. Beginning one to two hours before bedtime, turn off bright lights and use only dim lighting. Bright lights reduce melatonin secretion and stimulate neocortical activity and thereby inhibit sleep.
- Have an evening ritual/pattern that helps the psyche recognize that the time for sleep has arrived. Such practices can include relaxing warm tea, meditation, prayer, and daily reflection.
- For patients with a pattern of falling asleep and then waking approximately 4-6 hours later with feelings of hunger or anxiety (nocturnal hypoglycemia), they should eat a small meal or snack of complex carbohydrates, protein, and fat before going to bed. For example, the combination of nuts (or nut butter) with whole fruit such as apples provides protein, fat, and complex carbohydrate with a low glycemic index to provide sustenance throughout the night. Protein powders and other sources of "predigested" amino acids should generally be avoided late at night because an excess consumption of high protein foods can reduce tryptophan entry into the brain and thus reduce serotonin and melatonin synthesis. Most amino acid-derived neurotransmitters such as dopamine, glutamate, and norepinephrine are excitatory/stimulatory in nature.
- Vitamin and mineral supplementation is commonly beneficial, particularly with thiamine[147], methylcobalamin (weak evidence[148]), and magnesium (particularly sleep disturbance associated with restless leg syndrome[149]). Vitamins should be taken earlier in the day (with breakfast and lunch; not before bed); however calcium and magnesium can be taken before bed.
- Earplugs, window covers, and a quiet, snore-free environment are generally conducive to better sleep. For patients with difficulty falling asleep, consider 5-hydroxytryptophan consumed with simple carbohydrate (50-200 mg for adults, up to 2 mg/kg[150] for children), melatonin (0.5-10 mg), valerian-hops tea or capsules[151] 60-90 minutes before bedtime.

---

[142] "In 6 patients exhibiting low serum levels of melatonin, the circadian melatonin rhythm was found to be abolished. In 8 patients a diminished nocturnal melatonin increase was observed compared with the controls (n = 40)." Schwarz W, Birau N, Hornstein OP, Heubeck B, Schonberger A, Meyer C, Gottschalk J. Alterations of melatonin secretion in atopic eczema. *Acta Derm Venereol.* 1988;68(3):224-9

[143] "Our results show that psoriatic patients had lost the nocturnal peak and usual circadian rhythm of melatonin secretion." Mozzanica N, Tadini G, Radaelli A, Negri M, Pigatto P, Morelli M, Frigerio U, Finzi A, Esposti G, Rossi D, et al. Plasma melatonin levels in psoriasis. *Acta Derm Venereol.* 1988;68(4):312-6

[144] "This hypothesis is supported by the observation that administration of melatonin (3 mg, orally) at 2:00 p.m., when the patient experienced severe blurring of vision, resulted within 15 minutes in a dramatic improvement in visual acuity and in normalization of the visual evoked potential latency after stimulation of the left eye." Sandyk R. Diurnal variations in vision and relations to circadian melatonin secretion in multiple sclerosis. *Int J Neurosci.* 1995 Nov;83(1-2):1-6

[145] Cagnoni ML, Lombardi A, Cerinic MC, Dedola GL, Pignone A. Melatonin for treatment of chronic refractory sarcoidosis. *Lancet.* 1995;346(8984):1229-30

[146] "This is the first report to demonstrate that low intensity activity in an elderly population can increase deep sleep and improve memory functioning." Naylor E, Penev PD, Orbeta L, Janssen I, Ortiz R, Colecchia EF, Keng M, Finkel S, Zee PC. Daily social and physical activity increases slow-wave sleep and daytime neuropsychological performance in the elderly. *Sleep.* 2000 Feb 1;23(1):87-95

[147] Wilkinson TJ, Hanger HC, Elmslie J, George PM, Sainsbury R. The response to treatment of subclinical thiamine deficiency in the elderly. *Am J Clin Nutr.* 1997;66(4):925-8

[148] "However, because the percentage of improvement was low and significant improvement was inconsistent, Met-12 might be considered to have a low therapeutic potency and possible use as a booster for other treatment methods of the disorders." Takahashi K, et al. Double-blind test on the efficacy of methylcobalamin on sleep-wake rhythm disorders. *Psychiatry Clin Neurosci.* 1999 Apr;53(2):211-3

[149] "Our study indicates that magnesium treatment may be a useful alternative therapy in patients with mild or moderate RLS-or PLMS-related insomnia." Hornyak M, Voderholzer U, et al. Magnesium therapy for periodic leg movements-related insomnia and restless legs syndrome: an open pilot study. *Sleep.* 1998 Aug 1;21(5):501-5

[150] Bruni O, Ferri R, Miano S, Verrillo E. 1-5-Hydroxytryptophan treatment of sleep terrors in children. *Eur J Pediatr.* 2004 May 14

[151] "Sleep improvements with a valerian-hops combination are associated with improved quality of life. Both treatments appear safe and did not produce rebound insomnia upon discontinuation during this study. Overall, these findings indicate that a valerian-hops combination and diphenhydramine might be useful adjuncts in the treatment of mild insomnia." Morin CM, Koetter U, Bastien C, Ware JC, Wooten V. Valerian-hops combination and diphenhydramine for treating insomnia: a randomized placebo-controlled clinical trial. *Sleep.* 2005 Nov 1;28(11):1465-71

### Exercise:

"The health rewards of exercise extend far beyond its benefits for specific diseases." Exercise reduces blood clotting, lowers blood pressure, lowers cholesterol, improves glucose tolerance and insulin sensitivity, enhances self-image, elevates mood, reduces stress, creates a feeling of well-being, reinforces other positive life-style changes, stimulates creative thinking, increases muscle mass, increases basal metabolic rate, promotes improved sleep, stimulates healthy intestinal function, promotes weight loss, and enhances appearance. "Furthermore, **the ability of exercise to restore function to organs, muscles, joints, and bones is not shared by drugs or surgery.**"[152]

Human existence has changed radically over the past few millennia, centuries, and decades, and one of the most profound changes has been in our relationship to physical activity. Paleologists and historical scientists agree that physical activity among humans is at its all-time historical low, and that levels of exertion that we now call "vigorous and frequent exercise" would have been *completely normal* in the daily lives of our ancestors, who engaged in at least four times more physical activity than their modern-day progeny.[153] It is interesting to fathom a time in which physical activity was such a normal part of daily life that there was no word for "exercise."

"Although modern technology has made physical exertion optional, it is still important to exercise as though our survival depended on it, and in a different way it still does. **We are genetically adapted to live an extremely physically active lifestyle.**"[154]

Our current mode of compulsory primary and secondary education prioritizes "being still" over physical exertion and physical expression for the vast majority of students' time. Thus having been separated from their inherent tendency to be physically active and emotionally expressive, many children grow into adults who have to be *retaught to inhabit their bodies* and to engage in physical activity on a daily basis. Basic science has proven that this is true: when animals are restrained, they show less activity when freed and no longer tied down. Conversely, when animals are rigorously exercised, they show higher levels of *spontaneous physical activity* when left to their own discretion. A probable sociological parallel is at work in human cultures where, under the guise of *work* and *entertainment*, people are corralled into lifestyles of physical inactivity in a wide range of apparently divergent activities. Watching television, driving a car, seeing a movie, doing computer/desk work at the office, attending a sports event or educational lecture, seeing the opera—all of these are simply different forms of *sitting*, of physical inactivity. Changing our social structure in a way that prioritizes *life* over *work*, such as moving toward a 4-day work week and/or a 6-hour work day, would allow people more time to live their lives, to pursue healthy diets and relationships, to be creative, and to engage in more physical activity; thus, "escape entertainment" such as fiction books and movies and processed "fast foods"—the latter of which are inherently unhealthy[155]—would become less necessary and less attractive.

---

[152] Harold Elrick, MD. Exercise is Medicine. *The Physician and Sportsmedicine* - Volume 24 - No. 2 - February 1996
[153] Eaton SB, Cordain L, Eaton SB. An evolutionary foundation for health promotion. *World Rev Nutr Diet* 2001; 90:5-12
[154] O'Keefe JH Jr, Cordain L. Cardiovascular disease resulting from a diet and lifestyle at odds with our Paleolithic genome: how to become a 21st-century hunter-gatherer. *Mayo Clin Proc.* 2004 Jan;79(1):101-8. Available on-line at http://www.thepaleodiet.com/articles/Hunter-Gatherer%20Mayo.pdf on May 19, 2004
[155] For an additional perspective see movie by Morgan Spurlock (director). Super Size Me. www.supersizeme.com released in 2004

| Inactivity | Minimally active | Active | Healthy | Athletic |
|---|---|---|---|---|
| • Bed-ridden<br>• Chair-ridden<br>• Minimal activity, such as walking to car or bathroom or to buy groceries<br>• Activity in this category is equivalent to or barely above that which is necessary to sustain life | • The performance of more activity than the minimal needed to sustain life, such as walking around the block after dinner, or taking a brief stroll at a park or at the beach | • Regular performance of low/moderate levels of activity at work or leisure, at least 30-60 minutes of physical activity per day | • 60-120 minutes of vigorous activity such as running, swimming, or cycling 4-7 days per week | • More than 2 hours devoted to conditioning, strengthening, and skill-building 4-7 days per week |

At least 30-45 minutes of exercise four days per week is the *absolute minimum*. Following a health assessment, patients who have been previously sedentary for many years can start slowly with their new exercise program, gradually increasing the duration and intensity. **With the simple addition of regular exercise to their routine, patients will have significantly reduced risk for problems such as depression, chronic pain, cancer, coronary artery disease, stroke, hypertension, diabetes, arthritis, osteoporosis, dyslipidemia, obesity, chronic obstructive pulmonary disease, constipation, and other problems.**[156] Furthermore, successful prevention and treatment of health problems with exercise and lifestyle modifications reduces dependency on pharmaceutical drugs, thereby further saving lives. O'Keefe and Cordain[157] report that **during the hunter-gatherer period, humans averaged 5-10 miles of daily running *and walking*.** Additionally, **other physical activities such as heavy lifting, digging, and climbing would have been considered "normal" aspects of daily life rather than "exercise" — an achievement for which modern people seek recognition.** Thus, when sedentary patients achieve the first-step goal of walking around the block after dinner, we can commend them for making a significant stride forward in ultimately attaining better health, but we cannot stop there nor delude them into believing that this is adequate.

*Notes*:

_____
_____
_____
_____
_____
_____

---

[156] Harold Elrick, MD. Exercise is Medicine. *The Physician and Sportsmedicine* - Volume 24 - No. 2 - February 1996
[157] O'Keefe JH Jr, Cordain L. Cardiovascular disease resulting from a diet and lifestyle at odds with our Paleolithic genome: how to become a 21st-century hunter-gatherer. *Mayo Clin Proc*. 2004 Jan;79(1):101-8. Available on line at http://www.thepaleodiet.com/articles/Hunter-Gatherer%20Mayo.pdf on May 19, 2004

## Common physical activities and exercises

- ☑ **Walking**: easy, accessible, virtually free; allows for conversation and exploration; allows for time outdoors
- ☑ **Jogging and running**: easy, accessible, virtually free; allows for conversation and exploration; increases endorphin production and promotes a sense of well-being; detoxification via sweating
- ☑ **Hiking**: virtually free of expense; allows for conversation, exploration, and time in nature; mountains required
- ☑ **Swimming**: requires access to a pool or suitable body of water; excellent for promoting fitness in a way that is generally easy on joints and muscles and is without impact; requires and thus promotes coordination and timing
- ☑ **Indoor aerobics**: excellent for cardiovascular fitness and weight loss, requires and thus promotes coordination and timing
- ☑ **Indoor cycling**: excellent for cardiovascular fitness and weight loss, easy on the joints; accessible during inclement weather
- ☑ **Outdoor cycling (road)**: same as above with added bonus of being outdoors; promotes independence from automobiles and petroleum products – thereby reducing pollution and sustaining the environment
- ☑ **Outdoor cycling (mountain and trail)**: same as above; requires more balance and coordination
- ☑ **Weight lifting, bodybuilding, and powerlifting**: excellent for increasing lean body mass – one of the primary determinants of basal metabolic rate; promotes bone strengthening
- ☑ **Tennis and racket sports**: requires more balance, coordination, timing, strategy, endurance; the rapid stops, starts, and turns can be hard on joints; upper body exertion is asymmetric and can promote muscle imbalance
- ☑ **Aerobic machines such as elliptical runners and stair-climbing machines**: easy on joints; accessible during inclement weather; easy to integrate with weight-lifting which is commonly available at the same facility
- ☑ **Rock-climbing (indoor and outdoor)**: requires upper body and grip strength; promotes agility, resourcefulness, courage, and trust; good for building stronger relationships assuming that your partner does not drop the rope or get distracted; carries some inherent risk
- ☑ **Volleyball**: good team activity; not highly exertional in terms of either aerobic fitness nor strength acquisition
- ☑ **Baseball**: requires some skill in throwing and batting, but otherwise this is a very inactive sport
- ☑ **Football**: much of the game is spent in inactivity; most of the fitness comes from preparation for the game, not the game itself; high impact activity wherein injuries are expected
- ☑ **Soccer**: excellent for lower-body conditioning, teamwork, and coordination, the rapid stops and turns can be hard on joints
- ☑ **Yoga, Pilates, Calisthenics**: inexpensive, can be done alone or in groups; does not require much/any equipment, therefore costs are low and access is near universal
- ☑ **Martial arts**: requires more balance, coordination, timing, strategy, endurance; injuries are to be expected
- ☑ **Surfing**: paddling requires upper body endurance and strength; some leg strength is required but is not strongly developed during the riding portion of surfing, which is mostly technique and "style"; excellent proprioceptive training
- ☑ **Kayaking and canoeing**: excellent combination of relaxation and exertion; develops upper body strength and balance
- ☑ **"Boot camp"-style aerobics classes**: excellent variety and fast-pace maintains oxygen debt for the entire session (generally 60 minutes) even among reasonably well trained "healthy" people

## Obesity:

Obesity is a major risk factor for cardiovascular disease, cancer, diabetes, depression, and joint pain. Obese people also commonly report difficulties with performing daily activities, and they also report higher rates of depression and social isolation than do people of normal weight.

> "The magnitude of the problem in the United States is perhaps greater than in any other country. Estimates of the number of overweight Americans range from 50 million to 200 million. **The average American is said to have 20 to 30 lb of excess body fat.**"[158]

To calculate the "Body Mass Index" simply chart height and weight to determine the BMI number. Numbers greater than 25 correlate with being "overweight" while numbers greater than 30 meet the criteria for "obesity." BMI determinations may not be reflective of disease risk for people who are pregnant, highly muscular, or for young children or the frail elderly.

### BODY MASS INDEX interpretation
- Underweight: Under 18.5
- **Normal: 18.5-24**
- Overweight: 25-29
- Obese: 30 and over
- Severe obesity: > 40
- Morbid obesity: >40.0–49.9

**WEIGHT in pounds**

| HEIGHT | 100 | 110 | 120 | 130 | 140 | 150 | 160 | 170 | 180 | 190 | 200 | 210 | 220 | 230 | 240 | 250 |
|---|---|---|---|---|---|---|---|---|---|---|---|---|---|---|---|---|
| 5'0" | 20 | 21 | 23 | 25 | 27 | 29 | 31 | 33 | 35 | 37 | 39 | 41 | 43 | 45 | 47 | 49 |
| 5'1" | 19 | 21 | 23 | 25 | 26 | 28 | 30 | 32 | 34 | 36 | 38 | 40 | 42 | 43 | 45 | 47 |
| 5'2" | 18 | 20 | 22 | 24 | 26 | 27 | 29 | 31 | 33 | 35 | 37 | 38 | 40 | 42 | 44 | 46 |
| 5'3" | 18 | 19 | 21 | 23 | 25 | 27 | 28 | 30 | 32 | 34 | 35 | 37 | 39 | 41 | 43 | 44 |
| 5'4" | 17 | 19 | 21 | 22 | 24 | 26 | 27 | 29 | 31 | 33 | 34 | 36 | 38 | 39 | 41 | 43 |
| 5'5" | 17 | 18 | 20 | 22 | 23 | 25 | 27 | 28 | 30 | 32 | 33 | 35 | 37 | 38 | 40 | 42 |
| 5'6" | 16 | 18 | 19 | 21 | 23 | 24 | 26 | 27 | 29 | 31 | 32 | 34 | 36 | 37 | 39 | 40 |
| 5'7" | 16 | 17 | 19 | 20 | 22 | 23 | 25 | 27 | 28 | 30 | 31 | 33 | 34 | 36 | 38 | 39 |
| 5'8" | 15 | 17 | 18 | 20 | 21 | 23 | 24 | 26 | 27 | 29 | 30 | 32 | 33 | 35 | 36 | 38 |
| 5'9" | 15 | 16 | 18 | 19 | 21 | 22 | 24 | 25 | 27 | 28 | 30 | 31 | 32 | 34 | 35 | 37 |
| 5'10" | 14 | 16 | 17 | 19 | 20 | 22 | 23 | 24 | 26 | 27 | 29 | 30 | 32 | 33 | 34 | 36 |
| 5'11" | 14 | 15 | 17 | 18 | 20 | 21 | 22 | 24 | 25 | 26 | 27 | 28 | 30 | 32 | 33 | 35 |
| 6'0" | 14 | 15 | 16 | 18 | 19 | 20 | 22 | 23 | 24 | 26 | 27 | 28 | 30 | 31 | 33 | 34 |
| 6'1" | 13 | 15 | 16 | 17 | 18 | 20 | 21 | 22 | 24 | 25 | 26 | 28 | 29 | 30 | 32 | 33 |
| 6'2" | 13 | 14 | 15 | 17 | 18 | 19 | 21 | 22 | 23 | 24 | 26 | 27 | 28 | 30 | 31 | 32 |
| 6'3" | 12 | 14 | 15 | 16 | 17 | 19 | 20 | 21 | 22 | 24 | 25 | 26 | 27 | 29 | 30 | 31 |
| 6'4" | 12 | 13 | 15 | 16 | 17 | 18 | 19 | 21 | 22 | 23 | 24 | 26 | 27 | 28 | 29 | 30 |

---

[158] Harold Elrick, MD. Exercise is Medicine. *The Physician and Sportsmedicine* - Volume 24 - No. 2 - February 1996

*Overview of the Proinflammatory and Endocrinologic Activity of Adipose Tissue*

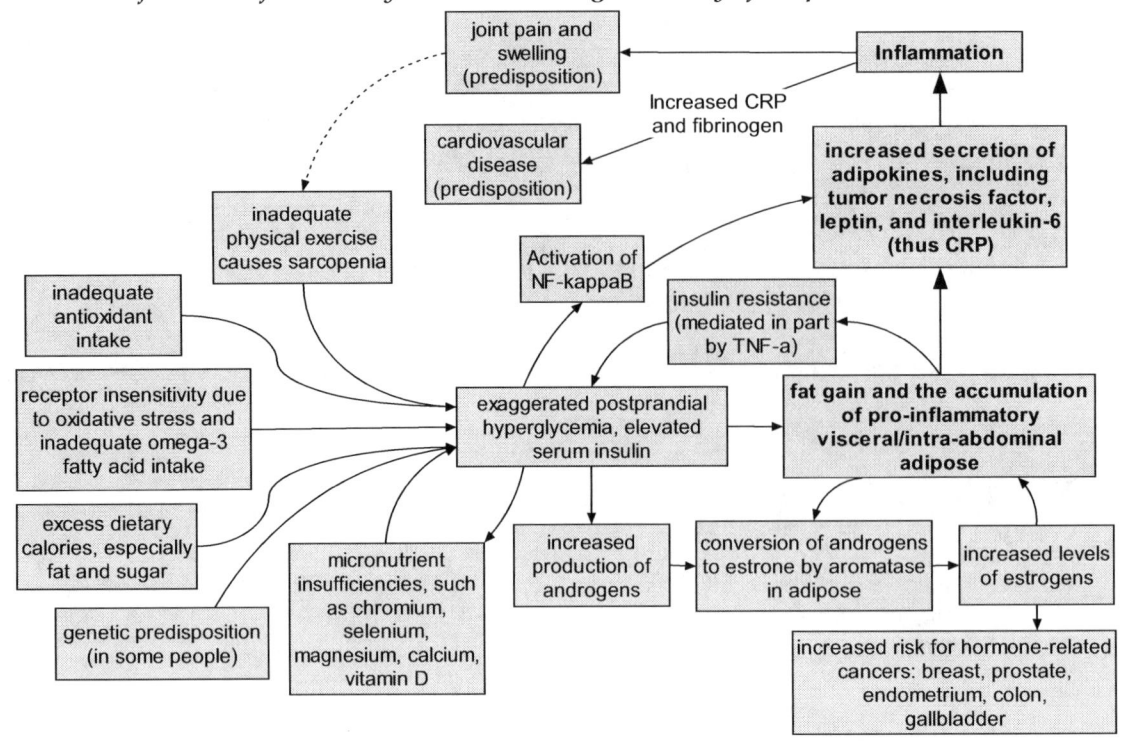

[Diagram showing relationships between factors contributing to proinflammatory and endocrinologic activity of adipose tissue, including: inadequate physical exercise causes sarcopenia; inadequate antioxidant intake; receptor insensitivity due to oxidative stress and inadequate omega-3 fatty acid intake; excess dietary calories, especially fat and sugar; genetic predisposition (in some people); micronutrient insufficiencies, such as chromium, selenium, magnesium, calcium, vitamin D; exaggerated postprandial hyperglycemia, elevated serum insulin; Activation of NF-kappaB; insulin resistance (mediated in part by TNF-a); fat gain and the accumulation of pro-inflammatory visceral/intra-abdominal adipose; increased production of androgens; conversion of androgens to estrone by aromatase in adipose; increased levels of estrogens; increased risk for hormone-related cancers: breast, prostate, endometrium, colon, gallbladder; increased secretion of adipokines, including tumor necrosis factor, leptin, and interleukin-6 (thus CRP); Increased CRP and fibrinogen; Inflammation; joint pain and swelling (predisposition); cardiovascular disease (predisposition).]

The old paradigm of fat (adipose) tissue as merely serving as an inert and inactive depot for lipid/energy storage is now replaced with the view that adipose tissue is biologically-active tissue that influences overall health via complex mechanisms that are biochemical-inflammatory-endocrinologic and not merely mechanical (i.e., excess weight, excess mass).[159] **Excess fat tissue creates a systemic proinflammatory state** evidenced most readily by elevations in C-reactive protein commonly seen in patients with obesity and the metabolic syndrome.[160] Adipokines are cytokines secreted by adipose tissue and include tumor necrosis factor-alpha, interleukin-6, adiponectin, and leptin—a cytokine derived from fat cells that promotes inflammation and immune activation; levels are higher in obese patients and decrease after weight loss. Obese patients also appear to have "leptin resistance" with regard to the suppression of appetite by leptin. **Adipose creates excess estrogens;** concomitant hyperglycemia increases androgen production[161], and these androgens are subsequently converted to estrogens by aromatase in the adipose tissue. For example, the adrenal gland makes androstenedione, which can be converted by aromatase in adipose tissue into estrone.[162] These proinflammatory and hormonal perturbations manifest clinically as an increased risk for breast, prostate, endometrial, colon and gallbladder cancers, and cardiovascular disease. This pattern of inflammation, reduced testosterone, and elevated estrogen is also a predisposition toward the development of autoimmune/inflammatory disease.

---

[159] "The fat cell is a true endocrine cell that secretes a variety of factors, including metabolites such as lactate, fatty acids, prostaglandin derivatives and a variety of peptides, including cytokines (leptin, tumor necrosis factor, interleukin-1 and -6, adiponectin), angiotensinogen, complement D (adipsin), plasminogen activator inhibitor-1 and undoubtedly many others." Bray GA. The underlying basis for obesity: relationship to cancer. *J Nutr*. 2002 Nov;132(11 Suppl):3451S-3455S
[160] "Our results indicate a strong relationship between adipocytokines and inflammatory markers, and suggest that cytokines secreted by adipose tissue could play a role in increased inflammatory proteins secretion by the liver." Maachi M, Pieroni L, Bruckert E, Jardel C, Fellahi S, Hainque B, Capeau J, Bastard JP. Systemic low-grade inflammation is related to both circulating and adipose tissue TNFalpha, leptin and IL-6 levels in obese women. *Int J Obes Relat Metab Disord*. 2004;28:993-7
[161] Christensen L, Hagen C, Henriksen JE, Haug E. Elevated levels of sex hormones and sex hormone binding globulin in male patients with insulin dependent diabetes mellitus. Effect of improved blood glucose regulation. *Dan Med Bull*. 1997 Nov;44(5):547-50
[162] "The conversion of androstenedione secreted by the adrenal gland into estrone by aromatase in adipose tissue stroma provides an important source of estrogen for the postmenopausal woman. This estrogen may play an important role in the development of endometrial and breast cancer." Bray GA. The underlying basis for obesity: relationship to cancer. *J Nutr*. 2002 Nov;132(11 Suppl):3451S-3455S

## Diet is a Powerful Intervention for the Prevention and Treatment of Disease

**Make "whole foods" the foundation of the diet—emphasize whole fruits, vegetables, and lean meats.** "Whole foods" are foods that are found in nature, and they should be eaten as closely as possible to their natural state—preferably *unprocessed* and *raw*. Creating a diet based on whole, natural foods by emphasizing the consumption of fruits, vegetables, and lean meats and excluding high-fat factory meats, high-sugar foods like white potatoes, and milled grains like wheat and corn is essential for our efforts of promoting health by matching the human *diet* with the human *genome*.[163] Our genetic make-up was co-created over a period of more than 2.6 million years with an environment that mandated daily physical activity and a diet that was exclusively composed of 1) fresh fruits, 2) fresh vegetables (mostly uncooked), 3) nuts, seeds, berries, roots, and 4) generous portions of lean meat that was rich in omega-3 fatty acids from free-living animals. Humans have deviated from this original diet for the sake of ease, conformity, and short-term satisfaction at the expense of health, power, and longevity. Peoples who consume traditional, natural diets have dramatically lower incidences *major* health disasters such as cancer, cardiovascular disease, diabetes, obesity and also suffer much less from *milder* problems such as acne, psoriasis, cavities, oral malocclusion, and chronic sinus congestion. Societies that are free of these disorders become overwhelmed with them—*within only one or two generations*—as soon as they adopt the American/Western style of eating. These facts were conclusively documented by Weston Price in his famous 1945 masterpiece *Nutrition and Physical Degeneration*[164] and have been reiterated recently in an excellent review by O'Keefe and Cordain in *Mayo Clinic Proceedings*.[165]

> My conclusion after reading several hundred articles on epidemiology, nutritional biochemistry, and dietary intervention studies is that the Paleo-Mediterranean pesco-vegetarian diet is the single most healthy dietary regimen for the broadest range of patients and for the prevention of the widest range of diseases including cancer, hypertension, diabetes, dermatitis, depression, obesity, arthritis and all inflammatory and autoimmune diseases. By definition, this is a diet that helps patients increase their intake of fruits and vegetables (fiber, antioxidants, phytonutrients), increases their intake of fish (for the anti-inflammatory omega-3 fats EPA and DHA) while reducing intake of the pro-cancer and pro-inflammatory omega-6 fats linoleic acid and arachidonic acid), and it is naturally low in sugars and cholesterol (for alleviating hyperglycemia and dyslipidemia). It helps patients avoid grains, particularly wheat (a common allergen), and it reduces the intake of the high-fermentation carbohydrates in breads, pasta, pastries, potatoes, and sucrose which promote overgrowth of bacteria and yeast in the intestines. Supplementing this pesco-vegetarian diet with vitamins, minerals, fatty acids such as fish oil and GLA (from borage oil), and protein from soy and whey makes this diet effective for both the treatment and prevention of many conditions; I call this **"the Supplemented Paleo-Mediterranean Diet."**

---

[163] O'Keefe JH Jr, Cordain L. Cardiovascular disease resulting from a diet and lifestyle at odds with our Paleolithic genome: how to become a 21st-century hunter-gatherer. *Mayo Clin Proc*. 2004 Jan;79(1):101-8. Available on line at http://www.thepaleodiet.com/articles/Hunter-Gatherer%20Mayo.pdf on May 19, 2004

[164] Price WA. *Nutrition and Physical Degeneration: A Comparison of Primitive and Modern Diets and Their Effects*. Santa Monica; Price-Pottinger Nutrition Foundation: 1945

[165] O'Keefe JH Jr, Cordain L. Cardiovascular disease resulting from a diet and lifestyle at odds with our Paleolithic genome: how to become a 21st-century hunter-gatherer. *Mayo Clin Proc*. 2004 Jan;79(1):101-8

**Most patients (and doctors) need to increase consumption of fruits and vegetables**: Encourage consumption of collard greens, broccoli, kale, spinach, chard, lettuce, onions, red peppers, green beans, carrots, apples, oranges, nuts, blueberries and other fruits and vegetables. Patients can find or make a good low-carbohydrate dressing (such as lemon garlic tahini[166]) to make these vegetables taste great. Fresh fruits and vegetables are best; but frozen fruits and vegetables are acceptable. Patients can buy a package of (organic) frozen vegetables; then when they are ready for a healthy-and-fast meal, simply warm/steam the vegetables on the stovetop. In just a few minutes and with only minimal effort, by regularly eating vegetables, they will have significantly reduced their risk for heart disease, diabetes, cancer, hemorrhoids, constipation, and many other chronic health problems. Using frozen vegetables and eating vegetables only twice per day is not *optimal*—it is *minimal*. For many patients, consuming two servings of vegetables per day is a major lifestyle change. **Ultimately, *the goal is for fresh fruits and vegetables to form a major portion of the diet*, to be the main course rather than simply a side dish**. A diet based on fruits and vegetables is a powerful nutritional strategy for reducing the risk for cancer, heart disease, and autoimmune and inflammatory disorders.[167]

**Phytochemicals—important antioxidant and anti-inflammatory nutrients from fruits and vegetables**: While we have all commonly thought of the benefits of fruits and vegetables as being derived from the vitamins, minerals, and fiber, we are learning from new research that many if not most of the health-promoting benefits of fruits and vegetables come from the phenolic chemicals that they contain. For example, while in the past we might have thought of the benefits of eating apples as being derived from the vitamin C content, we now know that vitamin C only provides 0.4% of the antioxidant action contained within a whole apple—obviously the other components of the apple, namely the phenolic compounds are responsible for most of an apple's antioxidant activity.[168] Recent research has shown that cranberries, apples, red grapes, and strawberries have the most antioxidant power of the fruits[169], while red peppers, broccoli, carrots, and spinach are the best antioxidant vegetables.[170] This is a very important concept to appreciate and remember: **the benefits derived from fruits and vegetables are not derived principally from the vitamins and therefore can never be obtained from the use of multivitamin pills as a substitute for whole foods.** Multivitamin and multimineral supplements are valuable and worthwhile *supplements* to a whole-foods diet but should not be used as *substitutes for* a whole-foods diet.

---

[166] Mollie Katzen. The New Moosewood Cookbook Ten Speed Press; page 103

[167] "…one of the most consistent research findings is that those who consume higher amounts of fruits and vegetables have lower rates of heart disease and stroke as well as cancer…" Seaman DR. The diet-induced proinflammatory state: a cause of chronic pain and other degenerative diseases? *J Manipulative Physiol Ther*. 2002;25(3):168-79

[168] "We propose that the additive and synergistic effects of phytochemicals in fruit and vegetables are responsible for their potent antioxidant and anticancer activities, and that the benefit of a diet rich in fruit and vegetables is attributed to the complex mixture of phytochemicals present in whole foods." Liu RH. Health benefits of fruit and vegetables are from additive and synergistic combinations of phytochemicals. *Am J Clin Nutr*. 2003 Sep;78(3 Suppl):517S-520S

[169] "Cranberry had the highest total antioxidant activity (177.0 +/- 4.3 micromol of vitamin C equiv/g of fruit), followed by apple, red grape, strawberry, peach, lemon, pear, banana, orange, grapefruit, and pineapple." Sun J, Chu YF, Wu X, Liu RH. Antioxidant and antiproliferative activities of common fruits. *J Agric Food Chem*. 2002 Dec 4;50(25):7449-54

[170] "Red pepper had the highest total antioxidant activity, followed by broccoli, carrot, spinach, cabbage, yellow onion, celery, potato, lettuce, and cucumber." Chu YF, Sun J, Wu X, Liu RH. Antioxidant and antiproliferative activities of common vegetables. *J Agric Food Chem*. 2002 Nov 6;50(23):6910-6

# Wellness Promotion: Re-Establishing the Foundation for Health

Fruits and vegetables contain more than 8,000 phytochemicals, most of which have anti-inflammatory, anti-proliferative, and anti-cancer benefits[171]—the best and only way to benefit from these chemicals is to change the diet in favor of relying principally on fruits and vegetables as the major component of the diet, and the easiest way to do this is to eliminate carbohydrate-rich antioxidant-poor foods such as bread, pasta, rice, sweets, crackers, chips and "junk foods."

| VEGETABLES | |
|---|---|
| **Phenolic content** | **Antioxidant capacity** |
| 1) Broccoli | 1. Red pepper |
| 2) Spinach | 2. Broccoli |
| 3) Yellow onion | 3. Carrot |
| 4) Red pepper | 4. Spinach |
| 5) Carrot | 5. Cabbage |
| 6) Cabbage | 6. Yellow onion |
| 7) Potato | 7. Celery |
| 8) Lettuce | 8. Potato |
| 9) Celery | 9. Lettuce |
| 10) Cucumber | 10. Cucumber |

Different fruits and vegetables contain different types, quantities, and ratios of vitamins, minerals, and phytochemicals, and *dietary diversity* will therefore help patients to obtain a broad spectrum of and maximum benefit from these different nutrients. The revelation that, in order to be as healthy as possible, we have to consume a diet that is derived principally from fruits and vegetables in order to obtain the diverse phytochemicals contained therein is somewhat problematic for at least two reasons. In the healthcare world, our policies, politics, and paradigms are centered around the pharmaceutical "silver bullet" model—the belief that single-drug interventions hold the promise to health. The reasons that this paradigm has dominated the American healthcare scene for the past 100 years are that 1) it is profitable for doctors and drug companies, and 2) because it exonerates patients from taking personal responsibly for their health by changing their lifestyles. Taking appropriate action with the data that a fruit/vegetable-based diet has powerful health-promoting benefits means that we as doctors and patients have to change our lifestyles with regard to how we plan our meals, what we buy, what we prepare, and what we eat. Behavior modification is a tremendous challenge for people, especially those who lack sufficient motivation or insight. This text is providing the *insight*—the data, references, and concepts. But without *motivation*—from doctors to help their patients attain the highest levels of health, and from patients to change their lifestyles to become as healthy as possible—the research itself does little to promote health. When *insight* is combined with *motivation* we have the *potential for change*, but the potential for change is meaningless until it is manifested into the world with *persistent, effective action*.

| FRUITS | |
|---|---|
| **Phenolic content** | **Antioxidant capacity** |
| 1. Cranberry | 1. Cranberry |
| 2. Apple | 2. Apple |
| 3. Red grape | 3. Red grape |
| 4. Strawberry | 4. Strawberry |
| 5. Pineapple | 5. Peach |
| 6. Banana | 6. Lemon |
| 7. Peach | 7. Pear |
| 8. Lemon | 8. Banana |
| 9. Orange | 9. Orange |
| 10. Pear | 10. Grapefruit |
| 11. Grapefruit | 11. Pineapple |

---

[171] Liu RH. Health benefits of fruit and vegetables are from additive and synergistic combinations of phytochemicals. *Am J Clin Nutr*. 2003 Sep;78(3 Suppl):517S-520S

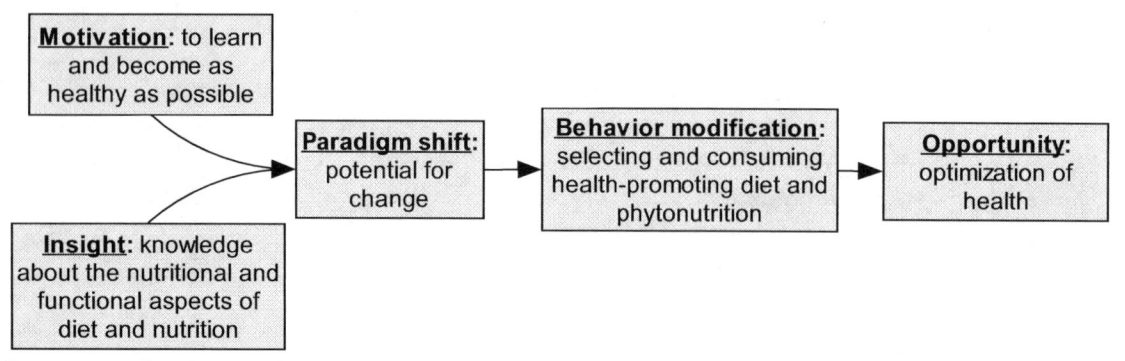

**Motivation:** to learn and become as healthy as possible

**Insight:** knowledge about the nutritional and functional aspects of diet and nutrition

**Paradigm shift:** potential for change

**Behavior modification:** selecting and consuming health-promoting diet and phytonutrition

**Opportunity:** optimization of health

Conceptualizations dictate behavior (action), and behavior (e.g., lifestyle, exercise, nutritional intake) is generally the strongest factor in determining health outcomes. Doctors influence patients' health outcomes by shaping patients' conceptualization of life.

<u>Eat the right amount of protein</u>: Dietary protein is eaten to provide the body with amino acids, which are the building blocks that the body uses to create new tissues, heal wounds, fight off infections, grow hair and fingernails, and to create specific hormones and neurotransmitters. Meats, eggs, and milk contain the types and amounts of essential amino acids that the human body requires and are thus said to provide more "complete protein" than do vegetable proteins. For most people (without kidney or liver problems) the goal should be ½ to ¾ gram of protein per pound of lean body weight, depending on activity level. Sufficient dietary protein is essential for patients with musculoskeletal injuries because tissue healing relies on the constant availability of amino acids and micronutrients[172], which should be supplied by a healthy, balanced, whole-foods diet that may be supplemented with specific nutraceuticals, as discussed later in this text. Low-protein diets suppress immune function, reduce muscle mass, and impair healing[173,174], whereas intakes of higher amounts of protein safely facilitate healing and the maintenance of muscle mass. Increased protein intake does not adversely affect bone health as long as dietary calcium intake is adequate.[175] According to the recent review by Lemon[176]:

> "Those involved in strength training might need to consume as much as …1.7 g protein x kg(-1) x day(-1)…while those undergoing endurance training might need about 1.2 to 1.6 g x kg(-1) x day(-1)… **…there is no evidence that protein intakes in the range suggested will have adverse effects in healthy individuals.**"

<u>For patients who are completely sedentary</u>: multiply body weight in pounds by 0.4 and this will give the number of grams of protein that should be eaten each day.[177]

<u>For patients who are very active (frequent weight lifting, or competitive athlete)</u>: multiply body weight in pounds by 0.7-0.9 and this will give the number of grams of protein that should be eaten each day.

---

[172] "Supplementation with protein and vitamins, specifically arginine and vitamins A, B, and C, provides optimum nutrient support of the healing wound." Meyer NA, Muller MJ, Herndon DN. Nutrient support of the healing wound. *New Horiz* 1994 May;2(2):202-14
[173] Castaneda C, Charnley JM, Evans WJ, Crim MC. Elderly women accommodate to a low-protein diet with losses of body cell mass, muscle function, and immune response. *Am J Clin Nutr* 1995 Jul;62(1):30-9 http://www.ajcn.org/cgi/reprint/62/1/30
[174] [No author listed]. Vegetarians and healing. *JAMA* 1995; 273: 910
[175] Heaney RP. Excess dietary protein may not adversely affect bone. *J Nutr* 1998 Jun;128(6):1054-7
[176] Lemon PW. Effects of exercise on dietary protein requirements. *Int J Sport Nutr 1998* Dec;8(4):426-47
[177] Pellet PL. Protein requirements in humans. *Am J Clin Nutr* 1990 May;51(5):723-37

Again, compared with sedentary people, *sick people, injured people,* and *athletes* **need more protein** to maintain weight, fight infections, repair injuries, and build and maintain muscle. Not only can insufficient protein intake cause muscle weakness and loss of weight, but recent articles have also suggested that low-protein diets can cause suppression of the immune system[178] and impairment of healing after injury or surgery.[179]

| Recommended Grams of Protein Per Pound of Body Weight Per Day[180] | |
|---|---|
| Infants and children ages 1-6 years[181] | 0.68-0.45 |
| RDA for sedentary adult and children ages 6-18 years[182] | 0.4 |
| **Adult recreational exerciser** | **0.5-0.75** |
| Adult competitive athlete | 0.6-0.9 |
| Adult building muscle mass | 0.7-0.9 |
| Dieting athlete | 0.7-1.0 |
| Growing teenage athlete | 0.9-1.0 |
| Pregnant women need additional protein | Add 15-30 grams/day[183] |

For example, in most instances, a person weighing 120 pounds should aim for at least 60 grams of protein per day, or 90 grams of protein per day if he/she is more physically active, ill, or injured. A can of tuna has 30 grams of protein; one egg has 6 grams of protein. If she is going to eat eggs as a source of protein for a meal, she might have to eat as many as five eggs to reach a target of 30 grams of protein per meal. When eating meat, visualize the amount of meat in a can of tuna to estimate the amount of protein being eaten—for example, if the portion of meat at a given meal is about the size of a half can of tuna, then we can estimate that the serving contains 15-20 grams of high-quality protein. By knowing the "target intake" for the day, and by estimating the amount of protein eaten with each meal, patients will be able to modify their protein intake to ensure that they reach their target intake.

**Protein supplements** can be used *in conjunction with a healthy diet*. Patients using a protein supplement should eat a healthy diet and then add protein supplements between regular meals. If they substitute a protein supplement for a regular meal, then they may not actually increase protein intake. Whole *real* foods should form the foundation for the diet—patients should not rely too heavily on *protein supplements* when patients can get better results *and improved overall health* with *whole foods*. Whey, casein, and lactalbumin are proteins from milk and dairy products, and may therefore be allergenic in people allergic to milk. Soy protein is safe and a source of high-quality protein for adults[184], and recent research indicates that consumption of soy protein

---

[178] Castaneda C, Charnley JM, Evans WJ, Crim MC. Elderly women accommodate to a low-protein diet with losses of body cell mass, muscle function, and immune response. *Am J Clin Nutr* 1995 Jul;62(1):30-9
[179] Vegetarians and healing. *Journal of the American Medical Association* 1995; 273: 910
[180] Slightly modified from Nancy Clark, MS, RD. The Power of Protein. *The Physician and Sportsmedicine* 1996, volume 24, number 4
[181] 1.5-1 g/kg/d (0.68-0.45 grams per pound of body weight. Younger people need proportionately more protein.) Brown ML (ed). Present Knowledge in Nutrition. Sixth Edition. Washington DC: International Life Sciences Institute Nutrition Foundation; 1990 page 68
[182] 0.83 g.kg-1.d-1 (equivalent to 0.37 grams per pound of body weight) Pellet PL. Protein requirements in humans. *Am J Clin Nutr* 1990 May;51(5):723-37
[183] Weinsier RL, Morgan SL (eds). Fundamentals of Clinical Nutrition. St. Louis: Mosby, 1993 page 50
[184] "These results indicate that for healthy adults, the isolated soy protein is of high nutritional quality, comparable to that of animal protein sources, and that the methionine content is not limiting for adult protein maintenance." Young VR, Puig M, Queiroz E, Scrimshaw NS, Rand WM. Evaluation of the protein quality of an isolated soy protein in young men: relative nitrogen requirements and effect of methionine supplementation. *Am J Clin Nutr.* 1984 Jan;39(1):16-24

can help reduce the risk of cancer and heart disease[185]; however, I do not recommend the use of large quantities of supplemental soy protein for pregnant women, or for children due to the potential for disrupting endocrine function. Patients may have to experiment with different products until they find one that "works" with regard to taste, texture, digestibility, hypoallergenicity, nutritional effects, and affordability.

Recall again that the goal is *improved health*, not simply *adequate protein intake*. If we focus solely on "grams of protein" then we might overlook adverse effects that are associated with certain protein sources. Cow's milk is a high quality protein, but it is commonly allergenic and can exacerbate joint pain in sensitive individuals.[186] Beef, liver, pork and other land animal meats are excellent sources of protein, but they are also rich sources of arachidonic acid[187] and iron[188], both of which have been shown to exacerbate joint pain and inflammation. Fish is an excellent source of protein, but fish are often poisoned with mercury and other toxicants, which are then ingested by humans with adverse effects.[189,190]

**Eat complex carbohydrates to stabilize blood sugar, mood, and energy**: Choose items with a "low glycemic index"[191] to stabilize blood sugar and—for many people—to lower triglycerides and cholesterol levels. Foods with a low Glycemic Index (GI < 55)[192] include yogurt, apple (36), whole orange (43), peach (28), legumes, lentils (28), and soybeans (18), cherries, dried apricots, nuts, most meats, and most vegetables. **Healthy foods that have both a low *glycemic index* as well as a low *glycemic load* include: apples, carrots, chick peas, grapes, green peas, kidney beans, oranges, peaches, peanuts, pears, pinto beans, red lentils, and strawberries.**[193]

**Reduce or eliminate simple sugars from the diet (as necessary)**: Nearly everyone should minimize intake of table sugar (sucrose), fructose and high-fructose corn syrup, and all artificial sweeteners. Chronic overconsumption of refined carbohydrates promotes disease by 1) increasing urinary excretion of magnesium and calcium, 2) inducing oxidative stress, 3) promoting fat deposition and obesity, which then generally leads to insulin resistance and hyperinsulinemia with an increase in production of cholesterol, triglycerides, and proinflammatory adipokines[194], and 4) reducing function of leukocytes.[195] Among sweeteners, honey is the best choice since it is the only natural sweetener available with a wide range of health-promoting benefits including anti-inflammatory, anticancer, antibacterial, antioxidant and anti-allergy effects. Also consider the herb *Stevia* as a non-caloric and nutritive sweetener.

---

[185] Lissin LW, Cooke JP. Phytoestrogens and cardiovascular health. *J Am Coll Cardiol*. 2000 May;35(6):1403-10
[186] Golding DN. Is there an allergic synovitis? *J R Soc Med* 1990 May;83(5):312-4
[187] Adam O, Beringer C, Kless T, Lemmen C, Adam A, Wiseman M, Adam P, Klimmek R, Forth W. Anti-inflammatory effects of a low arachidonic acid diet and fish oil in patients with rheumatoid arthritis. *Rheumatol Int* 2003 Jan;23(1):27-36
[188] Dabbagh AJ, Trenam CW, Morris CJ, Blake DR. Iron in joint inflammation. *Ann Rheum Dis* 1993; 52:67-73
[189] "These fish often harbor high levels of methylmercury, a potent human neurotoxin." Evans EC. The FDA recommendations on fish intake during pregnancy. *J Obstet Gynecol Neonatal Nurs* 2002 Nov-Dec;31(6):715-20
[190] "Geometric mean mercury levels were almost 4-fold higher among women who ate 3 or more servings of fish in the past 30 days compared with women who ate no fish in that period.." Schober SE, Sinks TH, Jones RL, Bolger PM, McDowell M, Osterloh J, Garrett ES, Canady RA, Dillon CF, Sun Y, Joseph CB, Mahaffey KR. Blood mercury levels in US children and women of childbearing age, 1999-2000. *JAMA* 2003 Apr 2;289(13):1667-74
[191] For more information on glycemic index, consult a nutrition book or website such as http://www.stanford.edu/~dep/gilists.htm last accessed August 16, 2003
[192] Janette Brand-Miller, Kaye Foster-Powell. Diets with a low glycemic index: from theory to practice. *Nutrition Today* 1999 March. Accessed on-line at: http://www.findarticles.com/cf_dls/m0841/2_34/54654508/p1/article.jhtml on August 16, 2003.
[193] Mendosa D. Glycemic Values of Common American Foods http://www.mendosa.com/common_foods.htm Accessed on August 4, 2004
[194] "Because visceral and subcutaneous adipose tissues are the major sources of cytokines (adipokines), increased adipose tissue mass is associated with alteration in adipokine production (eg, overexpression of tumor necrosis factor-a, interleukin-6, plasminogen activator inhibitor-1, and underexpression of adiponectin in adipose tissue)." Aldhahi W, Hamdy O. Adipokines, inflammation, and the endothelium in diabetes. *Curr Diab Rep*. 2003 Aug;3(4):293-8
[195] Sanchez A, Reeser JL, Lau HS, Yahiku PY, Willard RE, McMillan PJ, Cho SY, Magie AR, Register UD. Role of sugars in human neutrophilic phagocytosis. *Am J Clin Nutr*. 1973 Nov;26(11):1180-4

Occasional intake of sweets is likely to be of little consequence for people who are generally healthy and who are willing to sustain relatively short-term endothelial dysfunction[196], oxidative stress[197], increased LDL oxidation[198], and activation of NF-kappaB[199] as a result of their iatrogenic hyperglycemia. Postexertional hyperglycemia can be used to enhance athletic performance by sustaining and inducing glycogen storage following and during exercise (i.e., carbohydrate loading for glycogen "supercompensation"[200,201]). Similarly, consumption of "simple" carbohydrate without protein can be used to promote entry of tryptophan across the blood-brain barrier and into the brain to promote serotonin synthesis.[202] In summary, *habitual overconsumption* of simple carbohydrates promotes disease by oxidative and proinflammatory mechanisms, while conversely *periodic consumption* of simple carbohydrates can be used to promote athletic performance and to increase intracerebral serotonin synthesis for the promotion of enhanced mood and cognitive performance and for the regulation of food intake.

**Avoid artificial sweeteners, colors and other additives**: Absolutely never use **aspartame**—this is a synthetic chemical that is easily converted to the toxin formaldehyde.[203] Aspartame causes cancer in animals and is strongly linked to brain tumors in humans.[204,205] **Sodium benzoate** is a food preservative that can cause asthma[206] and skin rashes[207] in sensitive individuals. **Tartrazine (yellow dye #5)** is a food/drug coloring agent that can cause asthma and skin rashes in sensitive individuals.[208] **Carrageenan** is a naturally-occurring carbohydrate extracted from red seaweed.

---

[196] "Modest hyperinsulinemia, mimicking fasting hyperinsulinemia of insulin-resistant states, abrogates endothelium-dependent vasodilation in large conduit arteries, probably by increasing oxidant stress. These data may provide a novel pathophysiological basis to the epidemiological link between hyperinsulinemia/insulin-resistance and atherosclerosis in humans." Arcaro G, Cretti A, Balzano S, Lechi A, Muggeo M, Bonora E, Bonadonna RC. Insulin causes endothelial dysfunction in humans: sites and mechanisms. *Circulation*. 2002 Feb 5;105(5):576-82

[197] "Hyperglycemia increased plasma MDA concentrations, but the activities of GSH-Px and SOD were significantly higher after a larger dose of glucose only. Plasma catecholamines were unchanged. These results indicate that the transient increase of plasma catecholamine and insulin concentrations did not induce oxidative damage, while glucose already in the low dose was an important triggering factor for oxidative stress." Koska J, Blazicek P, Marko M, Grna JD, Kvetnansky R, Vigas M. Insulin, catecholamines, glucose and antioxidant enzymes in oxidative damage during different loads in healthy humans. *Physiol Res*. 2000;49 Suppl 1:S95-100

[198] "In conclusion, insulin at physiological doses is associated with increased LDL peroxidation independent of the presence of hyperglycemia." Quinones-Galvan A, Sironi AM, Baldi S, Galetta F, Garbin U, Fratta-Pasini A, Cominacini L, Ferrannini E. Evidence that acute insulin administration enhances LDL cholesterol susceptibility to oxidation in healthy humans. *Arterioscler Thromb Vasc Biol*. 1999 Dec;19(12):2928-32

[199] "These data show that the intake of a mixed meal results in significant inflammatory changes characterized by a decrease in IkappaBalpha and an increase in NF-kappaB binding, plasma CRP, and the expression of IKKalpha, IKKbeta, and p47(phox) subunit." Aljada A, Mohanty P, Ghanim H, Abdo T, Tripathy D, Chaudhuri A, Dandona P. Increase in intranuclear nuclear factor kappaB and decrease in inhibitor kappaB in mononuclear cells after a mixed meal: evidence for a proinflammatory effect. *Am J Clin Nutr*. 2004 Apr;79(4):682-90

[200] "A significant glycogen sparing, as well as supercompensation within 24 h of recovery, was observed after [carbohydrate] supplementation." Brouns F, Saris WH, Beckers E, Adlercreutz H, van der Vusse GJ, Keizer HA, Kuipers H, Menheere P, Wagenmakers AJ, ten Hoor F. Metabolic changes induced by sustained exhaustive cycling and diet manipulation. *Int J Sports Med*. 1989 May;10 Suppl 1:S49-62

[201] "The accepted method of increasing muscle glycogen stores is by "glycogen loading," which classically involves depletion of muscle glycogen, usually by exercise, followed by consumption of a high-CHO diet for several days (e.g., 3, 39). ...increase muscle glycogen concentrations ([glycogen]) to between 150 and 200% of normal resting levels." Robinson TM, Sewell DA, Hultman E, Greenhaff PL. Role of submaximal exercise in promoting creatine and glycogen accumulation in human skeletal muscle. *J Appl Physiol*. 1999 Aug;87(2):598-604

[202] "Our results suggest that high-carbohydrate meals have an influence on serotonin synthesis. We predict that carbohydrates with a high glycemic index would have a greater serotoninergic effect than carbohydrates with a low glycemic index." Lyons PM, Truswell AS. Serotonin precursor influenced by type of carbohydrate meal in healthy adults. *Am J Clin Nutr*. 1988 Mar;47(3):433-9

[203] Trocho C, Pardo R, Rafecas I, Virgili J, Remesar X, Fernandez-Lopez JA, Alemany M. Formaldehyde derived from dietary aspartame binds to tissue components in vivo. *Life Sci*. 1998;63(5):337-4949

[204] Compared to other environmental factors putatively linked to brain tumors, the artificial sweetener aspartame is a promising candidate to explain the recent increase in incidence and degree of malignancy of brain tumors. ...exceedingly high incidence of brain tumors in aspartame-fed rats compared to no brain tumors in concurrent controls..." Olney JW, Farber NB, Spitznagel E, Robins LN. Increasing brain tumor rates: is there a link to aspartame? *J Neuropathol Exp Neurol* 1996;55(11):1115-23

[205] Russell Blaylock MD. Excitotoxins. Health Press; December 1996 [ISBN: 0929173252] Pages 211-214

[206] "Adverse reactions to benzoate in this patient required avoidance of some drugs, some of those classically prescribed under the form of syrups in asthma." Petrus M, Bonaz S, Causse E, Rhabbour M, Moulie N, Netter JC, Bildstein G. [Asthma and intolerance to benzoates] [Article in French] *Arch Pediatr*. 1996;3(10):984-7

[207] Munoz FJ, Bellido J, Moyano JC, Alvarez M, Fonseca JL. Perioral contact urticaria from sodium benzoate in a toothpaste. *Contact Dermatitis*. 1996 Jul;35(1):51

[208] "Tartrazine sensitivity is most frequently manifested by urticaria and asthma... Vasculitis, purpura and contact dermatitis infrequently occur as manifestations of tartrazine sensitivity." Dipalma JR. Tartrazine sensitivity. *Am Fam Physician*. 1990 Nov;42(5):1347-50

Common sources of carrageenan are certain brands of "rice milk" and "soy milk." In addition to suppressing immune function[209], carrageenan causes intestinal ulcers and inflammatory bowel disease in animals[210] and some research indicates that carrageenan consumption is associated with an increased risk for cancer in humans.[211,212]

**Consume sufficient daily water in the form of water and health-promoting teas and juices**: Daily "water" intake should be approximately 30 ml/kg; thus, for a 150-lb (70-kg) person, fluid intake should be at least 2.1 liters, and for a person who weighs 220 lbs (100 kg) the daily intake should be approximately 3 liters. More fluids may be used during times of exercise, heat exposure, illness, or detoxification, while fluid restriction can be indicated in patients with heart failure or renal failure.

**Consider reducing or eliminating caffeine:** This is especially important for people with reactive hypoglycemia, insomnia, anxiety, hypertension, low-back pain, and for women with fibrocystic breast disease. Caffeine ingestion also leads to the activation of brain noradrenergic receptors, which can cause inhibition of dopaminergic pathways.[213] For people who are in good health, 1-3 servings of caffeine per day is not harmful. Herbal teas and green tea have many significant health-promoting effects due to their phytonutrient components.

**To the extent possible, eat "organic" foods rather than industrially-produced foods**: Organic foods (i.e., foods which are *naturally grown* rather than being treated with insect poisons, synthetic fertilizers, and chemicals to enhance shelf-life) tend to cost more than chemically-produced foods; but the increased phytonutrient content justifies the cost. Organic foods contain more nutrients than do chemically-produced foods.[214] More importantly, recent research has also indicated that organic foods are better able to prevent the genetic damage that can lead to cancer than are foods that have been grown in an environment of artificial fertilizers and pesticides.[215]

**Recognize the importance of avoiding food allergens**: Biomedical research has established that adverse food reactions, regardless of the underlying mechanisms or classification of allergy, intolerance, or sensitivity, can exacerbate a wide range of human illnesses, including thyroid disease[216], mental depression[217,218], asthma, rhinitis,[219] recurrent otitis media[220], migraine[221,222,223],

---

[209] "Impairment of complement activity and humoral responses to T-dependent antigens, depression of cell-mediated immunity, prolongation of graft survival and potentiation of tumour growth by carrageenans have been reported." Thomson AW, Fowler EF. Carrageenan: a review of its effects on the immune system. *Agents Actions*. 1981;11(3):265-73
[210] Watt J, Marcus R. Experimental ulcerative disease of the colon. *Methods Achiev Exp Pathol*. 1975;7:56-71
[211] Tobacman JK. Review of harmful gastrointestinal effects of carrageenan in animal experiments. *Environ Health Perspect*. 2001 Oct;109(10):983-94
[212] "However, the gum carrageenan which is comprised of linked, sulfated galactose residues has potent biological activity and undergoes acid hydrolysis to poligeenan, an acknowledged carcinogen." Tobacman JK, Wallace RB, Zimmerman MB. Consumption of carrageenan and other water-soluble polymers used as food additives and incidence of mammary carcinoma. *Med Hypotheses*. 2001 May;56(5):589-98
[213] "The results suggest that noradrenergic innervation of dopamine cells can directly inhibit the activity of dopamine cells. Paladini CA, Williams JT. Noradrenergic inhibition of midbrain dopamine neurons. *J Neurosci*. 2004 May 12;24(19):4568-75
[214] Smith B. Organic Foods versus Supermarket Foods: element levels. *Journal of Applied Nutrition* 1993; 45(1), p35-9
[215] "Against BaP, three species of OC vegetables showed 30-57% antimutagenecity, while GC ones did only 5-30%." Ren H, Endo H, Hayashi T. The superiority of organically cultivated vegetables to general ones regarding antimutagenic activities. *Mutat Res*. 2001 Sep 20;496(1-2):83-8
[216] Sategna-Guidetti C, Volta U, Ciacci C, Usai P, Carlino A, De Franceschi L, Camera A, Pelli A, Brossa C. Prevalence of thyroid disorders in untreated adult celiac disease patients and effect of gluten withdrawal: an Italian multicenter study. *Am J Gastroenterol*. 2001 Mar;96(3):751-7
[217] "The detection and treatment of psychological dysfunction related to food intolerance with particular reference to the problem of objective evaluation is discussed… Long-term follow-up revealed maintenance of marked improvements in psychological and physical functioning." Mills N. Depression and food intolerance: a single case study. *Hum Nutr Appl Nutr*. 1986 Apr;40(2):141-5
[218] "OBJECTIVE: To describe a patient with food intolerance probably contributing to depressive symptoms, intolerance to psychotropic medication and treatment resistance… RESULTS: The patient's course improved considerably with an elimination diet." Parker G, Watkins T. Treatment-resistant depression: when antidepressant drug intolerance may indicate food intolerance. *Aust N Z J Psychiatry*. 2002 Apr;36(2):263-5
[219] Speer F. The allergic child. *Am Fam Physician*. 1975 Feb;11(2):88-94
[220] Juntti H, Tikkanen S, Kokkonen J, Alho OP, Niinimaki A. Cow's milk allergy is associated with recurrent otitis media during childhood. *Acta Otolaryngol*. 1999;119(8):867-73

attention deficit and hyperactivity disorders[224], epilepsy[225,226,227], gastrointestinal inflammation[228], hypertension[229], joint pain and inflammation[230,231,232,233,234,235,236,237] and a wide range of other health problems. Any program of health promotion and health maintenance must include consideration of food allergies, food intolerances, and food sensitivities.

**Supplement the healthy diet with specific vitamins, minerals, and fatty acids**: Despite the fact that America is one of the richest nations on earth, and that we produce more than enough food to feed ourselves and many other nations with a healthy diet, Americans tend to have poor dietary habits and inadequate levels of nutritional intake that do not meet the minimal standards, such as the Recommended Daily Allowance (RDA, now Daily Reference Intake (DRI)).[238] Many people are under the misperception that if they appear healthy or are even overweight then they could not possibly have nutritional deficiencies. The truths of this matter are that 1) gross/obvious nutritional deficiencies are common among "apparently healthy" individuals, 2) common situations like stress, poor diets, and use of medications predispose people to nutritional deficiencies, 3) hereditary/genetic disorders affect a large portion of the population and lead to an increased need for nutritional intake which can generally only be met with supplementation in addition to a healthy whole-foods diet. Taking a "one-a-day" multivitamin is insufficient for people who truly desire significant benefit from supplementation. These one-a-day preparations generally only provide the minimum daily allowance—this dose is not large enough to provide truly preventive medicine results.

---

[221] "Foods which provoked migraine in 9 patients with severe migraine refractory to drug therapy were identified… These observations confirm that a food-allergic reaction is the cause of migraine in this group of patients." Monro J, Carini C, Brostoff J. Migraine is a food-allergic disease. *Lancet*. 1984 Sep 29;2(8405):719-21
[222] Egger J, Carter CM, Wilson J, et al. Is migraine food allergy? A double-blind controlled trial of oligoantigenic diet treatment. *Lancet*. 1983 Oct 15;2(8355):865-9
[223] Monro J, Brostoff J, Carini C, Zilkha K. Food allergy in migraine. Study of dietary exclusion and RAST. *Lancet*. 1980 Jul 5;2(8184):1-4
[224] Boris M, Mandel FS. Foods and additives are common causes of the attention deficit hyperactive disorder in children. *Ann Allergy*. 1994 May;72(5):462-8
[225] Egger J, Carter CM, Soothill JF, Wilson J. Oligoantigenic diet treatment of children with epilepsy and migraine. *J Pediatr*. 1989;114(1):51-8
[226] Pelliccia A, Lucarelli S, Frediani T, D'Ambrini G, Cerminara C, Barbato M, Vagnucci B, Cardi E. Partial cryptogenetic epilepsy and food allergy/intolerance. A causal or a chance relationship? Reflections on three clinical cases. *Minerva Pediatr*. 1999 May;51(5):153-7
[227] Frediani T, Lucarelli S, Pelliccia A, Vagnucci B, et al. Allergy and childhood epilepsy: a close relationship? *Acta Neurol Scand*. 2001;104(6):349-52
[228] Marr HY, Chen WC, Lin LH. Food protein-induced enterocolitis syndrome: report of one case. *Acta Paediatr Taiwan*. 2001;42(1):49-52
[229] Grant EC. Food allergies and migraine. *Lancet*. 1979 May 5;1(8123):966-9
[230] "Food allergy appeared to be responsible for the joint symptoms in three patients and in one it was possible to precipitate swelling of a knee due to synovitis with effusion by drinking milk a few hours beforehand, the synovial fluid having mildly inflammatory features and a relatively high eosinophil count." Golding DN. Is there an allergic synovitis? *J R Soc Med*. 1990 May;83(5):312-4
[231] Panush RS. Food induced ("allergic") arthritis: clinical and serologic studies. *J Rheumatol*. 1990 Mar;17(3):291-4
[232] Pacor ML, Lunardi C, Di Lorenzo G, Biasi D, Corrocher R. Food allergy and seronegative arthritis: report of two cases. *Clin Rheumatol*. 2001;20(4):279-81
[233] Schrander JJ, Marcelis C, de Vries MP, van Santen-Hoeufft HM. Does food intolerance play a role in juvenile chronic arthritis? *Br J Rheumatol*. 1997 Aug;36(8):905-8
[234] van de Laar MA, van der Korst JK. Food intolerance in rheumatoid arthritis. I. A double blind, controlled trial of the clinical effects of elimination of milk allergens and azo dyes. *Ann Rheum Dis*. 1992 Mar;51(3):298-302
[235] Haugen MA, Kjeldsen-Kragh J, Forre O. A pilot study of the effect of an elemental diet in the management of rheumatoid arthritis. *Clin Exp Rheumatol*. 1994;12(3):275-9
[236] van de Laar MA, Aalbers M, Bruins FG, et al. Food intolerance in rheumatoid arthritis. II. Clinical and histological aspects. *Ann Rheum Dis*. 1992;51(3):303-6
[237] Panush RS, Stroud RM, Webster EM. Food-induced (allergic) arthritis. Inflammatory arthritis exacerbated by milk. *Arthritis Rheum*1986; 29(2): 220-6
[238] "Most people do not consume an optimal amount of all vitamins by diet alone. Pending strong evidence of effectiveness from randomized trials, it appears prudent for all adults to take vitamin supplements." Fletcher RH, Fairfield KM. Vitamins for chronic disease prevention in adults: clinical applications. *JAMA* 2002 Jun 19;287(23):3127-9

For people still not convinced of the importance of a multi-vitamin/mineral supplement as part of the basic foundation of the health plan, please consider the following data from the medical research:
- Many people think that eating a "healthy diet" will supply them with the nutrients that they need and that they do not need to take a vitamin supplement. This may have been true 200 years ago, but today's industrially produced "foods" are generally stripped of much of their nutritional value long before they leave the factory. Industrially-produced fruits and vegetables contain less nutrients than naturally raised "organic" produce.[239]
- The reason that people can be of normal weight or can even be overweight and obese and still have nutrient deficiencies is that the body lowers the metabolic rate when the intake of vitamins and minerals is low. This is referred to as the "physiologic adaptation to marginal malnutrition." Even though people may eat enough calories and protein, they can still suffer from growth retardation and behavioral problems as a result of malnutrition, even though they *appear* nourished.[240]
- Most nutrition-oriented doctors will agree that magnesium is one of the most important nutrients, especially for helping prevent heart attack and stroke. **Magnesium deficiency is an epidemic in so-called "developed" nations, with 20-40% of different populations showing objective serologic/cytologic evidence of magnesium deficiency.**[241,242,243,244]
- Add to the above that every day we are confronted with more chronic emotional stress and toxic chemicals than has ever before existed on the planet, and it becomes easy to see that basic nutritional support and an organic whole foods diet is just the start of attaining improved health.

### Putting it all together with "the supplemented Paleo-Mediterranean diet":

The health-promoting diet of choice for the majority of people is a diet based on abundant consumption of fruits, vegetables, seeds, nuts, omega-3 and monounsaturated fatty acids, and lean sources of protein such as lean meats, fatty cold-water fish, soy and whey proteins. This diet prohibits and obviates overconsumption of chemical preservatives, artificial sweeteners, and carbohydrate-dominant foods such as candies, pastries, breads, potatoes, grains, and other foods with a high glycemic load and high glycemic index. This "Paleo-Mediterranean Diet" is a combination of the "Paleolithic" or "Paleo diet" and the well-known "Mediterranean diet", both of which are well described in peer-reviewed journals and the lay press. The Mediterranean diet is characterized by increased proportions of legumes, nuts, seeds, whole grain products, fruits, vegetables (including potatoes), fish and lean meats, and monounsaturated and n-3 fatty acids.[245] Consumption of this diet is consistently associated with improvements in insulin sensitivity and

---

[239] Smith B. Organic Foods versus Supermarket Foods: element levels. *Journal of Applied Nutrition* 1993; 45(1), p35-9. I recently found that this article is also available on-line at http://journeytoforever.org/farm_library/bobsmith.html as of June 19, 2004
[240] Allen LH. The nutrition CRSP: what is marginal malnutrition, and does it affect human function? *Nutr Rev* 1993 Sep;51(9):255-67
[241] "The American diet is low in magnesium, and with modern water systems, very little is ingested in the drinking water." Innerarity S. Hypomagnesemia in acute and chronic illness. *Crit Care Nurs Q*. 2000 Aug;23(2):1-19
[242] "Altogether 43% of 113 trauma patients had low magnesium levels compared to 30% of noninjured cohorts." Frankel H, Haskell R, Lee SY, Miller D, Rotondo M, Schwab CW. Hypomagnesemia in trauma patients. *World J Surg*. 1999 Sep;23(9):966-9
[243] "There was a 20% overall prevalence of hypomagnesemia among this predominantly female, African American population." Fox CH, Ramsoomair D, Mahoney MC, Carter C, Young B, Graham R. An investigation of hypomagnesemia among ambulatory urban African Americans. *J Fam Pract*. 1999 Aug;48(8):636-9
[244] "Suboptimal levels were detected in 33.7 per cent of the population under study. These data clearly demonstrate that the Mg supply of the German population needs increased attention." Schimatschek HF, Rempis R. Prevalence of hypomagnesemia in an unselected German population of 16,000 individuals. *Magnes Res*. 2001 Dec;14(4):283-90
[245] Curtis BM, O'Keefe JH Jr. Understanding the Mediterranean diet. Could this be the new "gold standard" for heart disease prevention? *Postgrad Med*. 2002 Aug;112(2):35-8, 41-5 http://www.postgradmed.com/issues/2002/08_02/curtis.htm

reductions in cardiovascular disease, diabetes, cancer, and all-cause mortality.[246] The Paleolithic diet detailed by collaborators Eaton[247], O'Keefe[248], and Cordain[249] is similar to the Mediterranean diet except for stronger emphasis on fruits and vegetables (preferably raw or minimally cooked), omega-3-rich lean meats, and reduced consumption of starchy foods such as potatoes and grains, the latter of which were not staples in the human diet until the last few thousand years. Emphasizing the olive oil and red wine of the Mediterranean diet and the absence of grains and potatoes per the Paleo diet appears to be the way to get the best of both dietary worlds; the remaining diet is characterized by fresh whole fruits, vegetables, nuts (especially almonds), seeds, olive oil, lean meats rich in n-3 fatty acids, and red wine in moderation. In sum, this dietary plan along with the inclusion of garlic and dark chocolate (a rich source of cardioprotective, antioxidative, and anti-inflammatory polyphenolic flavonoids[250,251]) is expected to reduce adverse cardiovascular events by more than 76%.[252] Biochemical justification for this type of diet is ample and is well supported by numerous long-term studies in humans wherein both Mediterranean and Paleolithic diets result in dramatic reductions in disease-specific and all-cause mortality.[253,254,255,256] Diets rich in fruits and vegetables are sources of more than 5,000 phytochemicals, many of which have antioxidant, anti-inflammatory, and anti-cancer properties.[257] Oleic acid, squalene, and phenolics in olive oil and phenolics and resveratrol in red wine have antioxidant, anti-inflammatory, and anti-cancer properties and also protect against cardiovascular disease.[258] N-3 fatty acids have numerous health benefits via multiple mechanisms as described in the sections that follow. Increased intake of dietary fiber from fruits and vegetable favorably modifies gut flora, promotes xenobiotic elimination (via flora modification, laxation, and overall reductions in enterohepatic recirculation), and is associated with reductions in morbidity and mortality. Such a "Paleolithic diet" can also lead to urinary alkalinization (average urine pH of ≥ 7.5 according to Sebastian et al[259]) which increases renal *retention of minerals* for improved musculoskeletal health[260,261,262] and which increases *urinary*

---

[246] Knoops KT, de Groot LC, Kromhout D, Perrin AE, Moreiras-Varela O, Menotti A, van Staveren WA. Mediterranean diet, lifestyle factors, and 10-year mortality in elderly European men and women: the HALE project. *JAMA*. 2004 Sep 22;292(12):1433-9

[247] Eaton SB, Shostak M, Konner M. The Paleolithic Prescription: A program of diet & exercise and a design for living, New York: Harper & Row, 1988

[248] O'Keefe JH Jr, Cordain L. Cardiovascular disease resulting from a diet and lifestyle at odds with our Paleolithic genome: how to become a 21st-century hunter-gatherer. *Mayo Clin Proc.* 2004 Jan;79(1):101-8

[249] Cordain L. The Paleo Diet: Lose Weight and Get Healthy by Eating the Food You Were Designed to Eat. Indianapolis; John Wiley and Sons, 2002

[250] Schramm DD, Wang JF, Holt RR, Ensunsa JL, Gonsalves JL, Lazarus SA, Schmitz HH, German JB, Keen CL. Chocolate procyanidins decrease the leukotriene-prostacyclin ratio in humans and human aortic endothelial cells. *Am J Clin Nutr.* 2001;73(1):36-40

[251] Engler MB, Engler MM, Chen CY, et al. Flavonoid-rich dark chocolate improves endothelial function and increases plasma epicatechin concentrations in healthy adults. *J Am Coll Nutr*. 2004;23(3):197-204

[252] Franco OH, Bonneux L, de Laet C, Peeters A, Steyerberg EW, Mackenbach JP. The Polymeal: a more natural, safer, and probably tastier (than the Polypill) strategy to reduce cardiovascular disease by more than 75%. *BMJ*. 2004;329(7480):1447-50

[253] de Lorgeril M, Salen P, Martin JL, Monjaud I, Boucher P, Mamelle N. Mediterranean dietary pattern in a randomized trial: prolonged survival and possible reduced cancer rate. *Arch Intern Med*. 1998 Jun 8;158(11):1181-7

[254] Knoops KT, de Groot LC, Kromhout D, Perrin AE, Moreiras-Varela O, Menotti A, van Staveren WA. Mediterranean diet, lifestyle factors, and 10-year mortality in elderly European men and women: the HALE project. *JAMA*. 2004 Sep 22;292(12):1433-9

[255] Lindeberg S, Cordain L, and Eaton SB. Biological and clinical potential of a Paleolithic diet. *J Nutri Environ Med* 2003; 13:149-160

[256] O'Keefe JH Jr, Cordain L, Harris WH, Moe RM, Vogel R. Optimal low-density lipoprotein is 50 to 70 mg/dl: lower is better and physiologically normal. *J Am Coll Cardiol*. 2004 Jun 2;43(11):2142-6

[257] Liu RH. Health benefits of fruit and vegetables are from additive and synergistic combinations of phytochemicals. *Am J Clin Nutr*. 2003;78(3 Sup):517S-520S

[258] Alarcon de la Lastra C, Barranco MD, Motilva V, Herrerias JM. Mediterranean diet and health: biological importance of olive oil. *Curr Pharm Des*. 2001;7:933-50

[259] Sebastian A, Frassetto LA, Sellmeyer DE, Merriam RL, Morris RC Jr. Estimation of the net acid load of the diet of ancestral preagricultural Homo sapiens and their hominid ancestors. *Am J Clin Nutr* 2002;76:1308-16

[260] Sebastian A, Harris ST, Ottaway JH, Todd KM, Morris RC Jr. Improved mineral balance and skeletal metabolism in postmenopausal women treated with potassium bicarbonate. *N Engl J Med*. 1994;330(25):1776-81

[261] Tucker KL, Hannan MT, Chen H, Cupples LA, Wilson PW, Kiel DP. Potassium, magnesium, and fruit and vegetable intakes are associated with greater bone mineral density in elderly men and women. *Am J Clin Nutr*. 1999;69(4):727-36

[262] Whiting SJ, Boyle JL, Thompson A, Mirwald RL, Faulkner RA. Dietary protein, phosphorus and potassium are beneficial to bone mineral density in adult men consuming adequate dietary calcium. *J Am Coll Nutr*. 2002;21(5):402-9

*elimination of many toxicants and xenobiotics* for a tremendous reduction in serum levels and thus adverse effects from chemical exposure or drug overdose.[263] Furthermore, therapeutic alkalinization was recently shown in an open trial with 82 patients to reduce symptoms and disability associated with low-back pain and to increase intracellular magnesium concentrations by 11%.[264] **Ample intake of amino acids via dietary proteins supports phase-2 detoxification** (amino acid and sulfate conjugation) for proper xenobiotic elimination[265,266], **provides amino acid precursors for neurotransmitter synthesis** and maintenance of mood, memory, and cognitive performance[267,268,269,270], **and prevents the immunosuppression and decrements in musculoskeletal status caused by low-protein diets**.[271] Described originally by the current author[272], the "supplemented Paleo-Mediterranean diet" provides patients the best of current knowledge in nutrition by relying on a foundational diet plan of fresh nuts, seeds, fruits, vegetables, fish, and lean meats which is adorned with olive oil for its squalene, phenolic antioxidant/anti-inflammatory and monounsaturated fatty acid content. Inclusive of medical foods such as red wine, garlic, and dark chocolate which may synergize to effect at least a 76% reduction in cardiovascular disease[273], this diet also reduces the risk for cancer[274] and can be an integral component of a health-promoting lifestyle.[275] Competitive athletes are allowed increased carbohydrate consumption before and after training and competition.[276]

*Implementation Notes*:

---

[263] Proudfoot AT, Krenzelok EP, Vale JA. Position Paper on urine alkalinization. *J Toxicol Clin Toxicol*. 2004;42(1):1-26

[264] "The results show that a disturbed acid-base balance may contribute to the symptoms of low back pain. The simple and safe addition of an alkaline multimineral preparate was able to reduce the pain symptoms in these patients with chronic low back pain." Vormann J, Worlitschek M, Goedecke T, Silver B. Supplementation with alkaline minerals reduces symptoms in patients with chronic low back pain. J Trace Elem Med Biol. 2001;15:179-83

[265] Liska DJ. The detoxification enzyme systems. *Altern Med Rev*. 1998;3:187-9

[266] Anderson KE, Kappas A. Dietary regulation of cytochrome P450. *Annu Rev Nutr*. 1991;11:141-67

[267] Rogers RD, Tunbridge EM, Bhagwagar Z, Drevets WC, Sahakian BJ, Carter CS. Tryptophan depletion alters the decision-making of healthy volunteers through altered processing of reward cues. *Neuropsychopharmacology*. 2003;28:153-62 Accessed at http://www.acnp.org/sciweb/journal/Npp062402336/default.htm on November 10, 2004

[268] Arnulf I, Quintin P, Alvarez JC, Vigil L, Touitou Y, Lebre AS, Bellenger A, Varoquaux O, Derenne JP, Allilaire JF, Benkelfat C, Leboyer M. Mid-morning tryptophan depletion delays REM sleep onset in healthy subjects. *Neuropsychopharmacology*. 2002;27(5):843-51 Accessed at http://www.acnp.org/sciweb/journal/Npp042502293/default.htm on November 10, 2004

[269] Thomas JR, Lockwood PA, Singh A, Deuster PA. Tyrosine improves working memory in a multitasking environment. *Pharmacol Biochem Behav*. 1999;64:495-500

[270] Markus CR, Olivier B, Panhuysen GE, Van Der Gugten J, Alles MS, Tuiten A, Westenberg HG, Fekkes D, Koppeschaar HF, de Haan EE. The bovine protein alpha-lactalbumin increases the plasma ratio of tryptophan to the other large neutral amino acids, and in vulnerable subjects raises brain serotonin activity, reduces cortisol concentration, and improves mood under stress. *Am J Clin Nutr*. 2000;71:1536-44

[271] Castaneda C, Charnley JM, Evans WJ, Crim MC. Elderly women accommodate to a low-protein diet with losses of body cell mass, muscle function, and immune response. *Am J Clin Nutr*. 1995;62:30-9

[272] **Vasquez A**. Five-Part Nutritional Protocol that Produces Consistently Positive Results. *Nutritional Wellness* 2005 Sept. http://optimalhealthresearch.com/protocol

[273] Franco OH, Bonneux L, de Laet C, Peeters A, Steyerberg EW, Mackenbach JP. The Polymeal: a more natural, safer, and probably tastier (than the Polypill) strategy to reduce cardiovascular disease by more than 75%. *BMJ*. 2004;329(7480):1447-50

[274] "The combination of 4 low risk factors lowered the all-cause mortality rate to 0.35 (95% CI, 0.28-0.44). In total, lack of adherence to this low-risk pattern was associated with a population attributable risk of 60% of all deaths, 64% of deaths from coronary heart disease, 61% from cardiovascular diseases, and 60% from cancer." Knoops KT, de Groot LC, Kromhout D, et al. Mediterranean diet, lifestyle factors, and 10-year mortality in elderly European men and women: the HALE project. *JAMA*. 2004 Sep 22;292(12):1433-9

[275] Orme-Johnson DW, Herron RE. An innovative approach to reducing medical care utilization and expenditures. *Am J Manag Care*. 1997;3(1):135-44

[276] Cordain L, Friel J. The Paleo Diet for Athletes : A Nutritional Formula for Peak Athletic Performance: Rodale Books (September 23, 2005)

## Profile of The Supplemented Paleo-Mediterranean Diet[277]

| Foods to consume: whole, natural, minimally processed foods include: | Foods to avoid: factory products, high-sugar foods, and chemicals |
|---|---|
| ☺ <u>Lean sources of protein</u><br>• Fish (avoiding tuna which is commonly loaded with mercury)<br>• Chicken and turkey<br>• Lean cuts of free-range grass-fed meats: beef, buffalo, lamb are occasionally acceptable<br>• Soy protein[278] and whey protein[279,280]<br>☺ <u>Fruits and fruit juices</u><br>☺ <u>Vegetables and vegetable juices</u><br>☺ <u>Nuts, seeds, berries</u><br>☺ <u>Generous use of olive oil</u>: On sautéed vegetables and fresh salads<br>☺ <u>Daily vitamin/mineral supplementation</u>: With a high-potency broad-spectrum multivitamin and multimineral supplement[281]<br>☺ <u>Sun exposure or vitamin D3 supplementation</u>: To ensure provision of 2,000-5,000 IU of vitamin D3 per day for adults[282]<br>☺ <u>Balanced broad-spectrum fatty acid supplementation</u>: With ALA, GLA, EPA, and DHA[283]<br>☺ <u>Water, tea, home-made fruit/vegetable juices</u>: Commercial vegetable juices are commonly loaded with sodium chloride; choose appropriately. Fruit juices can be loaded with natural and superfluous sugars. Herbal teas can be selected based on the medicinal properties of the plant that is used. | ☒ Avoid as much as possible fat-laden arachidonate-rich meats like beef, liver, pork, and lamb, as well as high-fat cream and other dairy products with emulsified, readily absorbed saturated fats and arachidonic acid<br>☒ <u>High-sugar pseudofoods</u>:<br>• Corn syrup<br>• Cola and soda<br>• Donuts, candy, etc…."junk food"<br>☒ <u>Grains such as wheat, rye, barley</u>: These have only existed in the human diet for less than 10,000 years and are consistently associated with increased prevalence of degenerative diseases due to the allergic response they invoke and because of their high glycemic load and high glycemic index.<br>☒ <u>Potatoes and rice</u>: High in sugar, low in phytonutrients<br>☒ <u>Avoid allergens</u>: Determined per individual<br>☒ <u>Chemicals</u>:<br>• <u>Pesticides, Herbicides, Fungicides</u><br>• <u>Carcinogenic sweeteners</u>: aspartame[284]<br>• <u>Artificial flavors</u><br>• <u>Artificial colors</u>: tartrazine<br>• <u>Preservatives</u>: benzoate<br>• <u>Flavor enhancers</u>: carrageenan and monosodium glutamate |

---

[277] **Vasquez A**. Five-Part Nutritional Protocol that Produces Consistently Positive Results. *Nutritional Wellness* 2005 Sept. http://optimalhealthresearch.com/protocol
[278] "These results indicate that for healthy adults, the isolated soy protein is of high nutritional quality, comparable to that of animal protein sources, and that the methionine content is not limiting for adult protein maintenance." Young VR, Puig M, Queiroz E, Scrimshaw NS, Rand WM. Evaluation of the protein quality of an isolated soy protein in young men: relative nitrogen requirements and effect of methionine supplementation. *Am J Clin Nutr*. 1984 Jan;39(1):16-24
[279] Bounous G. Whey protein concentrate (WPC) and glutathione modulation in cancer treatment. *Anticancer Res*. 2000 Nov-Dec;20(6C):4785-92
[280] Markus CR, Olivier B, Panhuysen GE, Van Der Gugten J, Alles MS, Tuiten A, Westenberg HG, Fekkes D, Koppeschaar HF, de Haan EE. The bovine protein alpha-lactalbumin increases the plasma ratio of tryptophan to the other large neutral amino acids, and in vulnerable subjects raises brain serotonin activity, reduces cortisol concentration, and improves mood under stress. *Am J Clin Nutr*. 2000 Jun;71(6):1536-44 http://www.ajcn.org/cgi/content/full/71/6/1536
[281] "Most people do not consume an optimal amount of all vitamins by diet alone. …it appears prudent for all adults to take vitamin supplements." Fletcher RH, Fairfield KM. Vitamins for chronic disease prevention in adults: clinical applications. *JAMA*. 2002;287:3127-9
[282] **Vasquez A**, Manso G, Cannell J. The clinical importance of vitamin D (cholecalciferol): a paradigm shift with implications for all healthcare providers. *Altern Ther Health Med*. 2004 Sep-Oct;10(5):28-36 http://optimalhealthresearch.com/monograph04
[283] **Vasquez A**. Reducing Pain and Inflammation Naturally. Part 2: New Insights into Fatty Acid Supplementation and Its Effect on Eicosanoid Production and Genetic Expression. *Nutritional Perspectives* 2005; January: 5-16 www.optimalhealthresearch.com/part2
[284] "In the past two decades brain tumor rates have risen in several industrialized countries, including the United States... Compared to other environmental factors putatively linked to brain tumors, the artificial sweetener aspartame is a promising candidate to explain the recent increase in incidence and degree of malignancy of brain tumors." Olney JW, Farber NB, Spitznagel E, Robins LN. Increasing brain tumor rates: is there a link to aspartame? *J Neuropathol Exp Neurol* 1996 Nov;55(11):1115-23

# Biochemical Individuality and Orthomolecular Medicine

"**Biochemical individuality**" was the term coined by biochemist Dr. Roger Williams of the University of Texas[285] to describe the genetic and physiologic variations in human beings that produced different nutritional needs among individuals. Because we all have different genes, each of our bodies therefore creates different protein enzymes, and many of these enzymes—which are essential for proper cellular function—are adversely affected by defects in their construction (i.e., amino acid sequence) that reduce their efficiency. Dr. Linus Pauling[286] noted that single amino acid substitutions could produce dramatic alterations in protein function. Pauling discovered that sickle cell disease was caused by a single amino acid substitution in the hemoglobin molecule, and for this discovery he won the Nobel Prize in Chemistry in 1954.[287] With recognition of the importance of individual molecules in determining health or disease, Pauling coined the phrase "**orthomolecular medicine**" based on his thesis that many diseases could be effectively prevented and treated if we used the "**right molecules**" to correct abnormal physiologic function. Pauling contrasted the clinical use of nutrients for the improvement of physiologic function (orthomolecular medicine) with the use of chemical drugs, which generally work by interfering with normal physiology (toximolecular medicine). Since nutrients are the fundamental elements of the human body from which all enzymes, chemicals, and cellular structures are formed, Pauling advocated that the use of customized nutrition and nutritional supplements could promote optimal health by optimizing cellular function and efficiency. More recently, Dr. Bruce Ames has thoroughly documented the science of the orthomolecular precepts[288] and has advocated **optimal diets along with nutritional supplementation** as a highly efficient and cost-effective method for preventing disease and optimizing health.[289,290] In sum, we see that 1) the foundational diet must be formed from whole foods such as fruits, nuts, seeds, vegetables, and lean meats, 2) processed and artificial foods should be

> **Orthomolecular precepts**
> - The functions of the body are dependent upon thousands of enzymes. Because of genetic defects that are common in the general population, some of these enzymes are commonly defective – even if only slightly – in large portions of the human population.
> - Enzyme defects reduce the function and efficiency of important chemical reactions. Because enzymes are so important for normal function and the prevention of disease, defects in enzyme function can result in disruptions in physiology and the creation of what later manifests as "disease."
> - Rather than treating these diseases with synthetic chemical drugs, it is commonly possible to prevent and treat disease with high-doses of vitamins, minerals, and other nutrients to compensate for or bypass metabolic dysfunctions, thus allowing for the promotion of optimal health by promoting optimal physiologic function.

---

[285] "Every individual organism that has a distinctive genetic background has distinctive nutritional needs which must be met for optimal well-being. …[N]utrition applied with due concern for individual genetic variations…offers the solution to many baffling health problems." Williams RJ. Biochemical Individuality : The Basis for the Genetotrophic Concept. Austin and London: University of Texas Press, 1956. Page x

[286] "…the concentration of coenzyme [vitamins and minerals] needed to produce the amount of active enzyme required for optimum health may well be somewhat different for different individuals. …many individuals may require a considerably higher concentration of one or more coenzymes than other people do for optimum health…" Pauling L. On the Orthomolecular Environment of the Mind: Orthomolecular Theory. In: Williams RJ, Kalita DK. A Physician's Handbook on Orthomolecular Medicine. New Cannan; Keats Publishing: 1977. Page 76

[287] http://www.nobel.se/chemistry/laureates/1954/pauling-bio.html on April 4, 2004

[288] "About 50 human genetic dis-eases due to defective enzymes can be remedied or ameliorated by the administration of high doses of the vitamin component of the corresponding coenzyme, which at least partially restores enzymatic activity." Ames BN, Elson-Schwab I, Silver EA. High-dose vitamin therapy stimulates variant enzymes with decreased coenzyme binding affinity (increased K(m)): relevance to genetic disease and polymorphisms. *Am J Clin Nutr*. 2002 Apr;75(4):616-58

[289] "An optimum intake of micronutrients and metabolites, which varies with age and genetic constitution, would tune up metabolism and give a marked increase in health, particularly for the poor and elderly, at little cost." Ames BN. The metabolic tune-up: metabolic harmony and disease prevention. *J Nutr*. 2003 May;133(5 Suppl 1):1544S-8S

[290] "Optimizing micronutrient intake [through better diets, fortification of foods, or multivitamin-mineral pills] can have a major impact on public health at low cost." Ames BN. Cancer prevention and diet: help from single nucleotide polymorphisms. *Proc Natl Acad Sci* U S A. 1999 Oct 26;96(22):12216-8

avoided, and 3) the use of nutritional supplements is necessary to provide sufficiently high levels of nutrition to overcome defects in enzymatic activity.

---

**Molecular basis for high-dose nutrient supplementation**

"As many as **one-third of mutations** in a gene result in the corresponding enzyme having an increased Michaelis constant, or Km, (decreased binding affinity) for a coenzyme, resulting in a lower rate of reaction. **About 50 human genetic dis-eases due to defective enzymes can be remedied or ameliorated by the administration of high doses of the vitamin component of the corresponding coenzyme**, which at least partially restores enzymatic activity."

"**High doses of vitamins are used to treat many inheritable human diseases**. The molecular basis of disease arising from as many as one-third of the mutations in a gene is an increased Michaelis constant, or Km, (decreased binding affinity) of an enzyme for the vitamin-derived coenzyme or substrate, which in turn lowers the rate of the reaction."

Ames BN, Elson-Schwab I, Silver EA. High-dose vitamin therapy stimulates variant enzymes with decreased coenzyme binding affinity (increased K(m)): relevance to genetic disease and polymorphisms. *Am J Clin Nutr*. 2002 Apr;75(4):616-58
http://www.ajcn.org/cgi/content/full/75/4/616

---

## Nutrigenomics: Nutritional Genomics

> "The fundamental concepts of [nutrigenomics] are that **the progression from a healthy phenotype to a chronic disease phenotype must occur by changes in gene expression** or by differences in activities of proteins and enzymes and that **dietary chemicals directly or indirectly regulate the expression of genomic information**."[291]

"Genome" refers to all of the genetic material in an organism, and "genomics" is the field of study of this information. The field of nutritional genomics—nutrigenomics—refers to the clinical synthesis of 1) research on the human genome (e.g., the Human Genome Project[292]), and 2) the advancing science of clinical nutrition, including research on nutraceuticals (nutritional medicines) and phytomedicinals (botanical medicines). Nutrigenomics represents a major advance in our understanding of the underlying biochemical and physiologic mechanisms of the effects of nutrition. Nutrition is far more than "fuel" for our biophysiologic machine; we know now that nutrition—the consumption of specific proteins, amino acids, vitamins, minerals, fatty acids, and phytochemicals—can alter genetic expression and can thus either promote health or disease at the very fundamental level of genetic expression. The commonly employed excuse that many patients use—"I just have bad genes"—now takes on a whole new meaning; it may be that these patients suffer from the expression of "bad genes" *because of the food that they eat*. The concept and phenomenon of nutrigenomics can be described by saying that each of us has the

---

[291] Kaput J, Rodriguez LR. Nutritional genomics: the next frontier in the postgenomic era. *Physiol Genomics* 16: 166–177 http://physiolgenomics.physiology.org/cgi/content/full/16/2/166
[292] "Begun formally in 1990, the U.S. Human Genome Project is a 13-year effort coordinated by the U.S. Department of Energy and the National Institutes of Health. The project originally was planned to last 15 years, but rapid technological advances have accelerated the expected completion date to 2003. Project goals are to identify all the approximate 30,000 genes in human DNA..." See the official Human Genome website at http://www.ornl.gov/sci/techresources/Human_Genome/home.shtml

genes for health, as well as the genes for disease; what largely determines our level of health is how we treat our genes with environmental inputs, especially nutrition. We appear able, to a large extent, to "turn on" disease-promoting genes with poor nutrition and a pro-inflammatory lifestyle[293,294], while, to a lesser extent, we are able to activate or "turn on" health-promoting genes with a healthy diet[295] and with proper nutritional supplementation.[296] For additional details, see the literature cited in this section and the review article by Vasquez available on-line.[297]

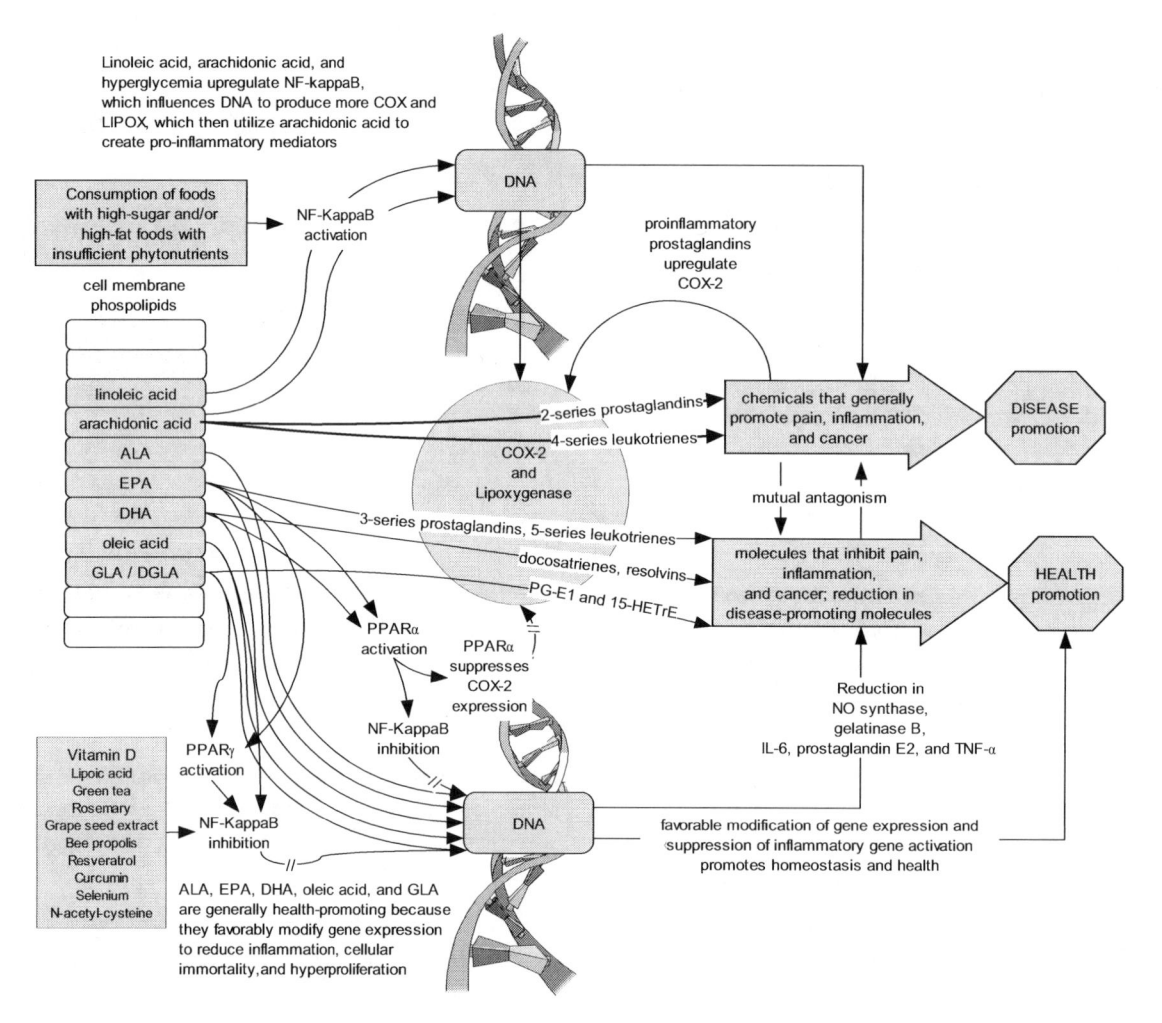

**Nutrigenomics--a conceptual diagram**: Nutrients strongly influence genetic expression as well as post-transcriptional/translational metabolism.

---

[293] Rusyn I, Bradham CA, Cohn L, Schoonhoven R, Swenberg JA, Brenner DA, Thurman RG. Corn oil rapidly activates nuclear factor-kappaB in hepatic Kupffer cells by oxidant-dependent mechanisms. *Carcinogenesis*. 1999 Nov;20(11):2095-100 http://carcin.oxfordjournals.org/cgi/content/full/20/11/2095
[294] Aljada A, Mohanty P, Ghanim H, Abdo T, Tripathy D, Chaudhuri A, Dandona P. Increase in intranuclear nuclear factor kappaB and decrease in inhibitor kappaB in mononuclear cells after a mixed meal: evidence for a proinflammatory effect. *Am J Clin Nutr*. 2004 Apr;79(4):682-90
[295] O'Keefe JH Jr, Cordain L. Cardiovascular disease resulting from a diet and lifestyle at odds with our Paleolithic genome. *Mayo Clin Proc*. 2004 Jan;79(1):101-8
[296] Kaput J, Rodriguez LR. Nutritional genomics: the next frontier in the postgenomic era. *Physiol Genomics* 16: 166–177 http://physiolgenomics.physiology.org/cgi/content/full/16/2/166
[297] **Vasquez A**. Reducing pain and inflammation naturally - Part 4: Nutritional and Botanical Inhibition of NF-kappaB, the Major Intracellular Amplifier of the Inflammatory Cascade. A Practical Clinical Strategy Exemplifying Anti-Inflammatory Nutrigenomics. *Nutritional Perspectives* 2005; July: 5-12 www.OptimalHealthResearch.com/part4

# General Guidelines for the Safe Use of Nutritional Supplements

Supplementation with vitamins and minerals is generally safe, especially if the following guidelines are followed:

- **Iron is potentially harmful**: Iron promotes the formation of "free radicals" and is thus implicated in several diseases, such as infections, cancer, liver disease, diabetes, and cardiovascular disease. Iron supplements should not be consumed except by people who have been definitively diagnosed with iron deficiency by measurement of serum ferritin.

- **Vitamins and minerals should generally be taken with food in order to eliminate the possibility of nausea and to increase absorption**: Most vitamins and other supplements should be taken with food so that nausea is avoided.

- **Vitamin A is one of the only vitamins with the potential for serious toxicity even at low doses**: Attention should be given to vitamin A intake so that toxicity is avoided. Add vitamin A amounts from all sources—foods, fish oils, and vitamin supplements. Manifestations of vitamin A toxicity include: skin problems (dry skin, flaking skin, chapped or split lips, red skin rash, hair loss), joint pain, bone pain, headaches, anorexia (loss of appetite), edema (water retention, weight gain, swollen ankles, difficulty breathing), fatigue, and/or liver damage.
    - Adults: Women who are pregnant or might become pregnant and who are planning to carry the baby to full term delivery should not ingest more than 10,000 IU of vitamin A per day. Vitamin A toxicity is seen with chronic ingestion of therapeutic doses (for example: 25,000 IU per day for 6 years, or 100,000 IU per day for 2.5 years[298]). Most patients should not consume more than 20,000 IU of vitamin A per day for more than 2 months without express supervision by a healthcare provider. Vitamin A is present in some multivitamins, in cod liver oil, and in other supplements—read labels to ensure that the total daily intake is not greater than 20,000 IU per day.
    - Infants and Children: Different studies have used either daily or monthly schedules of vitamin A supplementation. In a study with extremely low-birth weight infants, 5,000 IU of vitamin A per day for 28 days was safely used.[299] In another study conducted in sick children, those aged less than 12 months received 100,000 IU on two consecutive days, while children between ages 12-60 months received a larger dose of 200,000 IU on two consecutive days.[300]

- **Preexisting kidney problems (such as renal failure) increase the risks associated with nutritional supplementation**: Supplementation with vitamins and minerals does not cause kidney damage. However, if a patient already has kidney problems, then vitamin/mineral/protein supplementation may become hazardous. Assessment of renal

---

[298] "The smallest continuous daily consumption leading to cirrhosis was 25,000 IU during 6 years, whereas higher daily doses (greater than or equal to 100,000 IU) taken during 2 1/2 years resulted in similar histological lesions. ... The data also indicate that prolonged and continuous consumption of doses in the low "therapeutic" range can result in life-threatening liver damage." Geubel AP, De Galocsy C, Alves N, Rahier J, Dive C. Liver damage caused by therapeutic vitamin A administration: estimate of dose-related toxicity in 41 cases. *Gastroenterology*. 1991 Jun;100(6):1701-9

[299] "Infants with birth weight < 1000 g were randomised at birth to receive oral vitamin A supplementation (5000 IU/day) or placebo for 28 days." Wardle SP, Hughes A, Chen S, Shaw NJ. Randomised controlled trial of oral vitamin A supplementation in preterm infants to prevent chronic lung disease. *Arch Dis Child Fetal Neonatal Ed*. 2001 Jan;84(1):F9-F13 Available on-line at http://adc.bmjjournals.com/cgi/content/full/fetalneonatal%3b84/1/F9

[300] "Children were assigned to oral doses of 200 000 IU vitamin A (half that dose if <12 months) or placebo on the day of admission, a second dose on the following day, and third and fourth doses at 4 and 8 months after discharge from the hospital, respectively." Villamor E, Mbise R, Spiegelman D, Hertzmark E, Fataki M, Peterson KE, Ndossi G, Fawzi WW. Vitamin A supplements ameliorate the adverse effect of HIV-1, malaria, and diarrheal infections on child growth. *Pediatrics*. 2002 Jan;109(1):E6

function with serum or urine tests is encouraged before beginning an aggressive plan of supplementation. Conditions which cause kidney damage include:
- Use of specific medications—acetaminophen, aspirin, contrast and chemotherapy agents
- Hypertension, high blood pressure
- Diabetes mellitus
- Use of recreational drugs, such as cocaine[301]
- Other diseases, such as lupus (SLE) and polycystic kidney disease

- **Several drugs/medications may adversely interact with vitamin/mineral supplements and with botanical medicines**: Vitamins/minerals may reduce the effectiveness of some prescription medications. For example, taking certain antibiotics such as Cipro or tetracycline with calcium reduces absorption of the drugs, therefore rendering the drugs much less effective. Taking botanical medicines with medications may make the drugs dangerously less effective (such as when St. John's Wort is combined with protease inhibitor drugs[302]) or may make the drug dangerously more effective (such when Kava is combined with the anti-anxiety drug alprazolam[303]). If vitamin D is used in doses greater than 1,000 IU/d in patients taking hydrochlorothiazide or other calcium-retaining drugs, serum calcium should be monitored at least monthly until safety (i.e., lack of hypercalcemia) has been established per patient.[304] Patients should not combine nutritional or botanical medicines with chemical/synthetic drugs without specific advice from a knowledgeable doctor. Do not increase vitamin K consumption from supplements or dietary improvements in patients taking coumadin/warfarin. A reasonable recommendation is that nutritional supplements be taken 2 hours away from pharmaceutical medications to avoid complications such as intraintestinal drug-nutrient binding.

- **Pre-existing medical conditions may make supplementation unsafe**: A few rare medical conditions may cause nutritional supplementation to be unsafe, including severe liver disease, renal failure, electrolyte imbalances, hyperparathyroidism and other vitamin D hypersensitivity syndromes.

*Notes*:

---

[301] Horowitz BZ, Panacek EA, Jouriles NJ. Severe rhabdomyolysis with renal failure after intranasal cocaine use. *J Emerg Med*. 1997 Nov-Dec;15(6):833-7
[302] Piscitelli SC, Burstein AH, Chaitt D, Alfaro RM, Falloon J. Indinavir concentrations and St John's wort. *Lancet*. 2000 Feb 12;355(9203):547-8
[303] Almeida JC, Grimsley EW. Coma from the health food store: interaction between kava and alprazolam. *Ann Intern Med*. 1996 Dec 1;125(11):940-1
[304] **Vasquez A**, Manso G, Cannell J. The clinical importance of vitamin D (cholecalciferol): a paradigm shift with implications for all healthcare providers. *Altern Ther Health Med*. 2004 Sep-Oct;10(5):28-36 http://optimalhealthresearch.com/monograph04

## Emotional, Mental, and Social Health

### Stress management and authentic living

Mental, emotional, and physical "stress" describes any unpleasant living condition which can lead to negative effects on health, such as increased blood pressure, depression, apathy, increased muscle tension, and, according to some research, increased risk of serious health problems such as early death from cardiovascular disease and cancer. Many people find that their modern lives are characterized by excess amounts of multitasking, job responsibilities, family responsibilities, commuter traffic, expenses and an insufficient amount of relaxation, sleep, community support, exercise, time in nature, healthy nutrition, and time to simply *be* rather than *do*. Stress comes in many different forms and includes malnutrition, trauma, insufficient exercise (epidemic), excess exercise (rare), sleep deprivation, emotional turmoil, and exposure to chemicals and radiation. When most people talk about "stress" they are referring to either chronic anxiety (such as with high-pressure work situations or dysfunctional interpersonal relationships) or the acute stress reaction that is typical of unpredictable rapid-onset events such as an injury, accident, or other physically threatening situation. These **"different types of stress" are not separate from each other**; emotional stress causes nutritional depletion[305]; sleep deprivation alters immune response[306], chemical exposure can disrupt endocrine function.[307] Therefore, **any type of stress can cause other types of stress**. Avoiding stressful situations is, of course, an effective way to avoid being bothered or harmed by them. If work-related stress is the problem, then finding a new position or occupation is certainly an option worth considering and implementing. High-stress jobs are often high-paying jobs; but if in the process of making money, a person ruins her health and loses years from her life, then no one would ever say, "It was worth it." Money, success, and freedom only have value for the person alive and healthy to enjoy them. ***Toxic relationships***, whether at home or work, are relationships that cause more harm than good by re-injuring old emotional wounds and by creating new emotional injuries. We can all benefit from affirming our right to a happy and healthy life by minimizing/eliminating contact with people who cause emotional harm to us—this requires conscious effort[308]; Engel[309] provides a clear articulation and description of abusive relationships, along with checklists for their recognition and exercises for their remediation.

> "Good relationships make you feel loved, wanted, and cared for."
>
> Malcolm LL. Health Style. London; Thorsons: 2001, p 133

---

[305] Ingenbleek Y, Bernstein L. The stressful condition as a nutritionally dependent adaptive dichotomy. *Nutrition* 1999 Apr;15(4):305-20
[306] Heiser P, Dickhaus B, Opper C, Hemmeter U, Remschmidt H, Wesemann W, Krieg JC, Schreiber W. Alterations of host defense system after sleep deprivation are followed by impaired mood and psychosocial functioning. *World J Biol Psychiatry* 2001 Apr;2(2):89-94
[307] "Evidence suggests that environmental exposure to some anthropogenic chemicals may result in disruption of endocrine systems in human and wildlife populations." http://www.epa.gov/endocrine on March 7, 2004
[308] Bryn C. Collins. *How to Recognize Emotional Unavailability and Make Healthier Relationship Choices*. [Mjf Books; ISBN: 1567313442] Recently reprinted as: Emotional Unavailability: Recognizing It, Understanding It, and Avoiding Its Trap [McGraw Hill - NTC (April 1998); ISBN: 0809229145]
[309] Engel B. *The Emotionally Abusive Relationship: How to Stop Being Abused and How to Stop Abusing*. Wiley Publishers: 2003

|  | *Mental/emotional* | *Physical* | *Nutritional/biochemical* |
|---|---|---|---|
| *Therapeutic considerations* | • Social support<br>• Re-parenting<br>• Conversational style[310]<br>• Meditation, prayer<br>• Healthy boundaries<br>• Books, tapes, groups<br>• Expressive writing[311]<br>• Time to simply experience and otherwise "do nothing" | • Yoga<br>• Massage<br>• Exercise<br>• Stretching<br>• Swimming<br>• Resting<br>• Biking<br>• Hiking<br>• Affection | • Vitamins, including vitamin C[312]<br>• Fish oil[313]<br>• Hormones, cytokines, neurotransmitters, and eicosanoids<br>• Botanical medicines such as *kava*[314], *Ashwaganda,* and *Eleutherococcus* |

An important concept is that **stress is a "whole body" phenomenon**: affecting the mind, the brain, emotional state, the physical body (including musculoskeletal, immune, and cardiovascular systems), as well as the nutritional status of the individual. The adverse effects of stress can be reduced with an integrated combination of therapeutics that addresses each of the major body systems affected by stress, which are 1) mental/emotional, 2) physical, and 3) nutritional/biochemical.

**Stress affects the whole body.**

Therefore, a complete stress management program must address the whole body:

*Physical*
*Structural*

*Biochemical*
*Hormonal*
*Nutritional*

*Mental*
*Emotional*
*Spiritual*

- Mental / Emotional / Neurological / Spiritual
- Chemical / Nutritional / Hormonal
- Physical / Structural / Exercise

---

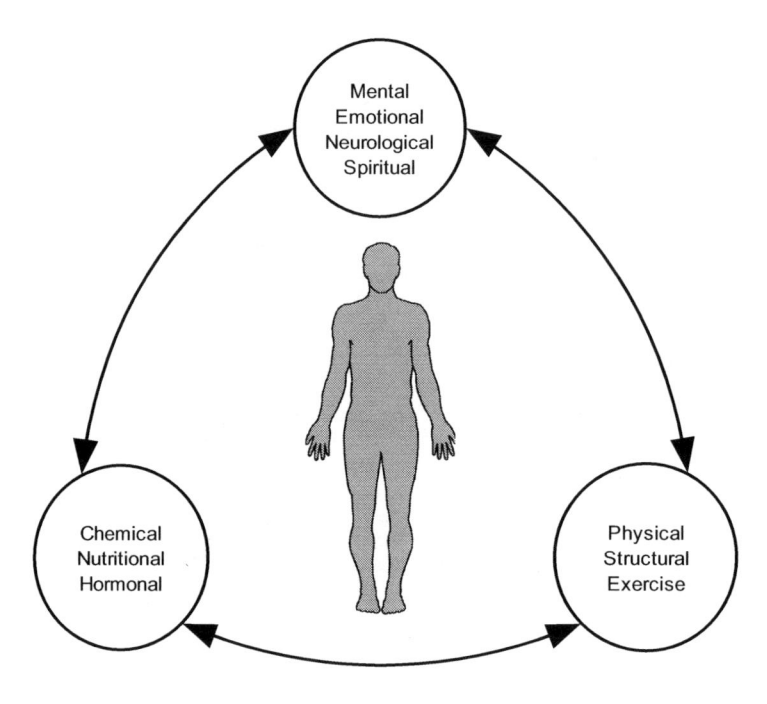

[310] Rick Brinkman ND and Rick Kirschner ND. *How to Deal With Difficult People* [Audio Cassette. Career Track, 1995]
[311] Smyth JM, Stone AA, Hurewitz A, Kaell A. Effects of writing about stressful experiences on symptom reduction in patients with asthma or rheumatoid arthritis: a randomized trial. *JAMA*. 1999 Apr 14;281(14):1304-9
[312] Brody S, Preut R, Schommer K, Schurmeyer TH. A randomized controlled trial of high dose ascorbic acid for reduction of blood pressure, cortisol, and subjective responses to psychological stress. *Psychopharmacology* (Berl). 2002 Jan;159(3):319-24
[313] Hamazaki T, Itomura M, Sawazaki S, Nagao Y. Anti-stress effects of DHA. *Biofactors*. 2000;13(1-4):41-5
[314] Cagnacci A, et al. Kava-Kava administration reduces anxiety in perimenopausal women. *Maturitas*. 2003 Feb 25;44(2):103-9

Sometimes a stressful situation can be modified into one that is less stressful or dysfunctional, so that the benefits are retained, yet the negative aspects are reduced. Of course, the best example of this is interpersonal relationships, which easily lend themselves to improvement with the application of conscious effort. Many audiotapes, books, and seminars are available for people interested in having improved interpersonal relationships. Selected resources are listed here:

- <u>Men & Women: Talking Together</u> by Deborah Tannen and Robert Bly [Sound Horizons, 1992. ISBN: 1879323095] A lively discussion of the different communication and relationship styles of men and women by two respected experts in their fields.
- <u>How to Deal with Difficult People</u> by Drs. Rick Brinkman and Rick Kirschner. [Audio Cassette. Career Track, 1995] An entertaining format with solutions to common workplace and situational difficulties. Authored and performed by two naturopathic physicians.
- <u>Men are From Mars, Women are From Venus</u> by John Gray. [Audio Cassette and Books]. Phenomenally popular concepts in understanding, accepting, and effectively integrating the differences between men and women.
- <u>The ManKind Project</u> (<u>www.mkp.org</u>). An international organization hosting events for men and women. The men's events, formats, and groups are authentic, clear, and healthy. The ManKind Project has an organization for women called The WomanWithin (<u>www.womanwithin.org</u>). No book or tape can substitute for the dynamics and personal attention that can be experienced by a conscious, empowered, and well-intended group.

When "the problem" cannot be avoided, and the interaction/relationship with the problem cannot be improved, a remaining option is to supplement the internal environment so that it is somewhat "strengthened" to deal with the stress of the bothersome event or situation. For example, when dealing with emotional stress, we can use counseling, support groups, or various relaxation techniques.[315] If we determine that the emotional stress has a biochemical component, then we can use specific botanical and nutritional supplementation to safely and naturally support and restore normal function. Moving deeper into the issue of "stress management" requires that we ask why a person is in a stressful situation to begin with. Of course, with *random acts of chaos* like car accidents, we cannot always ascribe the problem to the person, unless the accident resulted from their own negligence. But **when people are chronically stressed and unhappy about their jobs and/or relationships, then we need to employ more than stress reduction techniques**, and as clinicians we need to offer more than the latest adaptogen. **We have to ask why a person would subject himself/herself to such a situation, and what fears or limitations (self-imposed and/or externally applied) keep him/her from breaking free into a life that works.**[316,317,318,319]

---

[315] Martha Davis PhD, Matthew McKay MSW, Elizabeth Robbins Eshelman PhD. <u>The Relaxation & Stress Reduction Workbook 5th edition</u>. New Harbinger Publishers; 2000. [ISBN: 1572242140]
[316] Rick Jarow. <u>Creating the Work You Love: Courage, Commitment and Career</u>; Inner Traditions Intl Ltd; 1995 [ISBN: 0892815426]
[317] Breton D and Largent C. <u>The Paradigm Conspiracy: Why Our Social Systems Violate Human Potential-And How We Can Change Them</u>. Hazelden: 1998
[318] Dominguez JR. <u>Transforming Your Relationship With Money</u>. Sounds True; Book and Cassette edition: 2001 Audio tape.
[319] Gatto JT. <u>Dumbing us down: the hidden curriculum of compulsory education</u>. Gabriola Island, Canada; New Society Publishers: 2005

**Stress always has a biochemical/physiologic component**: Regardless of its origins, stress always takes a toll on the body—*the whole body*. Well-documented effects of stress include:
1. Increased levels of cortisol—higher levels are associated with osteoporosis, memory loss, slow healing
2. Reduced function of thyroid hormones[320]
3. Reduced levels of testosterone (in men)
4. Increased intestinal permeability and "leaky gut"[321]
5. Increased excretion of minerals in the urine
6. Increased need for vitamins and amino acids
7. Suppression of immune function and of natural killer cells that fight viral infections and tumors
8. Decreased production of sIgA—the main defense of the lungs, gastrointestinal tract, and genitourinary tract
9. Increased populations of harmful bacteria in the intestines and an associated increased rate of lung and upper respiratory tract infections
10. Increased incidence of food allergies[322]
11. Sleep disturbance

**The body functions as a whole—not as independent, autonomous organ systems**: Problems with one aspect of health create problems in other aspects of health. Treatment of disease and promotion of wellness must therefore improve overall health and functioning while simultaneously addressing the disease or presenting complaint.

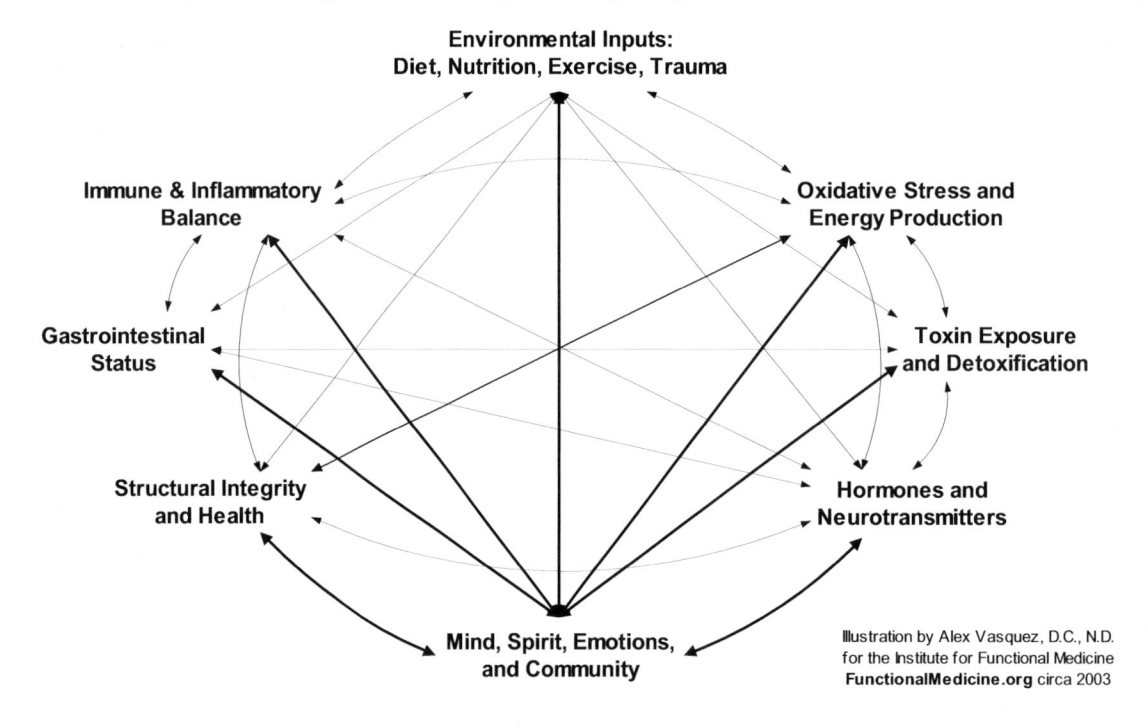

Illustration by Alex Vasquez, D.C., N.D. for the Institute for Functional Medicine
FunctionalMedicine.org circa 2003

---

[320] Ingenbleek Y, Bernstein L. The stressful condition as a nutritionally dependent adaptive dichotomy. *Nutrition* 1999 Apr;15(4):305-20
[321] Hart A, Kamm MA. Review article: mechanisms of initiation and perpetuation of gut inflammation by stress. *Aliment Pharmacol Ther* 2002;16(12):2017-28
[322] Anderzen I, Arnetz BB, Soderstrom T, Soderman E. Stress and sensitization in children: a controlled prospective psychophysiological study of children exposed to international relocation. *Journal of Psychosomatic Research* 1997; 43: 259-69

## **Autonomization, intradependence, emotional literacy, corrective experience**:

> "None of us are completely developed people when we reach adulthood.
> We are each incomplete in our own way."   Merle Fossum[323]

Consciousness-raising is a keystone gift that holistic physicians can impart to their patients and one which may be necessary for true healing to be manifested and maintained. Healthcare providers are quick to enlighten their patients to the details of diet, exercise, nutrition, medications, surgeries, and other *biomechanical* and *biochemical* aspects of health, but are routinely negligent when it comes to sharing with patients the emotional tools that may be necessary to repair or construct the "self" which is supposed to implement the treatment plan that the doctor has designed. Passivity and ignorance are not hindrances to the success of the *medical paradigm*, which requires that patients are "compliant" rather than self-directed; however, for *authentic, holistic healthcare* to be successful, it must empower the patient sufficiently such that he/she attains/regains appropriate *autonomy*—an "internal locus of control"—sufficient for lifelong internally-driven health maintenance. Health implications of autonomy (or its absence) are obvious and intuitive. For example, patients with an underdeveloped internal locus of control appear to experience greater degrees of social stress which can lead to hypercortisolemia and hippocampal atrophy.[324] Additionally, internal locus of control correlates strongly with the success of weight-loss programs, and for nonautonomous patients it is necessary to encourage the development of autonomous self-care behavior in addition to the provision of information about diet and exercise.[325]

Completely formed internal identities are the natural result of the *continuum* of positive childhood experiences (inclusive of stability, "unconditional love", healthy parenting, and active, conscious intergenerational social contact) which are ideally segued into adolescent and adulthood experiences of success, acceptance, inclusion, independence, interdependence, and intradependence with the end result being a socially-conscious adult with an internal locus of control. Where the patient has experienced a relative absence of these natural and expected prerequisites, there can only exist a truncated self. This largely explains why so many adult patients feign that they are incapable of action, "can't exercise", and "can't leave" their abusive jobs and relationships, and "can't resist" the dietary habits which daily contribute to their physical and psychoemotional decline. Thus, for more than a few patients, a therapeutic path must be explored which helps to re-create the foundation from which an autonomous adult and authentic self can grow—it is a *process* (not an event) of **emotional recovery**.[326] To this extent, interventional or therapeutic *autonomization* resembles a *recovery program* that can include various forms of conscious action, including goal-setting, positive reinforcement, developing **emotional literacy**[327] and **emotional intelligence**[328], and consciousness-raising experiences such as therapy and group work—all of which serve to intentionally (re)create the necessary climate

---

[323] Fossum M. Catching Fire: Men Coming Alive in Recovery. New York; Harper/Hazelden: 1989, 4-7

[324] "Cumulative exposure to high levels of cortisol over the lifetime is known to be related to hippocampal atrophy... Self-esteem and internal locus of control were significantly correlated with hippocampal volume in both young and elderly subjects." Pruessner JC, Baldwin MW, Dedovic K, Renwick R, Mahani NK, Lord C, Meaney M, Lupien S. Self-esteem, locus of control, hippocampal volume, and cortisol regulation in young and old adulthood. *Neuroimage*. 2005 Dec;28(4):815-26

[325] "Their weight loss was significant and associated with an internal locus of control orientation (P < 0.05)... Participants with an internal orientation could be offered a standard weight reduction programme. Others, with a more external locus of control orientation, could be offered an adapted programme, which also focused on and encouraged the participants' internal orientation." Adolfsson B, Andersson I, Elofsson S, Rossner S, Unden AL. Locus of control and weight reduction. *Patient Educ Couns*. 2005 Jan;56(1):55-61

[326] Bradshaw J. Healing the Shame that Binds You [Audio Cassette (April 1990) Health Communications Audio; ISBN: 1558740430]

[327] Dayton T. Trauma and Addiction: Ending the Cycle of Pain Through Emotional Literacy. Deerfield Beach; Health Communications, 2000

[328] Goleman D. Emotional Intelligence. New York; Bantam Books: 1995. Although the book as a whole was considered pioneering for its time, and the book continues to make a valuable contribution, a few of the concepts and author's personal stories are embarrassingly simplistic.

for selfhood. Therewith, the patient can accept challenges to further develop an *empowered self* by participating in exercises of intentional intradependence (self-reliance)—situations in which the ability to decide, choose, and act responsibly and appropriately are reinforced to eventually become second nature, replacing passivity, inaction, and ineffectiveness.[329] "Empowerment" can only be authentic if it is built on the foundation of a developed self. Thus while *recovery* and *empowerment* are separate spheres of activity and attention, they are not mutually exclusive and indeed are synergistic. However, *empowerment* cannot succeed without *recovery* because otherwise so-called "empowerment" is simply a complex defense mechanism that "protects" against pain and thereby blocks the development of an authentic self. In the words of Janov[330], **"Anything that builds a stronger defense system deepens the neurosis."**

**Primary, secondary, and tertiary means for developing an autonomous, authentic self**: Ideally, positive childhood experiences (A) segue into adolescent and adult experiences of confidence and maturity (B) for the development of a true adult (C). If A or B are lacking or insufficient, the result is an incomplete self often incapable of *effective* and *appropriate* action. **Corrective experiences must then be pursued to re-establish the foundation from which an authentic self can arise**.

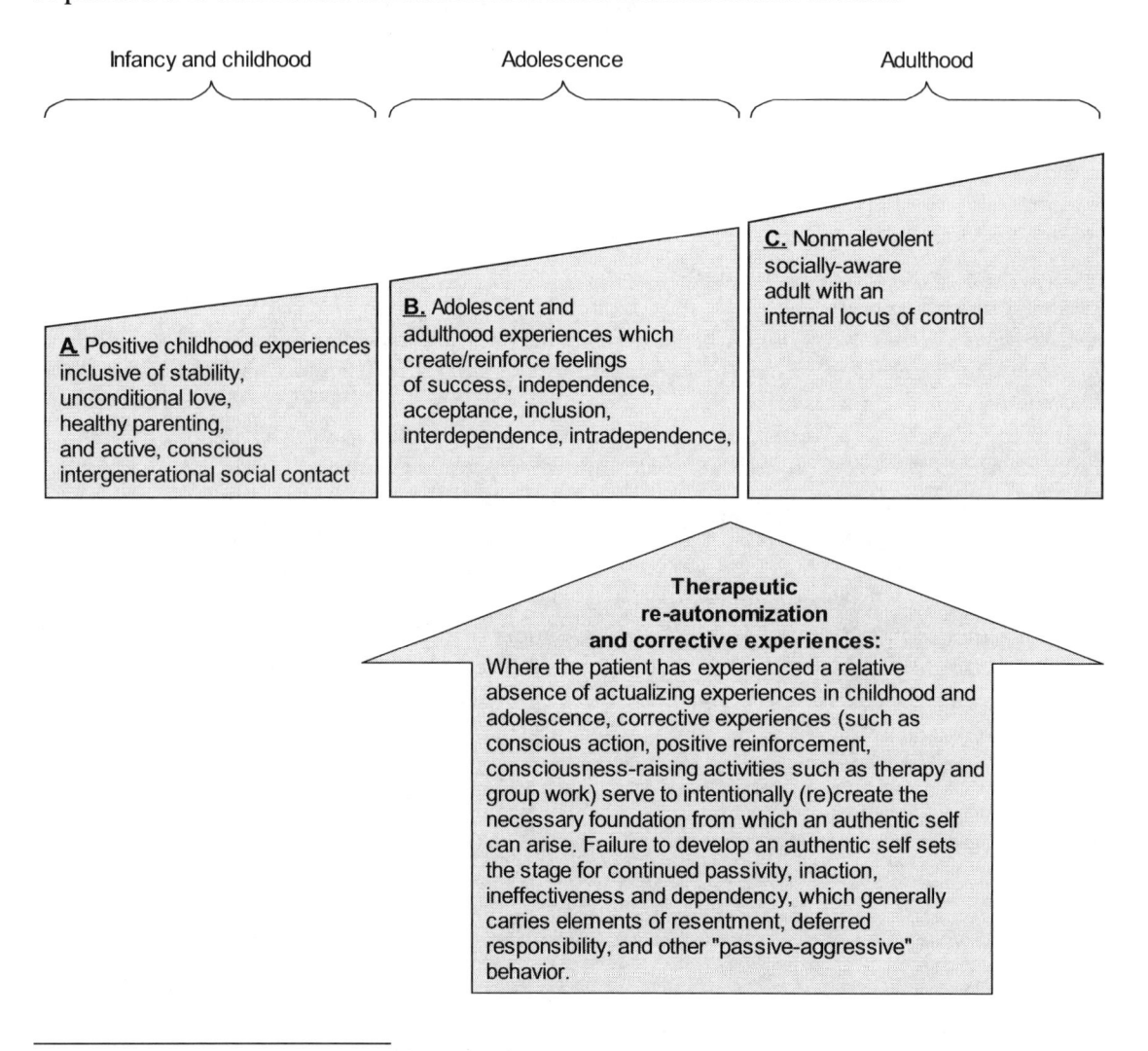

Infancy and childhood | Adolescence | Adulthood

**A.** Positive childhood experiences inclusive of stability, unconditional love, healthy parenting, and active, conscious intergenerational social contact

**B.** Adolescent and adulthood experiences which create/reinforce feelings of success, independence, acceptance, inclusion, interdependence, intradependence,

**C.** Nonmalevolent socially-aware adult with an internal locus of control

**Therapeutic re-autonomization and corrective experiences:** Where the patient has experienced a relative absence of actualizing experiences in childhood and adolescence, corrective experiences (such as conscious action, positive reinforcement, consciousness-raising activities such as therapy and group work) serve to intentionally (re)create the necessary foundation from which an authentic self can arise. Failure to develop an authentic self sets the stage for continued passivity, inaction, ineffectiveness and dependency, which generally carries elements of resentment, deferred responsibility, and other "passive-aggressive" behavior.

---

[329] Gatto JT. A Schooling Is Not An Education: interview by Barbara Dunlop. http://www.johntaylorgatto.com/bookstore/index.htm
[330] Janov A. The Primal Scream. New York; GP Putnam's Sons: 1970, page 20

> "The object of healing is…to move closer to wholeness."
>
> Albert Kreinheder, PhD, Jungian analyst[331]

Patients lacking an internal locus of control are much more likely to succumb to the tantalizing barrage of direct-to-consumer drug advertising[332] which infantilizes patients by 1) oversimplifying diseases, their causes, and treatments, 2) telling them that the disease is not their fault, and 3) encouraging a dependent, passively receptive role by telling patients that they have no proactive role other than to "ask your doctor if a prescription is right for you." It is no accident that Americans consume more prescription and OTC medications per capita than people in any other country.[333,334] With the combined and synergistic effects of 1) the dissolution of first the extended family and now the nuclear family[335], 2) a society-wide famine of mentors, elders, and community[336,337,338], 3) a dearth of autonomous, genuine exploration from childhood to adulthood, and 4) primary and secondary "educational" institutions designed to squelch independence and autonomy in favor of the more efficient, predictable, and controllable conformity and "standardization"[339,340], **industrialized societies have raised generations of people who lack completely formed internal identities**. Lacking an internal locus of control and identity from which to think independently and critically, these "adults" are easy prey for slick and flashy drug advertisements that promise the illusion of perfect health in exchange for passivity, abdication, and lifelong medicalization. It's bad enough that on average each American watches 4 hours of television per day[341] but what's worse is that "Americans who watch average amounts of television may be exposed to more than 30 hours of direct-to-consumer drug advertisements each year, far surpassing their exposure to other forms of health communication."[342] Thus, the pharmaceutical companies are the main source of "health education" for Americans, and—as we would expect—the solutions they propose for all health problems is drugs, drugs, drugs. It is obvious that if we are to wean our suckling culture from undue dependence on the pharmaceutical industry, we have to address our patient population directly and transform them from *passive, nonautonomous, and ignorant about health and disease* to pro-active, autonomous, and well-informed about health and the means required to obtain and sustain it.

> "…like most prospective consumers of therapy, I made up a bunch of excuses for why I could handle this on my own…
> I was smiling like an idiot…"
>
> Jeffrey Kottler, *The Compleat Therapist*[343]

Insight into a patient's internal dynamic can provide the clinician with an understanding that explains the phenomena of *non-compliance* and *disease identification*. Rather than seeing non-compliance as "weakness of will", non-compliance as a form of "disobedience" may be a

---

[331] Kreinheder A. Body and soul: the other side of illness. Toronto, Canada; Inner City Books: 1991, page 38
[332] Aronson E. The Social Animal. San Fransisco; WH Freeman and company: 1972: 21-22, 53
[333] America the medicated. http://www.cbsnews.com/stories/2005/04/21/health/printable689997.shtml and http://www.msnbc.msn.com/id/7503122/ . See also http://usgovinfo.about.com/od/healthcare/a/usmedicated.htm Accessed September 17, 2005.
[334] Kivel P. You Call This a Democracy? Apex Press (August, 2004). ISBN: 1891843265 http://www.paulkivel.com/
[335] Bly R. Iron John. Reading, Mass.: Addison Wesley, 1990
[336] Bly R. The Sibling Society. Vintage Books USA; Reprint edition (June 1, 1997) ISBN: 0679781285 (Abridged audio edition (May 1, 1996), ASIN: 0679451609)
[337] Bly R. Where have all the parents gone? A talk on the Sibling Society. New York: Sound Horizons, 1996 Highly recommended.
[338] Bly R, Hillman J, Meade M. Men and the Life of Desire. Oral Tradition Archives. ISBN: 1880155001. Audio Cassette
[339] Gatto JT. Dumbing Us Down: the Hidden Curriculum of Compulsory Education. Gabriola Island, Canada; New Society Publishers: 2005
[340] Gatto JT. The Paradox of Extended Childhood. [From a presentation in Cambridge, Mass. October 2000] http://www.johntaylorgatto.com/bookstore/index.htm
[341] "American children view over 23 hours of television per week. * Teenagers view an average of 21 to 22 hours of television per week. * By the time today's children reach age 70, they will have spent 7 to 10 years of their lives watching television." American Academy of Pediatrics http://www.aapcal.org/aapcal/tv.html See also TV-Turnoff Network. Facts and Figures About our TV Habit http://www.tvturnoff.org/factsheets.htm Accessed September 17, 2005
[342] Brownfield ED, Bernhardt JM, Phan JL, Williams MV, Parker RM. Direct-to-consumer drug advertisements on network television: an exploration of quantity, frequency, and placement. J Health Commun. 2004 Nov-Dec;9(6):491-7
[343] Kottler JA. The Compleat Therapist. San Francisco; Jossey-Bass publishers; 1991, pages 2-3

reflection of the patient's unconscious need to wrestle with and resolve parental introjects. For example, if a patient had a rejecting, nonaffirming parent, he/she may need to find another rejecting authority figure in order to continue playing the role of the child; by assuming this role and "setting the stage", the patient is unconsciously attempting to create a situation wherein the primary relationship can be healed.[344] Complicating this is *disease identification*—in which patients use their disease as a source of identity and secondary gain for martyrdom, social support, group participation, acceptance, admiration, purpose, excitement, and drama.

---

### Helping Patients (Re)Create Themselves: Practical Applications, Exercises, and Concepts

An absent or underdeveloped locus of control is the key problem that underlies many anxiety disorders, addictive behavioral traits such as overeating, overworking, codependency, as well as chronic ineffectiveness in the pursuit of one's goals. The solutions to this problem are logical, practical, and accessible to everyone; the major costs associated with each are open-mindedness, attentiveness, discipline and persistence. There is scant mention of this concept and its intervention in the biomedical literature; however, it is well described in the psychological literature, particularly that which focuses on various types of "recovery" such as that from addiction, co-dependence, and low self-esteem, the latter two of which are virtually synonymous with an insufficient internal locus of control.

There is no single path here. There are many paths. The goal is not to choose the right path; rather the goal is to travel several paths to the degree necessary, implement what has been learned, travel other paths, and return to the same path again to retrace one's steps in new ways. The process is similar to that of *ceremonial initiation*, the purpose of which is to formally mark the *beginning* of a process that is *ongoing* and *infinite*.[345] Each path and each process has its gifts, significance, and limitations. However, the ultimate goal of each must be a tangible and positive change in the ways which the patient either feels and/or behaves in and interacts with the world on a day-to-day basis.

In no particular order (since the proper sequence will have to be customized to the situation and willingness of the patient), the following are some of the more commonly cited exercises, processes, and sources of additional information:

**_Apprenticeship and Mentoring: books, tapes, and lectures_**: Children and non-autonomous adults are pulled into authentic adulthood by mentors, elders, and true adults. The therapeutic encounters thus provided—whether interpersonal or vicarious in the form of lectures, books, or audiotapes— serve as sources of information from which new possibilities can be gleaned, and these therefore serve as infinitely valuable resources for expanding the narrow horizons that characterize an underdeveloped internal locus of control. In essence, books, tapes, and lectures allow the patient to become a student and to choose a vicarious mentor. *Advantages*: Books and tapes allow access to many of the best minds in psychology; books and tapes are inexpensive; allow patients to explore and benefit from many different perspectives; books and tapes are always available and are therefore amenable to various schedules of work and responsibility. *Disadvantages*: Books and tapes do not re-create the interpersonal bridge which is essential for authentic recovery; do not provide a direct and objective means of accountably, thus potentially allowing patients to delude themselves about the effectiveness (or lack thereof) of their recovery process. Examples of better-known books, tapes and recorded lectures on the *process* of emotional recovery:

---

[344] Miller A. The Drama of the Gifted Child: The Search for the True Self. Basic Books: 1981, page 88
[345] Hillman J, Meade M, Some M. Images of initiation. Oral Tradition Archives; 1992

- **_Healing the Shame that Binds You_** by John Bradshaw [Audio Cassette (April 1990) Health Communications Audio; ISBN: 1558740430] Available as book and cassette with identical titles and different content.
- **_A Little Book on the Human Shadow_** by Robert Bly. Certainly among the most concise, accessible, and complete books ever written on the processes involved in losing and recovering the self.
- **_The Drama of the Gifted Child_** by Alice Miller. This internationally acclaimed book is considered a true classic among therapists and patients alike. Available as book and a brilliantly performed audio cassette.
- **_You Can Heal Your Life_** by Louise Hay. Another standard for recovery; very "new age."
- **_Codependent No More: How to Stop Controlling Others and Start Caring for Yourself_** by Melody Beattie. Pioneering for its time.
- **_The Artist's Date Book_** by Julia Cameron. Each page has a new creative idea for creative expression and "creative recovery."

**_Therapy_**: "_Therapy is a conversation that matters._" Therapy in this context specifically means face-to-face, active interaction, either one-on-one or in a group setting, with the specific intention to give and/or provide support for personal growth. Whether 12-step groups such as Codependents Anonymous qualify as a form of therapy depends entirely upon the level of engagement of the participant; sitting in a room while _other people_ do _their_ work provides slow or no benefit for the passive observer. **Recovery is an _active_ process, which is why it is antithetical to depression, which is a _passive_ state of being.** Patients should go in knowing that this is a _process_ and to not expect to be "fixed" after the first hour or even the first month. **_Advantages_**: Therapists can provide crucial support and insight while the client wrestles with undecipherable and convoluted emotional and psychic data. Therapists can help the client set goals ("stretches" and "homework") by which the client reaches beyond his/her comfort zone to attain the next expansion in being and experience. Therapists must create a safe space or "container" in which ideas and feelings can be brought forth to intermingle and be consciously appreciated. **_Disadvantages_**: Requires a flexible and disciplined schedule; costs money; bad therapists can do more harm than good if they misdirect their clients away from volatile and core issues and authentic expression.[346,347,348,349] Therapy can be disempowering if the patient continues to project his/her locus of control onto the therapist.

Some of the more commonly used tools of the psychotherapeutic trade include:
- **Active listening**
- **Insight, explanation of events**: their origins, reasons, and significance
- **Reminders** of previous conclusions and stories
- **Challenge old ideas and habits**: Therapy that generally or completely lacks confrontation and accountability is ineffective.
- **Encourage exploration and new modes of being and interacting**
- **Creating a safe container wherein the client can review the details, significance, and feelings associated with past events**
- **Modeling the expression of feeling**
- **Defining goals and helping the client focus on what is significant**
- **Correcting distortions of reality**
- **Asking patients to get in touch with and then express their feelings**
- **Support and encourage clients to take calculated risks for the sake of self-expansion**

---
[346] Lee J. Expressing Your Anger Appropriately (Audio Cassette). Sounds True (June 1, 1990); ISBN: 1564550338
[347] Bradshaw J. Healing the Shame that Binds You [Audio Cassette (April 1990) Health Communications Audio; ISBN: 1558740430]
[348] Miller A. The Drama of the Gifted Child: The Search for the True Self. Basic Books: 1981
[349] Miller A. The truth will set you free: overcoming emotional blindness and finding your true adult self. New York: Basic Books; 2001

- **Pointing out errors in logic**
- **Coaching patients in the proper and responsible use of emotional language**
- **Discouraging evasiveness; requiring accountability**[350]

**_Creativity_**: All types of self-expression reinforce and validate the patient's sense of self. Creative self-expression, such as writing about thoughts and feelings about significant experiences, can reduce symptomatology in patients with rheumatoid arthritis and asthma.[351]

**_Experiential_**: Corrective experiences can be obtained in therapy, with friends and family, in integration groups, and during "experiential" retreats. **_Advantages_**: Experiential events orchestrated by therapists and various groups such as ManKind Project (mkp.org) and WomanWithin.org can rapidly facilitate personal growth while also providing an ongoing container and support system that encourages self-development rather than the ego-inflation that accompanies short-term events. **_Disadvantages_**: "Adventures" like driving across the nation or climbing a mountain are unconscious and largely impotent attempts at self-initiation; authentic initiation has always been supervised by community elders. However, once a well-founded initiation has taken place, preferably with an on-going community that facilitates continued refinement and self-exploration, then "adventures" can be undertaken consciously to maintain and reinforce the experience of autonomy and competent selfhood. Eventually, transformative and sustentative experiences can be integrated and created in the daily life experience so that dramatic adventures become unnecessary for the continued renewal and "recharging" of the self.

**Creating and Re-creating the Self**: An on-going process that involves various types of "therapy" such as healthy formal/informal interpersonal and group relationships, creative expression and exploration, the periodic infusion of new ideas from teachers and mentors, attendance in workshops and seminars (or other forms of on-going consciousness-raising), reflection, and the integration of transformative and sustentative significance into everyday life, in such a way that daily life itself becomes _therapeutic_ and _affirmative_.

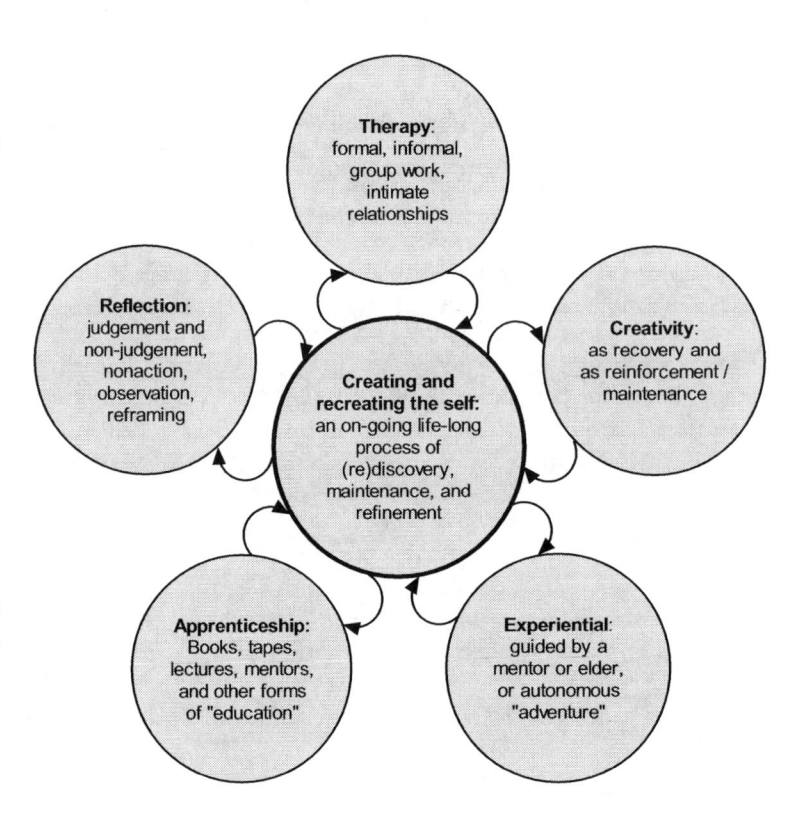

---

[350] Kottler JA. The Compleat Therapist. San Francisco; Jossey-Bass publishers; 1991, pages 134-174
[351] Smyth JM, Stone AA, Hurewitz A, Kaell A. Effects of writing about stressful experiences on symptom reduction in patients with asthma or rheumatoid arthritis: a randomized trial. _JAMA_. 1999 Apr 14;281(14):1304-9

## Sequence of events for effective, lasting, and authentic autonomization

The caterpillar does not blossom into a butterfly without spending time in its cocoon. The airborne seed descends into the earth for its nourishment before it sprouts and searches for the sun. Similarly, gratification of our ascentionist and impatient ego must be deferred for the sake of allowing the *time* and *descent* that provide "grounding", which allows the formation of a solid foundation from which authentic growth can arise. The Western view of "personal development" idealizes a life course of constant ascension that is generally inconsistent with living in a real world fraught with imperfections; two of the major complications arising from such a perfectionistic paradigm are 1) that it causes people to feel anxious and ashamed when confronted with otherwise *normal* delays and failures, and 2) that it biases people into believing that improvement comes only from *advancement* rather than also from the *return* and short-term *regression* that are characteristic of nearly all authentic healing traditions. With modification of the stepwise model proposed by Bradshaw[352], here I propose the following sequence:

1. **Short-term behavior modification**: For people whose behavior is acutely dysfunctional or harmful to themselves or others, they must stop the "acting out" that is the symptom of the underlying emotional injury or schism. Accepting abuse—at work or home—is a form of **acting out** that perpetuates old wounds and saps the strength required for recovery.

2. **Emotional recovery**: Complete healing is only possible when consciously pursued, and conscious healing can only be pursued after one has become conscious of the wounds, injuries, absences, dynamics, and events that lead to the current state. This process of recovery is referred to mythologically as the "descent" or the time of "eating ashes" that is a recurrent theme in various fairy tales ("Cinderella" literally means "ash girl") and cultural-religious histories (such as Jesus' descent into the tomb).[353] The biggest blockades to this process are 1) the ego, which prefers to ascend and to deny intrapersonal "negativity"[354], and 2) the challenge in finding elders and mentors in a society that constantly perpetuates and encourages immaturity, materialism, and superficiality.[355] In the words of famed psychologist Carl Gustav Jung, "One does not become enlightened by imagining figures of light, but by making the darkness *conscious*. The latter procedure, however, is disagreeable, and therefore unpopular." Recovery and the courage to relinquish the illusion of control must be an active process, often portrayed in ancient myths as "the hero's journey."[356]

3. **Long-term behavior modification and integration**: Insight allows for an illumination of the internal mental-emotional landscape, and effective insight must then be manifested externally by changes/modifications in behavior, habits, and interaction in the world. **Externalized behaviors simultaneously reflect and reinforce thoughts and feelings.** According to Grieneeks[357], patients (and their healthcare providers!) can "*think* their way into new ways of *acting*" and "*act* their way into new ways of *thinking*." Eventually, a consciously designed life can be created so that actions, interactions, thoughts, and feelings are melded together in such ways that everyday life itself becomes simultaneously *therapeutic, affirmative, sustentative,* and *empowering*. In this way, the person and his/her life are unified in such ways

---

[352] Bradshaw J. Healing the Shame that Binds You [Audio Cassette (April 1990) Health Communications Audio; ISBN: 1558740430]
[353] Bly R, Hillman J, Meade M. Men and the Life of Desire. Oral Tradition Archives. ISBN: 1880155001
[354] Robert Bly. The Human Shadow. Sound Horizons, New York 1991 [ISBN: 1879323001] and Bly R. A Little Book on the Human Shadow.[ ISBN: 0062548476]
[355] Bly R. Where have all the parents gone? A talk on the Sibling Society. New York: Sound Horizons, 1996
[356] Campbell J, Moyers B. Joseph Campbell and the Power of Myth. The Hero's Adventure. Published in various years as book, audiotape, CD, and DVD.
[357] Keith Grieneeks PhD. "Psychological Assessment" taught in 1998 at Bastyr University.

as to become self-perpetuating and self-sustaining cycles of ascents and descents, thought-feeling and action, reflection and courage, independence and interdependence—in sum: "a wheel rolling from its own center."[358] At this point the self is established, though it must be maintained and developed with the continuous application of conscious effort, reflection, and effective action.

4. *Metapersonal involvement in community, religion, spirituality, and the world*: Many people are tempted to move from a state of woundedness, relative incompleteness and the feelings of shame and impotence to a state of *perfection*, *enlightenment* and *omnipotence* without doing the requisite hard work that makes personal growth possible. People with unhealed emotional wounds often seek to camouflage those deficiencies by becoming pious and projecting an image of completeness and of "having it all figured out" and "having it all together"; religion and the acquisition of power are often misused for this purpose. Many people are successful in wearing this mask for many years; but its crumbling—often manifested as the "midlife crisis"—heralds an opportunity for personal growth if not medicated with anti-depressants, vacations, or the purchase of a sports car and flashy clothes.[359] The temptation to bypass Steps 2 [emotional recovery] and 3 [integration] and leapfrog to Step 4 [spirituality] should be resisted because the religion or spirituality is then used as a shield *against authenticity* and as a tool for illusory control. Religion can be misused in this way by providing an "identity" and sense of redemption for people with incompletely formed identities and for those with incompletely reconciled shadows and unresolved childhood-parental introjects.[360,361,362] Nietzsche's[363] response to this problem was to encourage self-knowledge and self-reconciliation as prerequisites to religious devotion, hence his admonition, "By all means love your neighbor as yourself – but *first* be such that you love yourself." Historical and recent events remind us of how religion can be misused for misanthropic ends.[364] What is commonly referred to as "spiritual development"—a level of resolution, reconciliation, and autonomy that allows for compassionate interdependence with people, the planet and the larger "world"—is synergistic with and can be supported by religion; but the latter is not a substitute for the former.[365,366] Religion and other forms of metapersonal involvement (e.g., community participation and social generosity) are *important* and *necessary* extensions of self-development. In order for personal development to blossom from the germ of necessary narcissism into its flower of functional completeness, it must eventually manifest in the larger community and the world.

---

[358] Friedrich Wilhelm Nietzsche, Walter Kaufmann (Translator). Thus Spoke Zarathustra. Penguin USA; 1978, page 27
[359] Robinson JC. Death of a Hero, Birth of a Soul: Answering the Call of Midlife. Council Oak Books, March 1997 ISBN: 1571780432
[360] Bradshaw J. Healing the Shame that Binds You [Audio Cassette (April 1990) Health Communications Audio; ISBN: 1558740430]
[361] Miller A. The Drama of the Gifted Child: The Search for the True Self. Basic Books: 1981
[362] Miller A. The truth will set you free: overcoming emotional blindness and finding your true adult self. New York: Basic Books; 2001
[363] Nietzsche N. Thus spoke Zarathustra. Read by Jon Cartwright and Alex Jennings. Naxos AudioBooks: http://www.naxosaudiobooks.com/nabusa/pages/432512.htm
[364] Bonhoeffer. (movie documentary by director/writer Martin Doblmeier) http://www.bonhoeffer.com/
[365] Lozoff B. It's a Meaningful Life : It Just Takes Practice. March 1, 2001. ISBN: 0140196242
[366] Bradshaw J. Healing the Shame that Binds You [Audio Cassette (April 1990) Health Communications Audio; ISBN: 1558740430]

5. <u>*Acceptance of mortality and death*</u>: No individual person or any system of thought, whether scientific or religious, can feign completeness without accounting for the end of life and incorporating this account into its overarching paradigm. The event is too significant, and the fear and concerns it provokes are too weighty to not be addressed directly and held in consciousness on a frequent basis. This topic is of practical importance, too, not only in our own lives and those of our friends and family, but also to the national healthcare system, which currently spends the bulk of its money and resources vainly attempting to preserve life in the last few years and months after which disease or age call unrelentingly for the end of life; perhaps if we as individuals and as part of the healthcare system could accept and deal with our own deaths, then we would not have to panic and participate in such superfluous expenditures of time, energy, emotion, and money when death arrives, either for our patients, our friends and family, or ourselves. Proximal to the panic and aversion that characterizes the West's relationship to death is the "subclinical" panic and aversion that infiltrate the lives, practices, and policies that we experience every day. Surely, many unconscious events and subconscious influences contribute to the "lives of quiet desperation"[367] and "universal anxiety"[368] that subtly yet powerfully afflict most people; surely, lack of reconciliation with death is a major contributor. Especially in western cultures, death is commonly seen as some type of failure or shortcoming, either on behalf of the patient or his/her doctors, and the most common questions asked on the topic of death are "*how can this be avoided*?" before the event and "*who is to blame*?" after the event. Other cultures accept death as a natural part of life, and indeed, people are seen to have an obligation to die so that the next generations can have their turn in the cycle of life. Alternatives to western hysteria are founded on acceptance of death, and the prerequisites for the acceptance of death are 1) the dedication of sufficient time for its consideration (most people would rather watch a bad movie or attend spectator sports), 2) reframing the event in terms of its being a natural part of our lives, certainly nothing to be ashamed of (discussed below), 3) making necessary logistical preparations (e.g., writing of wills, providing for dependents, and other obvious technicalities), and 4) living as completely, consciously, compassionately, effectively, and authentically as possible so that remorse can be minimized, perhaps completely mitigated. Reframing the event of death begins with its description in general terms so that its enigma, from which its power over the hearts and minds of humanity is derived, can be deciphered and thus deflated. The main characteristics of death which precipitate its fear are 1) the unpredictability of its arrival, 2) the duration of the dying process, and 3) the quality of that process, for example whether it is painful or associated with or precipitated by severe illness or injury. The first characteristic of *timeliness*—the unpredictability of its arrival—stresses people because of their inadequate preparation and the feeling that they have only recently begun to live or have not quite yet begun to live their authentic lives. These concerns are allayed by preparation, both logistical and intrapersonal. Each of us has the responsibility to "become authentically whole" so that we do not inflict our

> "**The event of death is not a tragedy**—to rabbit, fox or man. But **the *concept* of death *is* a tragedy**, for man, and *indirectly* for poor fox, rabbit, bush, bird, just anything and everything in man's path."
>
> Pearce JC, <u>Exploring the Crack in the Cosmic Egg</u>. Washington Square Press; 1974, page 59

---

[367] Throeau HD, (Thomas O, ed). <u>Walden and Civil Disobedience</u>. New York: WW Norton and Company; 1966, page 5
[368] Becker E. <u>The Denial of Death</u>. New York: Free Press; 1973, pages 11 and 21

incompleteness onto others, either directly through various forms of transference or deprivation[369] or indirectly though the more subtle means of politics and cultural mores. If a person can live with vitality, authenticity, compassion and effectiveness then little is left to want, and fears of death and its untimely arrival are diminished. The remaining variables are both controllable and uncontrollable; they are uncontrollable to the extent that we are all subject to chaos and accidents, whether in cars, planes, or bathtubs. *Duration* and *quality* are both controllable on an inpatient setting to the extent that palliative care[370] and voluntary euthanasia are sufficiently available.[371]

> **"Once accepted, death is an integral component of every event, as the left hand to the right. The cultural death concept could only be instilled in a mind split from its own life flow."** *Joseph Chilton Pearce*[372]

Life can only be authentically and completely experienced after one has created an authentic self and has thereafter accepted life *as it is*. Since death is part of life, the full engagement of life requires *acceptance of* and *reconciliation with* death. Acceptance of death does not necessarily entail that life becomes permeated with nihilistic resignation; on the contrary, it infuses daily events with significance and makes all experiences rare and unique.

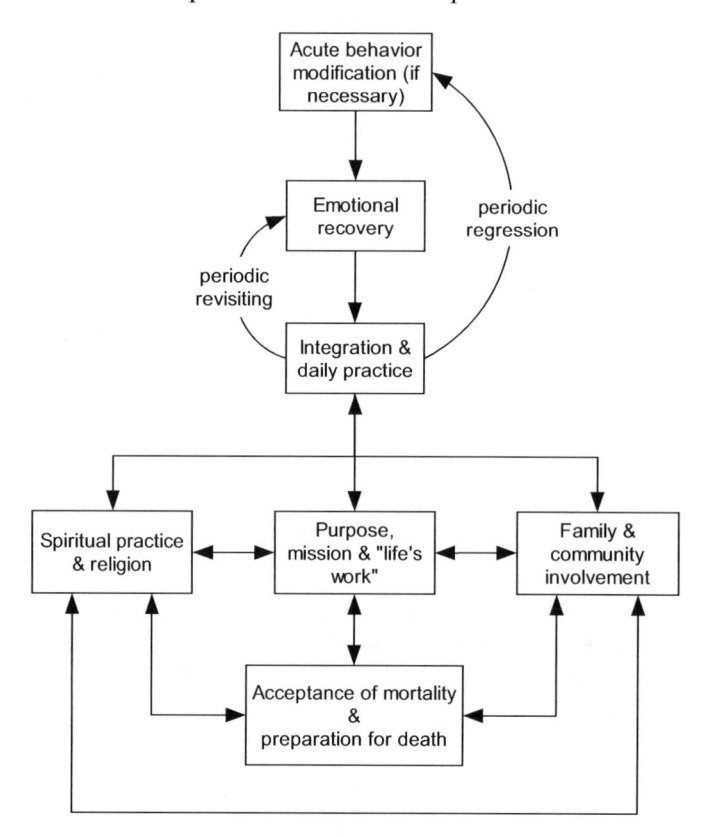

"They say there's no future for us. They're right, which is fine with us." *Rumi*[373]

---

[369] Miller A. The Drama of the Gifted Child: The Search for the True Self. Basic Books: 1981
[370] "Failure to give an effective therapy to seriously ill patients, either adults or children, violates the core principles of both medicine and ethics... Therefore, in the patient's best interest, patients and parents/surrogates, have the right to request medical marijuana under certain circumstances and physicians have the duty to disclose medical marijuana as an option and prescribe it when appropriate." Clark PA. Medical marijuana: should minors have the same rights as adults? *Med Sci Monit*.2003;9:ET1-9 www.medscimonit.com/pub/vol_9/no_6/3640.pdf
[371] Steinbrook R. Medical marijuana, physician-assisted suicide, and the Controlled Substances Act. *N Engl J Med*. 2004 Sep 30;351(14):1380-3
[372] Pearce JC. Exploring the Crack in the Cosmic Egg: Split Minds and Meta-Realities. New York: Washington Square Press; 1974, page 59
[373] Rumi in Barks C (translator). The Essential Rumi. HarperSanFransisco: 1995, page 2

# Environmental Health: Tribute to Rachel Carson[374] and Walter Crinnion, ND[375]

> "Man's attitude toward nature is today critically important simply because we have now acquired a fateful power to alter and destroy nature. But man is a part of nature, and his war against nature is inevitably a war against himself."
> 
> *Rachel Carson*[376]

**Environmental exposures to chemicals and toxic substances**:
Studies using blood tests and tissue samples from Americans across the nation have consistently shown that **all** Americans have toxic chemical **accumulation** whether or not they work in chemical factories or are exposed at home or work.[377,378] **The recent report from the CDC found toxic chemicals such as pesticides in all Americans, especially minorities, women, and children.**[379] Nearly all of these chemicals are known to contribute to health problems in humans—problems such as cancer, fatigue, poor memory, endocrinopathy, subfertility/infertility, Parkinson's disease, autoimmune diseases like lupus, and many other serious conditions. Therefore, *detoxification programs are a necessity—not a luxury*.

### Examples of common toxicants found in Americans

| Environmental pollutant (population frequency with elevated levels) | Biologic effects as quoted from HSDB: Hazardous Substances Data Bank. National Library of Medicine, NIH[380] or other reference as noted |
|---|---|
| **DDE (99% of Americans):** DDE is the main metabolite of DDT, a pesticide that was presumably banned in the US in 1972 | <ul><li>DDT is known to be immunosuppressive in animals. A study published in 2004 showed that increasing levels of DDE in African-American male farmers in North Carolina correlated with a higher prevalence of antinuclear antibodies and up to 50% reductions in serum IgG.[381]</li><li>Other studies in humans have suggested an estrogenic or anti-androgenic effect.[382]</li><li>All women have evidence of DDT accumulation. Women with higher levels of DDT show pregnancy and childbirth complications and have higher rates of infant mortality.[383]</li></ul> |

---

[374] Rachel Carson. *Silent Spring*. Boston, Houghton Mifflin Company (2002). ISBN: 0395683297
[375] Crinnion W. Results of a Decade of Naturopathic Treatment for Environmental Illnesses: A Review of Clinical Records. *J Naturopathic Medicine* vol.7 (2); 21-27
[376] Rachel Carson Dies of Cancer; 'Silent Spring' Author Was 56. New York Times 1956. http://www.rachelcarson.org/ on August 1, 2004
[377] "The average concentration of 2,3,7,8-tetrachlorodibenzo-p-dioxin in the adipose tissue of the US population was 5.38 pg/g, increasing from 1.98 pg/g in children under 14 years of age to 9.40 pg/g in adults over 45." Orban JE, Stanley JS, Schwemberger JG, Remmers JC. Dioxins and dibenzofurans in adipose tissue of the general US population and selected subpopulations. *Am J Public Health* 1994 Mar;84(3):439-45
[378] "Although the use of HCB as a fungicide has virtually been eliminated, detectable levels of HCB are still found in nearly all people in the USA." Robinson PE, Leczynski BA, Kutz FW, Remmers JC. An evaluation of hexachlorobenzene body-burden levels in the general population of the USA. *IARC Sci Publ* 1986;77:183-92
[379] "Many of the pesticides found in the test subjects have been linked to serious short- and long-term health effects including infertility, birth defects and childhood and adult cancers." http://www.panna.org/campaigns/docsTrespass/chemicalTrespass2004.dv.html July 25, 2004
[380] Primary source for this data is the Hazardous Substances Data Bank. National Library of Medicine, National Institutes of Health: http://toxnet.nlm.nih.gov/cgi-bin/sis/htmlgen?HSDB accessed on August 1, 2004
[381] Cooper GS, Martin SA, Longnecker MP, Sandler DP, Germolec DR. Associations between plasma DDE levels and immunologic measures in African-American farmers in North Carolina. *Environ Health Perspect.* 2004 Jul;112(10):1080-4
[382] Dalvie MA, Myers JE, Lou Thompson M, Dyer S, Robins TG, Omar S, Riebow J, Molekwa J, Kruger P, Millar R. The hormonal effects of long-term DDT exposure on malaria vector-control workers in Limpopo Province, South Africa. *Environ Res.* 2004 Sep;96(1):9-19
[383] "The findings strongly suggest that DDT use increases preterm births, which is a major contributor to infant mortality. If this association is causal, it should be included in any assessment of the costs and benefits of vector control with DDT." Longnecker MP, Klebanoff MA, Zhou H, Brock JW. Association between maternal serum concentration of the DDT metabolite DDE and preterm and small-for-gestational-age babies at birth. *Lancet.* 2001 Jul 14;358(9276):110-4

**Examples of common toxicants found in Americans**—*continued*

| Environmental pollutant (population frequency) | Biologic effects as quoted from HSDB: Hazardous Substances Data Bank. National Library of Medicine, NIH[384] or other reference as noted |
|---|---|
| **2,4-dichlorophenol** (87% of Americans): pesticide | - Human Toxicity Excerpts: same as for 2,5-dichlorophenol<br>- In males, significant increases in relative risk ratios for lung cancer, rectal cancer, and soft tissue sarcomas were reported; in females, there were increases in the relative risk of cervical cancer. |
| **2,5-dichlorophenol** (88% nationally and up to 96% in select children populations): Dichlorophenols can occur in tap water as a result of standard chlorination treatment; general population may be exposed to 2,5-dichlorophenol through oral consumption or dermal contact with chlorinated tap water; 2,5-Dichlorophenol was identified in 96% of the urine samples of children residing in Arkansas near a herbicide plant at concentrations of 4-1,200 ppb. The sole manufacturer for herbicide use is Sandoz (Clariant Corporation). | - Human Toxicity Excerpts: 1. Burning pain in mouth and throat. White necrotic lesions in mouth, esophagus, and stomach. Abdominal pain, vomiting ... and bloody diarrhea. 2. Pallor, sweating, weakness, headache, dizziness, tinnitus. 3. Shock: Weak irregular pulse, hypotension, shallow respirations, cyanosis, pallor, and a profound fall in body temperature. 4. Possibly fleeting excitement and confusion, followed by unconsciousness. ... 5. Stentorous breathing, mucous rales, rhonchi, frothing at nose and mouth and other signs of pulmonary edema are sometimes seen. Characteristic odor of phenol on the breath. 6. Scanty, dark-colored ... urine ... moderately severe renal insufficiency may appear. 7. Methemoglobinemia, Heinz body hemolytic anemia and hyperbilirubinemia have been reported. ... 8. Death from respiratory, circulatory or cardiac failure. 9. If spilled on skin, pain is followed promptly by numbness. The skin becomes blanched, and a dry opaque eschar forms over the burn. When the eschar sloughs off, a brown stain remains. |
| **Chlorpyrifos** (93% of Americans): insecticide used on corn and cotton and for termite control.<br><br>Conservative estimates hold that 80% of the chlorpyrifos in the US was produced directly or indirectly by Dow Chemical Corporation.[385] This pesticide is routinely used in schools and is thus found in blood and tissue samples of nearly all American children. | - Toxic if inhaled, in contact with skin and if swallowed.<br>- All the organophosphorus insecticides have a cumulative effect by progressive inhibition of cholinesterase.<br>- The symptoms of chronic poisoning due to organophosphorus pesticides include headache, weakness, feeling of heaviness in head, decline of memory, quick onset of **fatigue, disturbed sleep**, loss of appetite, and loss of orientation. **Psychic disorders**, nystagmus, trembling of the hands and other nervous system disorders can be observed in certain cases. Sometimes neuritis and paralysis develop. Other manifestations of accumulation include **tension, anxiety, restlessness, insomnia, headache, emotional instability, fatigue**...<br>- Chlorpyrifos is a suspected endocrine disruptor.[386] |

---

[384] Primary source for this data is the Hazardous Substances Data Bank, National Institutes of Health: http://toxnet.nlm.nih.gov/cgi-bin/sis/htmlgen?HSDB accessed on August 1, 2004
[385] Kristin S. Schafer, Margaret Reeves, Skip Spitzer, Susan E. Kegley. Chemical Trespass: Pesticides in Our Bodies and Corporate Accountability. Pesticide Action Network North America. May 2004 Available at http://www.panna.org/campaigns/docsTrespass/chemicalTrespass2004.dv.html on August 1, 2004
[386] http://www.panna.org/resources/documents/factsChlorpyrifos.dv.html accessed August 1, 2004

**Examples of common toxicants found in Americans**—*continued*

| Environmental pollutant (population frequency) | Biologic effects as quoted from HSDB: Hazardous Substances Data Bank. National Library of Medicine, NIH[387] or other reference as noted |
|---|---|
| **Mercury** (8% of American women of reproductive age have mercury levels high enough to cause brain damage to their fetuses) | • Mercury is a well-known neurotoxin, with damaging and deadly effects in adults and especially in children.<br>• A recent study published by the American Medical Association[388] noted that "**Humans are exposed to methylmercury, a well-established neurotoxin**, through fish consumption. The fetus is most sensitive to the adverse effects of exposure. … **approximately 8% of women had concentrations higher than the US EPA's recommended reference dose (5.8 microg/L),** below which exposures are considered to be without adverse effects." The most obvious interpretation of this data published in *JAMA* is that 8% of American women have mercury poisoning—poisoning in this case refers specifically to elevated blood levels of a known toxicant that consistently demonstrates adverse effects on human health. Logical deduction holds that such a high level of human poisoning should be unacceptable and should lead directly to legislative restrictions on corporate emissions to protect and salvage the health of the public. |

*Notes, Implications, Feelings, and Plans for Action:*

---

[387] Primary source for this data is the Hazardous Substances Data Bank, National Institutes of Health: http://toxnet.nlm.nih.gov/cgi-bin/sis/htmlgen?HSDB accessed on August 1, 2004
[388] Schober SE, Sinks TH, Jones RL, Bolger PM, McDowell M, Osterloh J, Garrett ES, Canady RA, Dillon CF, Sun Y, Joseph CB, Mahaffey KR. Blood mercury levels in US children and women of childbearing age, 1999-2000. *JAMA*. 2003 Apr 2;289(13):1667-74

Though a detailed clinical explanation of detoxification procedures will not be included here (see Chapter 4 of *Integrative Rheumatology*[389]), the general concepts for detoxification are as follows:

1. *Avoidance*: reduced exposure = reduced problem
   a. If there were less chemical pollution, then our environment would be less toxic and therefore we would not have such problems with environmental poisoning.
   b. Limit or eliminate exposure to paint fumes, car exhaust, new carpet, solvents, adhesives, artificial foods, synthetic chemical drugs, copier fumes, pesticides, herbicides, chemical fertilizers, etc.
2. *Depuration*: "The act or process of freeing from foreign or impure matter"[390]
   a. Exercise and sauna
   b. Bowel cleansing, fiber, probiotics, antibiotics, laxatives
   c. Liver and bile stimulators
   d. Cofactors for phase 1 oxidation and phase 2 conjugation
   e. Chelation for heavy metals
   f. Urine alkalinization
3. *Damage control*: managing the consequences of chemical and heavy metal toxicity
   a. Hormone replacement
   b. Antioxidant therapy
   c. Occupational and rehabilitative training
   d. Management of resultant diseases, particularly autoimmune diseases
4. *Political and social action*: Due in large part to corporate influence and government deregulation, environmental contamination with pesticides from American corporations has increased to such an extent over the past few decades that now all Americans show evidence of pesticide accumulation in their bodies. Failure to hold corporations to tight regulatory standards has jeopardized the future of humanity. Voter passivity combined with collusion between multinational corporations and government officials is the underlying problem. Political action is the solution. The past and recent history on this topic is clear and well documented for those who wish to access the facts.[391,392,393,394,395,396,397,398,399]

---

[389] **Vasquez A**. Integrative Rheumatology. IBMRC. http://optimalhealthresearch.com/textbooks/rheumatology.html
[390] Webster's 1913 Dictionary
[391] Robert Van den Bosch. The pesticide conspiracy. Garden City, NY: Doubleday, 1978. ISBN: 0385133847
[392] "Monsanto Corporation is widely known for its production of the herbicide Roundup and genetically engineered Roundup-ready crops... altered to survive a dousing of the toxic herbicide. ...glyphosate, is known to cause eye soreness, headaches, diarrhea, and other flu-like symptoms, and has been linked to non-Hodgkin's lymphoma." Bush Names Former Monsanto Executive as EPA Deputy Administrator. Daily News Archive From March 29, 2001 http://www.beyondpesticides.org/NEWS/daily_news_archive/2001/03_29_01.htm accessed on August 1, 2004
[393] "They pointed to budgets cuts for research and enforcement, to steep declines in the number of cases filed against polluters, to efforts to relax portions of the Clean Air Act, to an acceleration of federal approvals for the spraying of restricted pesticides and more." Patricia Sullivan. Anne Gorsuch Burford, 62, Dies; Reagan EPA Director. *Washington Post*. Thursday, July 22, 2004; Page B06 http://www.washingtonpost.com/wp-dyn/articles/A3418-2004Jul21.html on August 2, 2004
[394] "In fact, amongst the crimes of Reagan and Bush which will go down in history are their emasculation of Federal regulatory apparatus... But in 1988, under the Bush administration, the EPA - illegally, in our view - revoked the Dellaney Law..." Samuel Epstein MD, 1993. Professor of Occupational and Environmental Medicine at the School of Public Health, University of Illinois Medical Center Chicago. http://www.converge.org.nz/pirm/pestican.htm accessed August 1, 2004
[395] "The Environmental Protection Agency will be free to approve pesticides without consulting wildlife agencies to determine if the chemical might harm plants and animals protected by the Endangered Species Act, according to new Bush administration rules.... It also is intended to head off future lawsuits, the officials said." Associated Press. Bush Eases Pesticide Laws http://www.cbsnews.com/stories/2004/07/29/tech/main633009.shtml accessed August 1, 2004
[396] "The new policy also could bolster pesticide makers' contention that federal labeling insulates them from suits alleging that their products cause illness or environmental damage, Olson says. 'It . . . could really be disastrous for public health.'" Bush Exempts Pesticide Companies from Lawsuits. Law on Pesticides Reinterpreted: Government Alters Policy in Effort to Protect Manufacturers. Peter Eisler. USA TODAY. October 6, 2003 http://www.organicconsumers.org/foodsafety/bushpesticides100703.cfm Accessed August 1, 2004
[397] WASHINGTON (AP) — "The Environmental Protection Agency will be free to approve pesticides without consulting wildlife agencies to determine if the chemical might harm plants and animals protected by the Endangered Species Act, according to new Bush administration rules." Bush eases pesticide reviews for endangered species. http://www.usatoday.com/news/washington/2004-07-29-epa-pesticides_x.htm?csp=34 Accessed August 2004

## Wellness Promotion: Re-Establishing the Foundation for Health

> **"Your lack of interest in the past, your lack of involvement, your unwillingness to develop coherent strategies, your unwillingness to challenge authority - these have created a vacuum in decision-making, that has been filled by professional groups with close relationships with the chemical industries..."** *Samuel Epstein, M.D.* [400]

The recent findings that mercury poisoning can result from once-weekly consumption of tuna[401] and that the average American has 13 pesticides in his/her body[402] should be seen as an indication of how dangerously toxic our environment has become, largely due to irresponsible corporate and government policies that value profitability over sustainability. "Detoxification" is the micromanagment band-aid for the problem, and it is professionally and ethically inappropriate for healthcare professionals to limit their attention to clinical detoxification when the real problem is manifest on a much wider—national and worldwide—level. Focusing on *detoxification* only benefits a minute section of the population, namely those with the worst symptoms and/or the most money, leaving huge sections of the population untreated, unserved, underserved, and unrepresented.

*Personal plans for taking responsible action and avoiding political/social passivity that has created the opportunity for regulatory failure and corporate exploitation of the environment that threatens the sustainability of the human species:*

_____
_____
_____
_____
_____
_____
_____
_____
_____

---

[398] "It is simply intolerable that the EPA, instead of providing an example for open scientific discussion, has continuously violated key environmental legislation, stifling legitimate dissent. The failure of EPA to properly encourage and protect whistleblowing has undermined the ability of the EPA and state environmental agencies to enforce environmental laws." Letter to Carol Browner, Administrator U.S. Environmental Protection Agency from Stephen Kohn, Chair National Whistleblower Center Board of Directors dated March 23, 1999. Availble at http://www.whistleblowers.org/statements.htm on October 10, 2004

[399] "The Bush administration has imposed a gag order on the U.S. Environmental Protection Agency from publicly discussing perchlorate pollution, even as two new studies reveal high levels of the rocket-fuel component may be contaminating the nation's lettuce supply." Peter Waldman. Rocket Fuel Residues Found in Lettuce: Bush administration issues gag order on EPA discussions of possible rocket fuel tainted lettuce. *THE WALL STREET JOURNAL.* See http://www.organicconsumers.org/toxic/lettuce042903.cfm http://www.rhinoed.com/epa's_gag_order.htm http://www.peer.org/press/508.html http://yubanet.com/artman/publish/article_13637.shtml

[400] Samuel Epstein MD, 1993. Professor of Occupational and Environmental Medicine at the School of Public Health, University of Illinois Medical Center Chicago. http://www.converge.org.nz/pirm/pestican.htm accessed September 11, 2004

[401] "The neurobehavioral performance of subjects who consumed tuna fish regularly was significantly worse on color word reaction time, digit symbol reaction time and finger tapping speed (FT)." Carta P, Flore C, Alinovi R, Ibba A, Tocco MG, Aru G, Carta R, Girei E, Mutti A, Lucchini R, Randaccio FS. Sub-clinical neurobehavioral abnormalities associated with low level of mercury exposure through fish consumption. *Neurotoxicology.* 2003 Aug;24(4-5):617-23

[402] "A comprehensive survey of more than 1,300 Americans has found traces of weed- and bug-killers in the bodies of everyone tested, …. The survey, conducted by the U.S. Centers for Disease Control and Prevention, found that the body of the average American contained 13 of these chemicals." Martin Millestaedt. 13 pesticides in body of average American. *The Globe and Mail.* Friday, May 21, 2004 - Page A17 Available on-line at http://www.theglobeandmail.com/servlet/ArticleNews/TPStory/LAC/20040521/HPEST21/TPEnvironment/ on August 6, 2004

## *Overview of Toxicant Exposure and Detoxification/Depuration*

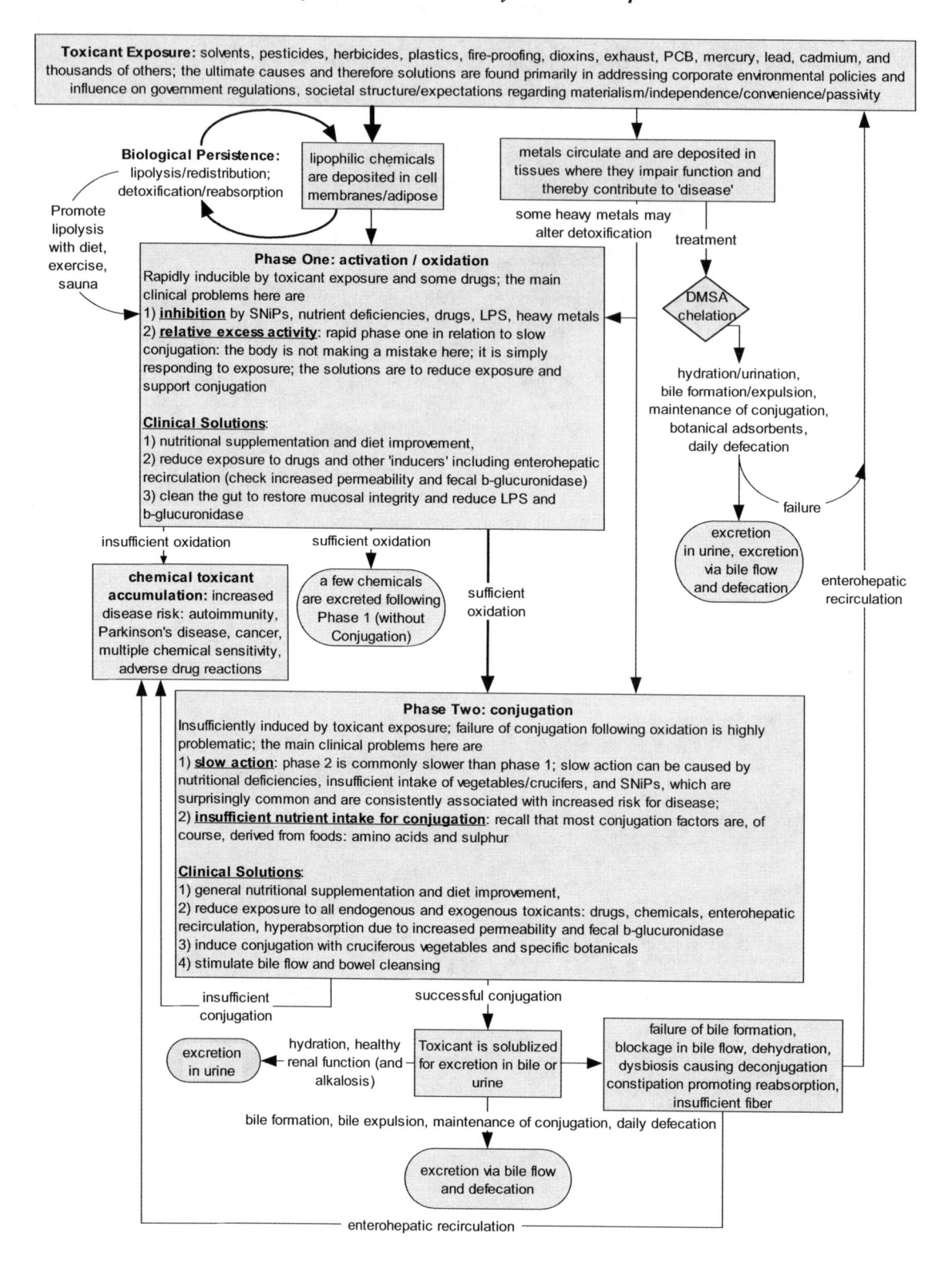

**Toxicant Exposure:** solvents, pesticides, herbicides, plastics, fire-proofing, dioxins, exhaust, PCB, mercury, lead, cadmium, and thousands of others; the ultimate causes and therefore solutions are found primarily in addressing corporate environmental policies and influence on government regulations, societal structure/expectations regarding materialism/independence/convenience/passivity

**Biological Persistence:** lipolysis/redistribution; detoxification/reabsorption

Promote lipolysis with diet, exercise, sauna

lipophilic chemicals are deposited in cell membranes/adipose

metals circulate and are deposited in tissues where they impair function and thereby contribute to 'disease'

some heavy metals may alter detoxification

treatment → DMSA chelation

### Phase One: activation / oxidation
Rapidly inducible by toxicant exposure and some drugs; the main clinical problems here are
1) **inhibition** by SNiPs, nutrient deficiencies, drugs, LPS, heavy metals
2) **relative excess activity**: rapid phase one in relation to slow conjugation: the body is not making a mistake here; it is simply responding to exposure; the solutions are to reduce exposure and support conjugation

**Clinical Solutions:**
1) nutritional supplementation and diet improvement,
2) reduce exposure to drugs and other 'inducers' including enterohepatic recirculation (check increased permeability and fecal b-glucuronidase)
3) clean the gut to restore mucosal integrity and reduce LPS and b-glucuronidase

hydration/urination, bile formation/expulsion, maintenance of conjugation, botanical adsorbents, daily defecation

failure → excretion in urine, excretion via bile flow and defecation

enterohepatic recirculation

insufficient oxidation → **chemical toxicant accumulation:** increased disease risk: autoimmunity, Parkinson's disease, cancer, multiple chemical sensitivity, adverse drug reactions

sufficient oxidation → a few chemicals are excreted following Phase 1 (without Conjugation)

sufficient oxidation →

### Phase Two: conjugation
Insufficiently induced by toxicant exposure; failure of conjugation following oxidation is highly problematic; the main clinical problems here are
1) **slow action**: phase 2 is commonly slower than phase 1; slow action can be caused by nutritional deficiencies, insufficient intake of vegetables/crucifers, and SNiPs, which are surprisingly common and are consistently associated with increased risk for disease;
2) **insufficient nutrient intake for conjugation**: recall that most conjugation factors are, of course, derived from foods: amino acids and sulphur

**Clinical Solutions:**
1) general nutritional supplementation and diet improvement,
2) reduce exposure to all endogenous and exogenous toxicants: drugs, chemicals, enterohepatic recirculation, hyperabsorption due to increased permeability and fecal b-glucuronidase
3) induce conjugation with cruciferous vegetables and specific botanicals
4) stimulate bile flow and bowel cleansing

insufficient conjugation

successful conjugation → Toxicant is solublized for excretion in bile or urine

hydration, healthy renal function (and alkalosis) → excretion in urine

failure of bile formation, blockage in bile flow, dehydration, dysbiosis causing deconjugation constipation promoting reabsorption, insufficient fiber

bile formation, bile expulsion, maintenance of conjugation, daily defecation → excretion via bile flow and defecation

enterohepatic recirculation

## Avoid chemical medications and medical procedures to the extent possible

- "In 1983, 2876 people died from medication errors... By 1993, this number had risen to 7,391 - a 2.57-fold increase." [403]
- "Recent estimates suggest that **each year more than 1 million patients are injured while in the hospital and approximately 180,000 die because of these injuries**. Furthermore, drug-related morbidity and mortality are common and are estimated to cost more than $136 billion a year."[404]
- "There is a substantial amount of injury to patients from medical management, and many injuries are the result of substandard care."[405]

Adverse effects of chemical medications and surgical procedures are a major cause of death and disability in America.[408] **Choose your drugs carefully**, and whenever possible choose natural treatments, which are generally safer, less expensive, and more effective for the long-term management and prevention of chronic health problems.[409] Chemical-pharmaceutical drugs are a significant cause of death in America[410], perhaps because they generally function by inhibiting or blocking the body's natural processes, e.g., calcium channel *blockers*, serotonin *antagonists*[411], HMG-CoA reductase *inhibitors*[412], and angiotensin converting enzyme (ACE) *inhibitors*. Chemical drugs are often necessary for patients with acute and life-threatening problems; but on a more frequent basis they are unnecessary and/or obfuscate true healthcare. In contrast to the illusion of efficacy portrayed by the medical-pharmaceutical industry, it is commonly appreciated that most pharmaceutical drugs are only partially effective or are almost ineffective for the conditions they are claimed to treat, as demonstrated in the table.

| Health condition[406] | Drug treatment efficacy* |
|---|---|
| Asthma | 60% |
| Cardiac arrhythmias | 60% |
| Depression (SSRI) | 62% |
| Diabetes | 57% |
| Hepatitis C (HCV) | 47% |
| Migraine (prophylaxis) | 50% |
| Oncology | 25% |
| Rheumatoid arthritis | 50% |
| Schizophrenia[407] | 60% |

\* *Drug treatment efficacy*: Note that a drug is generally considered "effective" if it elicits a "response"—most commonly *alleviation of symptoms* or *short-term improvement* or a *minor change that achieves "statistical significance" in a large-scale* trial rather than **correction of the underlying problem**. However, from a naturopathic perspective, we would often consider this a treatment *failure* since the underlying problem has not been addressed, the patient's overall health has not been improved, the patient has been disempowered and is now reliant upon a drug treatment when other integrative options may have well produced better long-term results at lower cost and would have retained or established the patient's autonomy. For life-threatening emergencies and conditions for which there are no natural effective treatments, pharmaceutical drugs are, of course, valuable.

---

[403] Phillips DP, Christenfeld N, Glynn LM. Increase in US medication-error deaths between 1983 and 1993. *Lancet*. 1998 Feb 28;351(9103):643-4
[404] Holland EG, Degruy FV. Drug-induced disorders. *Am Fam Physician*. 1997 Nov 1;56(7):1781-8, 1791-2. http://aafp.org/afp/971101ap/holland.html
[405] Brennan TA, Leape LL, Laird NM, Hebert L, Localio AR, Lawthers AG, Newhouse JP, Weiler PC, Hiatt HH. Incidence of adverse events and negligence in hospitalized patients: results of the Harvard Medical Practice Study I. 1991. *Qual Saf Health Care*. 2004;13(2):145-51; discussion 151-2
[406] "A senior executive with Britain's biggest drugs company has admitted that most prescription medicines do not work on most people who take them. Allen Roses, worldwide vice-president of genetics at GlaxoSmithKline, said fewer than half of the patients prescribed some of the most expensive drugs actually derived any benefit from them." Connor S. Glaxo Chief: Our Drugs Do Not Work on Most Patients. Published on Monday, December 8, 2003 by the Independent/UK. Available on-line at http://www.commondreams.org/headlines03/1208-02.htm on July 4, 2004
[407] See also: Whitaker R. The case against antipsychotic drugs: a 50-year record of doing more harm than good. *Med Hypotheses*. 2004;62(1):5-13
[408] Holland EG, Degruy FV. Drug-induced disorders. *Am Fam Physician*. 1997 Nov 1;56(7):1781-8, 1791-2. http://aafp.org/afp/971101ap/holland.html
[409] Orme-Johnson DW, Herron RE. An innovative approach to reducing medical care utilization and expenditures. *Am J Manag Care* 1997;3(1):135-44
[410] Phillips DP, Christenfeld N, Glynn LM. Increase in US medication-error deaths between 1983 and 1993. *Lancet*. 1998 Feb 28;351(9103):643-4
[411] "Lotronex was an early example of a new class of drug for irritable bowel, the 5-HT3 antagonists... At least five people had died after taking the drug... There had been 49 cases of ischemic colitis and ... 34 patients had required admission to hospital and ten needed surgery." Horton R. Lotronex and the FDA: a fatal erosion of integrity. *Lancet*. 2001 May 19;357(9268):1544-5
[412] "FDA has received reports of 31 U.S. deaths due to severe rhabdomyolysis associated with use of Baycol, 12 of which involved concomitant gemfibrozil use." US Food and Drug Administration. Bayer voluntarily withdraws Baycol. http://www.fda.gov/bbs/topics/ANSWERS/2001/ANS01095.html March 14, 2004

## Intestinal Health and Bowel Function:

We are not simply talking about the quantity of bowel movements (which must never average less than one per day, and should be at least 2 per day). Chronic constipation increases the circulation of toxins in the blood and may predispose to "minor" problems like fatigue and headaches while possibly contributing to an increased risk of colon cancer, too.[413] A study published in *The American Journal of Public Health* showed that women with mild constipation had an increased incidence of breast cancer.[414] More recently, research has shown and increased risk for Parkinson's disease in people with a life-long history of constipation; researchers have proposed that chronic constipation may contribute to neurodegeneration via toxins from the gut being absorbed into the vagus nerve and thereby transported directly into the central nervous system.[415,416] Additionally, we need to talk about the quality of digestion, absorption, and the presence or absence of harmful bacteria, yeasts, and parasites.

> "They also hypothesize that some yet undefined toxins break through the mucosal barrier of the intestine and are incorporated into the axon terminal of the vagus nerve and transported in a retrograde manner to the vagus nucleus [in the central nervous system]."
>
> Ueki A, Otsuka M. Life style risks of Parkinson's disease: association between decreased water intake and constipation. *J Neurol*. 2004 Oct;251 Suppl 7:vII18-23

- **Poor digestion—insufficient stomach acid or insufficient pancreatic enzymes**: For reasons that are not always clear, some people do not make enough stomach acid and pepsin[417] (this is especially true of older adults), and as a result they are not able to properly/completely digest their foods and they are less able to sterilize the foods that enter their intestines. As a result, people with low stomach acid often have nutritional deficiencies and excessive growth of bacteria and yeast in the intestines. It is well established that medications used to mask the symptom of gastrointestinal reflux disease by blocking acid production can cause such a severe degree of impaired digestion and bacterial overgrowth that vitamin deficiencies result.[418] Recent studies have shown that impairment of acid secretion by the use of antacid medications promotes bacterial overgrowth of the small bowel[419], exacerbation of nutritional deficiencies[420], and the development of food allergies (animal study).[421]
- **Malabsorption**: Once the food is digested, it must be absorbed into the body. Intestinal absorption can be assessed quantitatively with the lactulose-mannitol assay, as well as measuring fecal fat levels.
- **Harmful yeast, bacteria, and other parasites**: If you think parasites are rare, think again: in my own clinical practice I find patients with "parasites" (harmful gastrointestinal microorganisms) on a routine basis, even in patients with no specific or obvious gastrointestinal complaints such

---

[413] Talley NJ. Definitions, epidemiology, and impact of chronic constipation. *Rev Gastroenterol Disord*. 2004;4 Suppl 2:S3-S10 http://www.medreviews.com/pdfs/articles/RIGD_4Suppl2_S3.pdf on July 4, 2004
[414] Micozzi MS, Carter CL, Albanes D, Taylor PR, Licitra LM. Bowel function and breast cancer in US women. *Am J Public Health* 1989 Jan;79(1):73-5
[415] "The present results support previous findings that constipation precedes the onset of motor dysfunction in PD." Ueki A, Otsuka M. Life style risks of Parkinson's disease: association between decreased water intake and constipation. *J Neurol*. 2004 Oct;251 Suppl 7:vII18-23
[416] "...the disorder might originate outside of the central nervous system, caused by a yet unidentified pathogen that is capable of passing the mucosal barrier of the gastrointestinal tract and, via postganglionic enteric neurons, entering the central nervous system along unmyelinated praeganglionic fibers generated from the visceromotor projection cells of the vagus nerve." Braak H, Rub U, Gai WP, Del Tredici K. Idiopathic Parkinson's disease: possible routes by which vulnerable neuronal types may be subject to neuroinvasion by an unknown pathogen. *J Neural Transm*. 2003 May;110(5):517-36
[417] Williams RJ. Biochemical Individuality : The Basis for the Genetotrophic Concept. Austin/London: University of Texas Press, 1956 pages 60-61
[418] Ruscin JM, Page RL 2nd, Valuck RJ. Vitamin B(12) deficiency associated with histamine(2)-receptor antagonists and a proton-pump inhibitor. *Ann Pharmacother* 2002 May;36(5):812-6
[419] "CONCLUSION: Drug-induced hypochlorhydria causes high duodenal bacterial counts in the elderly but, in the short term, this bacterial overgrowth is not associated with malabsorption." Pereira SP, Gainsborough N, Dowling RH. Drug-induced hypochlorhydria causes high duodenal bacterial counts in the elderly. *Aliment Pharmacol Ther*. 1998 Jan;12(1):99-104
[420] Force RW, Nahata MC. Effect of histamine H2-receptor antagonists on vitamin B12 absorption. *Ann Pharmacother*. 1992 Oct;26(10):1283-6
[421] "CONCLUSIONS: When antacid medication impairs the gastric digestion, IgE synthesis toward novel dietary proteins is promoted, leading to food allergy." Untersmayr E, Scholl I, Swoboda I, Beil WJ, Forster-Waldl E, Walter F, Riemer A, Kraml G, Kinaciyan T, Spitzauer S, Boltz-Nitulescu G, Scheiner O, Jensen-Jarolim E. Antacid medication inhibits digestion of dietary proteins and causes food allergy: a fish allergy model in BALB/c mice. *J Allergy Clin Immunol*. 2003 Sep;112(3):616-23

as nausea, constipation, or diarrhea. A study of 197 patients published in *American Journal of Gastroenterology*[422] reported that 48% of people with irritable bowel syndrome (which affects an estimated 35 million Americans—more than 10% of the US population) and other chronic digestive complaints were infected with the parasite *Giardia lamblia*—getting rid of the parasite cured 90% of patients. Gastrointestinal infections with microbes such as *Blastocystis hominis* and *Entamoeba histolytica* can produce manifestations similar to irritable bowel syndrome, rheumatoid arthritis, fibromyalgia, food allergy, endogenous mental depression, chronic fatigue syndrome, or multiple chemical sensitivity and can exacerbate HIV infection.[423] While many of these people could probably benefit from other treatments as well, in many cases the most important treatment that they needed was a specific treatment to get rid of their parasites—treating the cause of the problem is always the most effective way to obtain health improvements for people with specific health complaints. Presence of intestinal overgrowth of harmful yeast, bacteria, and other "parasites" is currently referred to as dysbiosis and was previously referred to in the medical literature as "autointoxication"[424]; this critically important topic is detailed in <u>Integrative Rheumatology</u> within the context of treating systemic autoimmune diseases such as rheumatoid arthritis.

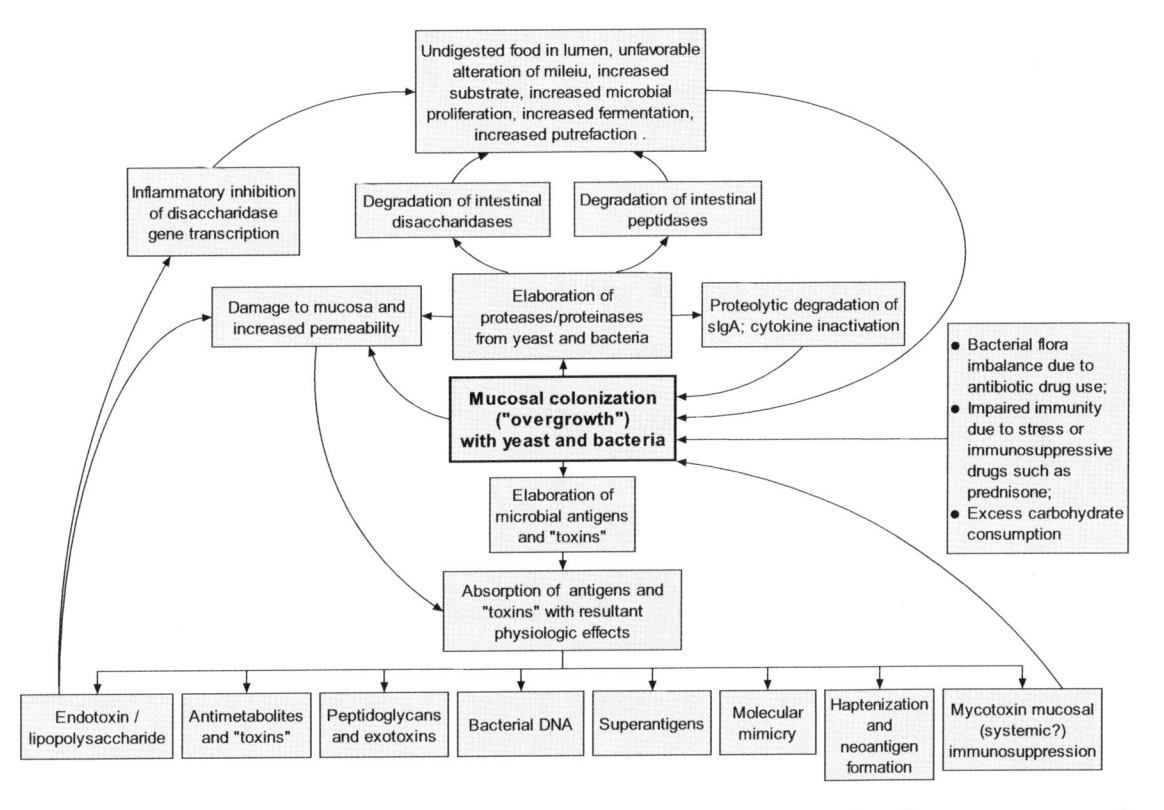

**Introduction to the Interconnected Vicious Cycles and Molecular Consequences of Intestinal Dysbiosis**: Partial diagram from <u>Integrative Rheumatology</u>

---

[422] Galland L, Lee M. #170 High frequency of giardiasis in patients with chronic digestive complaints. *Am J Gastroenterol* 1989;84:1181
[423] Galland L. Intestinal protozoan infection is a common unsuspected cause of chronic illness. *J Advancement Med.* 1989;2: 539-552
[424] "The writer has observed numerous cases suffering from such conditions as chronic arthritis, hypertension, coronary disease, chronic abdominal distention, constipation, and colitis, in which the element of constipation, auto-intoxication and possible colon infection seemed to play a prominent part, which responded very satisfactorily to colonic irrigations after failure to improve following the usual forms of medical treatment." Snyder RG. The value of colonic irrigations in countering auto-intoxication of intestinal origin. *Medical Clinics of North America* 1939; May: 781-788

# Preventive Health Screening: General Recommendations[425]

| ALL GROUPS | • Height and weight, blood pressure measurement at least every 1-2 years<br>• Screening lab tests with physical exams; special tests for specific concerns or family pattern of disease<br>• Regular dental care; periodic eye examinations<br>• Dietary advice; smoking cessation; limited alcohol consumption |
|---|---|
| 19 months to 6 years | • Eye examination for strabismus; regular clinical exams, vaccinations offered<br>• Consider hearing tests; consider testing for lead poisoning |
| 7-18 years: office visit every 3-5 years | • Physical examination for normal physical development<br>• Screening assessments including: cholesterol, blood glucose, and electrolytes; kidney and liver function should be performed at least once<br>• Sexually active adolescents should begin receiving periodic clinical examinations and blood tests to assess for STDs; additionally, sexually active females should receive a pelvic examination with Pap smear. Young men should be taught to perform self-testicular examination to assess for testicular cancer. |
| 19-39 years: office visit every 2-3 years | • Screening assessments including: cholesterol, blood glucose, and electrolytes, kidney and liver function should be performed at least every five years; men and women with high risk for or concern about cardiovascular disease should consider comprehensive risk factor analysis.<br>• Clinical skin examination<br>• MEN: All men over age 30 years should be tested for iron overload[426]; monthly testicular self-examination, and annual clinical testicular examination.<br>• WOMEN: monthly breast self-examination; clinical breast examination every 1-3 years beginning at age 30; annual pelvic examination with Pap smear beginning at age 18; consider assessments for developing osteoporosis if family history shows high risk. |
| 40-64 years: office visits at least every 1-2 years | • Screening assessments including: cholesterol, blood glucose, and electrolytes, kidney and liver function; men and women with high risk for or concern about cardiovascular disease should consider comprehensive risk factor analysis<br>• Clinical skin examination<br>• Cardiac assessment (ECG) can be considered for persons 1) with two or more risk factors for cardiovascular disease, 2) who are considering exercise after a long period of sedentary lifestyle, and 3) whose health affects public safety (e.g., pilots, police officers).<br>• Beginning at age 50: annual testing for fecal occult blood; begin sigmoidoscopy every 5 years.<br>• WOMEN: Annual clinical breast examination; mammogram every 1-2 years until age 50, annual mammogram between age 50-70 (controversial[427]: "…no large study has shown the effectiveness of breast cancer screening by either CBE or mammography for women whose risk of breast cancer is higher than the general population."[428]); assessments for osteoporosis are strongly recommended; thyroid hormone assessment every 5 years.<br>• MEN: consider annual digital examination of the prostate and baseline PSA. |

Wear your seatbelt. ♦ Don't smoke tobacco. ♦ Eat fruit/vegetables every day. ♦ Get regular exercise. ♦ Have people in your life who support you and listen to you. ♦ Get a massage. ♦ Practice safe sex. ♦ Brush and floss your teeth. ♦ Wear eye and ear protection when operating machinery. ♦ Get plenty of sleep.

---

[425] *American Family Physician* 1992; 45: 1917 et al; *Patient Care Archive* January 15, 1998; *Cleveland Clin J Med* 2000; 67: 521-30
[426] Baer DM, Simons JL, et al. Hemochromatosis screening in asymptomatic ambulatory men 30 years of age and older. *Am J Med.* 1995;98(5):464-8.
[427] Sellman S. Breast cancer awareness: seeing deception is your only protection. *Alternative Medicine* November 2001, pages 68-74
[428] *Patient Care Archive* January 15, 1998

# Wellness Promotion: Re-Establishing the Foundation for Health

## *Natural holistic healthcare empowers patients with the ability to understand and effectively participate in the course of their life and health*

| Allopathic chemical medicine | *Paradigm* | Holistic natural healthcare |
|---|---|---|
| • Doctor as "savior" and indifferent observer | *Role of the doctor* | • Doctor as "teacher" and active partner |
| • Helpless victim, disempowered, dependent | *Role of the patient* | • Active participant, empowered, responsible |
| • Illness is impossibly complex, and treating this with natural means is impossible<br>• Treatment is simple: you have this disease, and you need to take a drug for every problem<br>• You can change your diet and lifestyle but it won't make a big difference | *Nature of illness* | • Multifactorial: involving many different aspects of lifestyle, diet, exercise, genetic inheritance, and environment<br>• Many causes allows for many different treatment approaches and different ways of attaining health<br>• Illness can be modified via selective dietary and lifestyle changes and a custom-tailored treatment plan |
| • Disease-centered, drug-centered | *Viewpoint* | • Patient-centered, wellness-centered |
| • Drugs, including chemotherapy<br>• Surgery<br>• Radiation<br>• Electroconvulsive treatment | *Treatment and options* | • Diet and lifestyle improvement<br>• Relationship/emotional work<br>• Botanical and nutritional medicines<br>• Physical medicine, chiropractic, exercise<br>• Acupuncture<br>• *Selective* rather than *first-line* use of pharmaceuticals and medical procedures |
| • Symptom suppression<br>• Drug side-effects are a significant cause of death in the US<br>• Only *treats disease*, does not *promote health*; cannot reach optimal health by only reactively treating established health problems<br>• Enormous expense, often subsidized | *Long-term outcome* | • Improved health<br>• Potential for successful prevention, treatment or eradication of chronic disease<br>• Potential to become optimally healthy<br>• Proven cost-reduction |
| • For the most part, drugs are chemicals that have action in the body by interfering with the way that they body works<br>• Every drug has side-effects, some of which can be life-threatening<br>• Surgery causes irreparable changes to the body, many times for the worse.<br>• Radiation and chemotherapy can cause a secondary cancer to develop | *Risks* | • Minimal, since most of the botanical treatments and all of the nutritional medicines have been a major part of the human diet for centuries/millennia and have proven safety<br>• Most treatments are not fast-acting enough to be of value in traumatic or acutely life-threatening situations<br>• Patients must be willing to discard unhealthy lifestyles. |
| • Allows a doctor to see many patients within a short amount of time, thus increasing profitability<br>• Since drugs do not cure problems, patients must return for lifelong prescription renewals<br>• Therapeutic passivity: minimal action or effort required by patient and doctor<br>• The doctor holds all the power, and the patient is completely dependent on the doctor for treatment | *Benefits* | • Improved short-term and long-term health<br>• Empowerment<br>• Understanding of body processes as well as healthcare directions and goals<br>• Options |

*Opposite Influences of Health Promotion vs. Disease Promotion: Lifestyle Concept*

**Health-promoting:**
- Frequent exercise and physical activity
- Plenty of sleep
- Maintaining ideal body weight
- Avoiding exposure to chemicals, drugs, pollution, exhaust, tobacco smoke
- Daily consumption of fruits and vegetables
- Ideal protein intake for body size, physical activity, and health status
- Diet high in fiber and complex carbohydrates
- Use of health-promoting beverages such as green tea, fruit/vegetable juices, water, and light consumption of beer or red wine
- Increased intake of ALA, EPA, DHA, GLA, and oleic acid
- Multi-vitamin and multi-mineral supplementation
- Optimal vitamin D and iron status
- Beneficial gastrointestinal flora
- Natural and phytonutraceutical interventions to promote optimal health
- Pro-active healthcare
- Healthy and supportive relationships that foster responsibility, independence, interdependence, health and feelings of being wanted and cared for
- Work environments that promote collaboration and creativity and which appreciate personal time and allow for schedule flexibility

**Disease-promoting:**
- Physical inactivity and sedentary lifestyle
- Insufficient sleep
- Obesity
- Frequent exposure to chemicals, drugs, pollution, exhaust, tobacco smoke
- Daily consumption of processed and artificial foods
- Insufficient (common) or excessive (rare) protein
- Diet high in simple carbohydrates and sugars
- Use of disease-promoting beverages such as cola, artificially colored/flavored/sweetened drinks, and hard liquor
- Increased intake of linoleic acid (vegetable oils) and arachidonic acid (beef, liver, pork, lamb and most farm-raised land animals)
- Low intake of vitamins and minerals
- Excess iron and insufficient vitamin D
- Dysbiosis: intestinal overgrowth of yeast, parasites, and harmful bacteria
- Use of synthetic chemical drugs to suppress symptoms of poor health
- Reactive healthcare that only responds to problems after they have developed
- Dysfunctional relationships that enable and foster illness, dependency and isolation
- Work environments that promote isolation, pressure, perfectionism and which disapprove of creativity, personal time, and flexibility

Maximize factors that promote health ♦ Minimize factors that promote disease

Improved clinical outcomes will be attained when doctors and patients attend to both **prescription of health-promoting activities** and **proscription of disease-promoting activities**. Indeed, attention needs to be given to the **ratio** of these disparate and opposing forces, which ultimately influence genetic expression and physiologic function of many organ systems.

# A Five-Part Nutritional Wellness Protocol That Produces Consistently Positive Results: Brief Review of Scientific Rationale

*Alex Vasquez, DC, ND*

This article was originally published in *Nutritional Wellness*
http://www.nutritionalwellness.com/archives/2005/sep/09_vasquez.php

When I am lecturing here in the U.S., as well as in Europe, doctors often ask if I will share the details of my protocols with them. Thus, in 2004, I published a 486-page textbook for doctors that includes several protocols and important concepts for the promotion of wellness and treatment of musculoskeletal disorders.[429] In this article, I will share with you what I consider a basic protocol for wellness promotion. I've implemented this protocol as part of the treatment plan for a wide range of clinical problems. In my next column, I will provide several case reports of patients from my office to exemplify the effectiveness of this program and show how it can be the foundation upon which additional treatments can be added as necessary.

Nutrients are required in the proper amounts, forms, and approximate ratios for essential physiologic function; if nutrients are lacking, the body cannot function normally, let alone optimally. Impaired function results in subjective and objective manifestations of what is commonly labeled as "disease." Thus, a powerful and effective alternative to treating diseases with drugs is to re-establish normal/optimal physiologic function by replenishing the body with essential nutrients.

Of course, many diseases are multifactorial and therefore require multicomponent treatment plans, and some diseases actually require the use of drugs. However, while only a relatively small portion of patients actually need drugs for their problems, I am sure we all agree that everyone needs a foundational nutrition plan, as outlined and substantiated below.

1. Health-promoting diet: Following an extensive review of the research literature, I developed what I call the "supplemented Paleo-Mediterranean diet," which I have described in greater detail elsewhere.[430] In essence, this diet plan combines the best of the Mediterranean diet with the best of the Paleolithic diet, the latter of which has been detailed most recently by Dr. Loren Cordain in his book, The Paleo Diet, and his numerous scientific articles.[431] This diet places emphasis on fruits, vegetables, nuts, seeds, and berries that meet the body's needs for fiber, carbohydrates, and most importantly, the 8,000+ phytonutrients that have additive and synergistic health benefits.[432] Preferred protein sources are lean meats such as fish and poultry. In contrast to Cordain's Paleo diet, I also advocate soy and whey for their high-quality protein and anticancer, cardioprotective, and mood-enhancing benefits. Rice and

---

[429] **Vasquez A**. *Integrative Orthopedics: The Art of Creating Wellness While Managing Acute and Chronic Musculoskeletal Disorders*. 2004, 2007
[430] **Vasquez A**. The Importance of Integrative Chiropractic Health Care in Treating Musculoskeletal Pain and Reducing the Nationwide Burden of Medical Expenses and Iatrogenic Injury and Death: A Concise Review of Current Research and Implications for Clinical Practice and Healthcare Policy. *The Original Internist* 2005; 12(4): 159-182
[431] Cordain L. *The Paleo Diet*. (John Wiley and Sons, 2002). Also: Cordain L. Cereal grains: humanity's double edged sword. *World Rev Nutr Diet* 1999;84:19-73  Access to most of Dr Cordain's articles is available at http://thepaleodiet.com/
[432] Liu RH. Health benefits of fruit and vegetables are from additive and synergistic combinations of phytochemicals. *Am J Clin Nutr* 2003;78(3 Suppl):517S-520S

potatoes are discouraged due to their relatively high glycemic indexes and high glycemic loads, and their lack of fiber and phytonutrients (compared to other fruits and vegetables). Generally speaking, grains such as wheat and rye are discouraged due to the high glycemic loads/indexes of most breads and pastries, as well as the allergenicity of gluten, a protein that appears to help trigger disorders such as migraine, celiac disease, psoriasis, epilepsy, and autoimmunity. Sources of simple sugars such as high-fructose corn syrup (e.g., cola, soda) and processed foods (e.g., "TV dinners" and other manufactured snacks and convenience foods) are strictly forbidden. Chemical preservatives, colorants, sweeteners and carrageenan are likewise prohibited. In summary, this diet plan provides plenty of variety, as most dishes comprised of poultry, fish, soy, fruits, vegetables, nuts, berries, and seeds are allowed. The diet also provides plenty of fiber, phytonutrients, carbohydrates, potassium, and protein, while simultaneously being low in fat, sodium, arachidonic acid, and "simple sugars." The diet must be customized with regard to total protein and calorie intake, as determined by the size, status, and activity level of the patient, and individual food allergens should be avoided. Regular consumption of this diet has shown the ability to reduce hypertension, alleviate diabetes, ameliorate migraine headaches, and result in improvement of overall health and a lessening of the severity of many common "diseases." This diet is supplemented with vitamins, minerals, and fatty acids as described below.

2. <u>Multivitamin and multimineral supplementation</u>: Vitamin and mineral supplementation finally received endorsement from "mainstream" medicine when researchers from Harvard Medical School published a review article in Journal of the American Medical Association that concluded, "Most people do not consume an optimal amount of all vitamins by diet alone. ...It appears prudent for all adults to take vitamin supplements."[433] Long-term nutritional insufficiencies experienced by "most people" promote the development of "long-latency deficiency diseases" such as cancer, neuroemotional deterioration, and cardiovascular disease.[434] Impressively, the benefits of multivitamin/multimineral supplementation have been demonstrated in numerous clinical trials. Multivitamin/multimineral supplementation has been shown to improve nutritional status and reduce the risk for chronic diseases[435], improve mood[436], potentiate antidepressant drug treatment[437], alleviate migraine headaches (when used with diet improvement and fatty acids[438]), improve immune function and infectious disease outcomes in the elderly[439] (especially diabetics[440]), reduce morbidity and mortality in patients with HIV infection[441,442] alleviate premenstrual syndrome[443,444] and bipolar disorder[445], reduce violence and antisocial behavior in children[446] and incarcerated

---

[433] Fletcher RH, Fairfield KM. Vitamins for chronic disease prevention in adults: clinical applications. *JAMA* 2002;287:3127-9
[434] Heaney RP. Long-latency deficiency disease: insights from calcium and vitamin D. *Am J Clin Nutr* 2003;78:912-9
[435] McKay DL, Perrone G, Rasmussen H, Dallal G, Hartman W, Cao G, Prior RL, Roubenoff R, Blumberg JB. The effects of a multivitamin/mineral supplement on micronutrient status, antioxidant capacity and cytokine production in healthy older adults consuming a fortified diet. *J Am Coll Nutr* 2000;19(5):613-21
[436] Benton D, Haller J, Fordy J. Vitamin supplementation for 1 year improves mood. *Neuropsychobiology* 1995;32(2):98-105
[437] Coppen A, Bailey J. Enhancement of the antidepressant action of fluoxetine by folic acid: a randomised, placebo controlled trial. *J Affect Disord* 2000;60:121-30
[438] Wagner W, Nootbaar-Wagner U. Prophylactic treatment of migraine with gamma-linolenic and alpha-linolenic acids. *Cephalalgia* 1997;17:127-30
[439] Langkamp-Henken B, Bender BS, Gardner EM, Herrlinger-Garcia KA, Kelley MJ, Murasko DM, Schaller JP, Stechmiller JK, Thomas DJ, Wood SM. Nutritional formula enhanced immune function and reduced days of symptoms of upper respiratory tract infection in seniors. *J Am Geriatr Soc* 2004;52:3-12
[440] Barringer TA, Kirk JK, Santaniello AC, Foley KL, Michielutte R. Effect of a multivitamin and mineral supplement on infection and quality of life. A randomized, double-blind, placebo-controlled trial. *Ann Intern Med* 2003;138:365-71
[441] Fawzi WW, Msamanga GI, Spiegelman D, et al. A randomized trial of multivitamin supplements and HIV disease progression and mortality. *N Engl J Med* 2004;351:23-32
[442] Burbano X, Miguez-Burbano MJ, McCollister K, Zhang G, Rodriguez A, Ruiz P, Lecusay R, Shor-Posner G. Impact of a selenium chemoprevention clinical trial on hospital admissions of HIV-infected participants. *HIV Clin Trials* 2002;3:483-91
[443] Abraham GE. Nutritional factors in the etiology of the premenstrual tension syndromes. *J Reprod Med* 1983;28(7):446-64
[444] Stewart A. Clinical and biochemical effects of nutritional supplementation on the premenstrual syndrome. *J Reprod Med* 1987;32:435-41
[445] Kaplan BJ, Simpson JS, Ferre RC, Gorman CP, McMullen DM, Crawford SG. Effective mood stabilization with a chelated mineral supplement: an open-label trial in bipolar disorder. *J Clin Psychiatry* 2001;62:936-44
[446] Kaplan BJ, Crawford SG, Gardner B, Farrelly G. Treatment of mood lability and explosive rage with minerals and vitamins: two case studies in children. *J Child Adolesc Psychopharmacol* 2002;12(3):205-19

young adults (when used with essential fatty acids[447]), and improve scores of intelligence in children.[448] Vitamin supplementation has anti-inflammatory benefits, as evidenced by significant reduction in C-reactive protein, (CRP) in a double-blind, placebo-controlled trial.[449] The ability to safely and affordably deliver these benefits makes multimineral-multivitamin supplementation and essential component of any and all health-promoting and disease-prevention strategies. Vitamin A can result in liver damage with chronic consumption of 25,000 IU or more, and intake should generally not exceed 10,000 IU per day in women of childbearing age. Iron should not be supplemented except in patients diagnosed with iron deficiency by a blood test (serum ferritin). Additional vitamin D should be used, as described in the next section.

3. <u>Physiologic doses of vitamin D3</u>: The prevalence of vitamin D deficiency varies from 40 percent (general population) to almost 100 percent (patients with musculoskeletal pain) in the American population. I described the many benefits of vitamin D3 supplementation in the previous issue of *Nutritional Wellness* and in the major monograph published last year.[450] In summary, vitamin D deficiency causes or contributes to depression, hypertension, seizures, migraine, polycystic ovary syndrome, inflammation, autoimmunity, and musculoskeletal pain such as low-back pain. Clinical trials using vitamin D supplementation have proven the cause-and-effect relationship between vitamin D deficiency and these conditions by showing that each of these could be cured or alleviated with vitamin D supplementation. In our review of the literature, we concluded that daily vitamin D doses should be 1,000 IU for infants, 2,000 IU for children, and 4,000 IU for adults. Cautions and contraindications include the use of thiazide diuretics (e.g., hydrochlorothiazide) or any other medications that can promote hypercalcemia, as well as granulomatous diseases such as sarcoidosis, tuberculosis, and certain types of cancer, especially lymphoma. Effectiveness is monitored by measuring serum 25-OH-vitamin D, and safety is monitored by measuring serum calcium.

4. <u>Balanced and complete fatty acid supplementation</u>: A detailed survey of the literature shows there are at least five health-promoting fatty acids commonly found in the human diet.[451] These are alpha-linolenic acid (ALA; omega-3, from flaxseed oil), eicosapentaenoic acid (EPA; omega-3, from fish oil), docosahexaenoic acid (DHA; omega-3, from fish oil and algae), gamma-linolenic acid (GLA; omega-6, most concentrated in borage oil), and oleic acid (omega-9, from olive oil, also flaxseed and borage oils). Each of these fatty acids has health benefits that cannot be fully attained from supplementing a different fatty acid. The benefits of GLA (borage oil) are not attained by consumption of EPA and DHA (fish oil); in fact, consumption of fish oil can actually promote a deficiency of GLA.[452] Likewise, consumption of GLA alone can reduce EPA levels while increasing levels of proinflammatory arachidonic acid; both of these problems are avoided with co-administration of fish oil any time borage oil is used. Using ALA (flaxseed oil) alone only slightly increases EPA but generally leads to no improvement in DHA status and can lead to a reduction of oleic acid; thus, fish oil, olive

---

[447] Gesch CB, Hammond SM, Hampson SE, Eves A, Crowder MJ. Influence of supplementary vitamins, minerals and essential fatty acids on the antisocial behaviour of young adult prisoners. Randomised, placebo-controlled trial. *Br J Psychiatry* 2002;181:22-8
[448] Benton D. Micro-nutrient supplementation and the intelligence of children. *Neurosci Biobehav Rev* 2001;25:297-309
[449] Church TS, Earnest CP, Wood KA, Kampert JB. Reduction of C-reactive protein levels through use of a multivitamin. *Am J Med* 2003;115:702-7
[450] **Vasquez A**, Manso G, Cannell J. The clinical importance of vitamin D (cholecalciferol): a paradigm shift with implications for all healthcare providers. *Alternative Therapies in Health and Medicine* 2004;10:28-37 http://optimalhealthresearch.com/cholecalciferol.html
[451] **Vasquez A**. Reducing Pain and Inflammation Naturally. Part 2: New Insights into Fatty Acid Supplementation and Its Effect on Eicosanoid Production and Genetic Expression. *Nutritional Perspectives* 2005; January: 5-16 http://optimalhealthresearch.com/part2
[452] Cleland LG, Gibson RA, Neumann M, French JK. The effect of dietary fish oil supplement upon the content of dihomo-gammalinolenic acid in human plasma phospholipids. *Prostaglandins Leukot Essent Fatty Acids* 1990 May;40(1):9-12

oil (and borage oil) should be supplemented when flaxseed oil is used.[453] Obviously, the goal here is a balanced intake of all of the health-promoting fatty acids; using only one or two sources of fatty acids is not balanced and results in suboptimal improvement, at best. In clinical practice, I routinely use combination fatty acid therapy comprised of ALA, EPA, DHA, and GLA for essentially all patients. The product also contains a modest amount of oleic acid, and I encourage use of olive oil for salads and cooking. This approach results in complete and balanced fatty acid intake, and the clinical benefits are impressive.

5. <u>Probiotics /gut flora modification</u>: Proper levels of good bacteria promote intestinal health, proper immune function, and support overall health. Excess bacteria or yeast, or the presence of harmful bacteria, yeast, or "parasites" such as amoebas and protozoas, can cause "leaky gut," systemic inflammation, and a wide range of clinical problems. Intestinal flora can become imbalanced by poor diets, excess stress, immunosuppressive drugs, antibiotics, or exposure to contaminated food or water, all of which are common among American patients. Thus, as a rule, I reinstate the good bacteria by the use of probiotics (good bacteria and yeast), prebiotics (fiber, arabinogalactan, and inulin), and the use of fermented foods such as kefir (in patients not allergic to milk). Harmful yeast, bacteria, and other "parasites" can be eradicated with the combination of dietary change, drugs, and/or herbal extracts. For example, oregano oil in an emulsified, time-released form has proven safe and effective for the elimination of various parasites encountered in clinical practice.[454] Likewise, the herb Artemisia annua (sweet wormwood) commonly is used to eradicate specific bacteria and has been used for thousands of years in Asia for the treatment and prevention of infectious diseases, including malaria.[455]

## Conclusion:

In this brief review, I have outlined and scientifically substantiated a fundamental protocol that can serve as effective therapy for patients with a wide range of "diseases." Customizing the Paleo-Mediterranean diet to avoid food allergens, using vitamin-mineral supplements along with physiologic doses of vitamin D and broad-spectrum balanced fatty acid supplementation, and ensuring gastrointestinal health with the skillful use of probiotics, prebiotics, and antimicrobial treatments provides an excellent health-promoting and disease-eliminating foundation and lifestyle for many patients. Often, this simple protocol is all that is needed for the effective treatment of a wide range of clinical problems. For other patients with more complex illnesses, of course, additional interventions and laboratory assessments can be used to customize the treatment plan. However, we must always remember that the attainment and preservation of health requires that we meet the body's basic nutritional needs. This five-step protocol begins the process of meeting those needs. In my next article, I'll give you some examples from my clinical practice and additional references to show how safe and effective this protocol can be.

---

[453] Jantti J, Nikkari T, Solakivi T, Vapaatalo H, Isomaki H. Evening primrose oil in rheumatoid arthritis: changes in serum lipids and fatty acids. *Ann Rheum Dis* 1989;48(2):124-7
[454] Force M, Sparks WS, Ronzio RA. Inhibition of enteric parasites by emulsified oil of oregano in vivo. *Phytother Res* 2000;14:213-4
[455] Schuster BG. Demonstrating the validity of natural products as anti-infective drugs. *J Altern Complement Med* 2001;7 Suppl 1:S73-82

# Implementing the Five-Part Nutritional Wellness Protocol for the Treatment of Various Health Problems

*Alex Vasquez, DC, ND*

This article was originally published in *Nutritional Wellness*
http://www.nutritionalwellness.com/archives/2005/nov/11_vasquez.php

In my last article in *Nutritional Wellness* I described a 5-part nutritional protocol that can be used in the vast majority of patients without adverse effects and with major benefits. For many patients, the basic protocol consisting of 1) the Paleo-Mediterranean diet, 2) multivitamin/multimineral supplementation, 3) additional vitamin D3, 4) combination fatty acid therapy with an optimal balance of ALA, GLA, EPA, DHA, and oleic acid, and 5) probiotics (including the identification and eradication of harmful yeast, bacteria, and other "parasites") is all the treatment that they need. For patients who need additional treatment, this foundational plan still serves as the core of the biochemical aspect of their intervention. Of course, in some cases, we have to use other lifestyle modifications (such as exercise), additional supplements (such as policosanol or antimicrobial herbs), manual treatments (including spinal manipulation) and occasionally select medications (such has hormone modulators) to obtain our goal of maximum improvement.

The following examples show how the 5-part protocol serves to benefit patients with a wide range of conditions. For the sake of saving space, I will use only highly specific citations to the research literature, since I have provided the other references in the previous issue of *Nutritional Wellness* and elsewhere.[456]

- **A Man with High Cholesterol**: This patient is a 41-year-old slightly overweight man with very high cholesterol. His total cholesterol was 290 (normal < 200), LDL cholesterol was 212 (normal <130), and his triglycerides were 148 (optimal <100). I am quite certain that nearly every medical doctor would have put this man on cholesterol-lowering statin drugs for life. *Treatment*: In contrast, I advised a low-carb Paleo-Mediterranean diet because such diets have been shown to reduce cardiovascular mortality more powerfully that "statin" cholesterol-lowering drugs in older patients.[457] Likewise, fatty acid supplementation is more effective than statin drugs for reducing cardiac and all-cause mortality.[458] We added probiotics, because supplementation with *Lactobacillus* and *Bifidobacterium* has been shown to lower cholesterol levels in humans with high cholesterol.[459] Finally, I also prescribed 20 mg of policosanol for its well-known ability to favorably modify cholesterol levels.[460] *Results*: Within **one month** the patient had lost weight, felt better, and his total cholesterol had dropped to normal at 196 (from 290!), LDL was reduced to 141, and triglycerides were reduced to 80. Basically, this

---

[456] **Vasquez A**. Integrative Orthopedics. www.OptimalHealthResearch.com and Chiropractic and Naturopathic Medicine for the Promotion of Optimal Health and Alleviation of Pain and Inflammation. http://optimalhealthresearch.com/monograph05
[457] Knoops KT, et al. Mediterranean diet, lifestyle factors, and 10-year mortality in elderly European men and women: the HALE project. *JAMA*. 2004 Sep 22;292(12):1433-9
[458] Studer M, et al. Effect of different antilipidemic agents and diets on mortality: a systematic review. *Arch Intern Med*. 2005;165:725-30
[459] Xiao JZ, et al. Effects of milk products fermented by Bifidobacterium longum on blood lipids in rats and healthy adult male volunteers. *J Dairy Sci*. 2003;86:2452-61
[460] Cholesterol-lowering action of policosanol compares well to that of pravastatin and lovastatin. *Cardiovasc J S Afr*. 2003;14(3):161

treatment plan was "the protocol + policosanol." Drug treatment of this patient would have been more expensive, more risky, and would not have resulted in global health improvements.

- **A Child with Intractable Seizures**: This is a 4-year-old nonverbal boy with 3-5 seizures per day despite being on two anti-seizure medications and having previously had several other "last resort" medical and surgical procedures. He also had a history of food allergies. *Treatment*: Obviously, there was no room for error in this case. We implemented a moderately low-carb hypoallergenic diet since both carbohydrate restriction[461] and allergy avoidance[462] can reduce the frequency and severity of seizures. Since many "anti-seizure" medications actually cause seizures by causing vitamin D deficiency[463], I added 800 IU per day of emulsified vitamin D3 for its antiseizure benefit.[464] We used 1 tsp per day of a combination fatty acid supplement that provides balanced amounts of ALA, GLA, EPA, and DHA, since fatty acids appear to have potential antiseizure benefits.[465] Vitamin B-6 (250 mg of P5P) and magnesium (bowel tolerance) were also added to reduce brain hyperexcitability.[466] Stool testing showed an absence of *Bifidobacteria* and *Lactobacillus*; probiotics were added for their anti-allergy benefits.[467] *Results*: Within about 2 months seizure frequency reduced from 3-5 per day to one seizure every other day: *an 87% reduction in seizure frequency*. Patient was able to discontinue one of the anti-seizure medications. His parents also noted several global improvements: the boy started making eye contact with people, he was learning again, and intellectually he was "making gains every day." His parents considered this an "amazing difference." Going from 30 seizures per week to 4 seizures per week while reducing medication use by 50% is a major achievement. Notice that we simply used the basic wellness protocol with some additional B6 and magnesium. It is highly unlikely that B6 and magnesium alone would have produced such a favorable response.

- **A Young Woman with Full-Body Psoriasis Unresponsive to Drug Treatment**: This is a 17-year-old woman with head-to-toe psoriasis since childhood. She wears long pants and long-sleeved shirts year-round, and the psoriasis is a major interference to her social life. Medications have ceased to help. *Treatment*: The Paleo-Mediterranean diet was implemented with an emphasis on food allergy identification.[1] We used a multivitamin-mineral supplement with 200 mcg selenium to compensate for the nutritional insufficiencies and selenium deficiency that are common in patients with psoriasis; likewise 10 mg of folic acid was added to address the relative vitamin deficiencies and elevated homocysteine that are common in these patients.[468] Combination fatty acid therapy with EPA and DHA from fish oil and GLA from borage oil was used for the anti-inflammatory and skin-healing benefits.[469] Vitamin E (1200 IU of mixed tocopherols) and lipoic acid (1,000 mg per day) were added for their anti-inflammatory benefits and to combat the oxidative stress that is characteristic of psoriasis.[470] Of course, probiotics were used to modify gut flora, which is commonly deranged in patients

---

[461] Freeman JM, et al. The efficacy of the ketogenic diet-1998: a prospective evaluation of intervention in 150 children. *Pediatrics*. 1998;102:1358-63
[462] Egger J, Carter CM, Soothill JF, Wilson J. Oligoantigenic diet treatment of children with epilepsy and migraine. *J Pediatr*. 1989;114:51-8
[463] Ali FE, Al-Bustan MA, Al-Busairi WA, Al-Mulla FA. Loss of seizure control due to anticonvulsant-induced hypocalcemia. *Ann Pharmacother*. 2004;38:1002-5
[464] Christiansen C, Rodbro P, Sjo O."Anticonvulsant action" of vitamin D in epileptic patients? A controlled pilot study. *Br Med J*. 1974 May 4;2(913):258-9
[465] Yuen AW, et al. Omega-3 fatty acid supplementation in patients with chronic epilepsy: A randomized trial. *Epilepsy Behav*. 2005 Sep;7(2):253-8
[466] Mousain-Bosc M, et al. Magnesium VitB6 intake reduces central nervous system hyperexcitability in children. *J Am Coll Nutr*. 2004;23(5):545S-548S
[467] Majamaa H, Isolauri E.Probiotics: a novel approach in the management of food allergy. *J Allergy Clin Immunol*. 1997 Feb;99(2):179-85
[468] Vanizor Kural B, et al. Plasma homocysteine and its relationships with atherothrombotic markers in psoriatic patients. *Clin Chim Acta*. 2003 Jun;332(1-2):23-3
[469] **Vasquez A**. Reducing Pain and Inflammation Naturally. Part 2: New Insights into Fatty Acid Supplementation and Its Effect on Eicosanoid Production and Genetic Expression. *Nutritional Perspectives* 2005; January: 5-16 www.OptimalHealthResearch.com/part2
[470] Kokcam I, Naziroglu M. Antioxidants and lipid peroxidation status in the blood of patients with psoriasis. *Clin Chim Acta*. 1999 Nov;289(1-2):23-31

with psoriasis.[471] **Results**: Within a few weeks, this patient's "lifelong psoriasis" was essentially gone. Food allergy identification and avoidance played a major role in the success of this case. When I saw the patient again 9 months later for her second visit, she had no visible evidence of psoriasis. Her "medically untreatable" condition was essentially cured by the use of my basic protocol, with the addition of a few extra nutrients.

- **A Man with Fatigue and Recurrent Numbness in Hands and Feet**. This 40-year-old man had seen numerous neurologists and had spent tens of thousands of dollars on MRIs, CT scans, lumbar punctures, and other diagnostic procedures. No diagnosis had been found, and no effective treatment had been rendered by medical specialists. **Assessments**: We performed a modest battery of lab tests which revealed elevations of fibrinogen and C-reactive protein (CRP), two markers of acute inflammation. Assessment of intestinal permeability with the lactulose-mannitol assay showed major intestinal damage ("leaky gut"). Follow-up parasite testing on different occasions showed dysbiosis caused by *Proteus, Enterobacter, Klebsiella, Citrobacter,* and *Pseudomonas aeruginosa*—of course, these are gram-negative bacteria that can induce immune dysfunction and autoimmunity, as described elsewhere.[1] Specifically, *Pseudomonas aeruginosa* has been linked to the development of nervous system autoimmunity, such as multiple sclerosis.[472] **Treatment**: We implemented a plan of diet modification, vitamins, minerals, fatty acids, and probiotics. The dysbiosis was further addressed with specific antimicrobial herbs (including caprylic acid and emulsified oregano oil[473]) and drugs (such as tetracycline, Bactrim, and augmentin). The antibiotic drugs proved to be ineffective based on repeat stool testing. **Results**: Within one month we witnessed impressive improvements, both subjectively and objectively. Subjectively, the patient reported that the numbness and tingling almost completely resolved. Fatigue was reduced, and energy was improved. Objectively, the patient's elevated CRP plummeted from abnormally high at 11 down to completely normal at 1. Eighteen months later, the patient's CRP had dropped to less than 1 and fatigue and numbness were no longer problematic. Notice that this treatment plan was basically "the protocol" with additional attention to eradicating the dysbiosis we found with specialized stool testing.

- **A 50-year-old Man with Rheumatoid Arthritis**. This patient presented with a 3-year history of rheumatoid arthritis that had been treated unsuccessfully with drugs (methotrexate and intravenous Remicade). The first time I tested his CRP level, it was astronomically high at 124 (normal is <3). Because of the severe inflammation and other risk factors for sudden cardiac death, I referred this patient to an osteopathic internist for immune-suppressing drugs; the patient refused, stating that he was no longer willing to rely on immune-suppressing chemical medications. His treatment was entirely up to me. **Assessments and Treatments**: We implemented the Paleo-Mediterranean diet and a program of vitamins, minerals, optimal combination fatty acid therapy (providing ALA, GLA, EPA, DHA, and oleic acid), and 4000 IU of vitamin D in emulsified form to overcome defects in absorption that are seen in older patients and those with gastrointestinal problems.[474] Hormone testing showed abnormally low DHEA, low testosterone, and slightly elevated estrogen; these problems were corrected

---

[471] Waldman A, et al. Incidence of Candida in psoriasis--a study on the fungal flora of psoriatic patients. *Mycoses*. 2001 May;44(3-4):77-81
[472] Hughes LE, et al. Antibody responses to Acinetobacter spp. and Pseudomonas aeruginosa in multiple sclerosis: prospects for diagnosis using the myelin-acinetobacter-neurofilament antibody index. *Clin Diagn Lab Immunol*. 2001;8(6):1181-8
[473] Force M, Sparks WS, Ronzio RA. Inhibition of enteric parasites by emulsified oil of oregano in vivo. *Phytother Res*. 2000 May;14(3):213-4
[474] **Vasquez A**. Subphysiologic Doses of Vitamin D are Subtherapeutic: Comment on the Study by The Record Trial Group. *TheLancet.com* Accessed June 16, 2005

with DHEA supplementation and the use of a hormone-modulating drug (Arimidex) that lowers estrogen and raises testosterone. Specialized stool testing showed absence of *Lactobacillus* and *Bifidobacteria* and intestinal overgrowth of *Citrobacter* and *Enterobacter* which was corrected with probiotics and antimicrobial treatments including undecylenic acid and emulsified oregano oil. Importantly, I also decided to inhibit NF-kappaB (the primary transcription factor that upregulates the pro-inflammatory response[475]) by using a combination botanical formula that contains curcumin, piperine, lipoic acid, green tea extract, propolis, rosemary, resveratrol, ginger, and phytolens (an antioxidant extract from lentils that may inhibit autoimmunity[476])—all of these herbs and nutrients have been shown to inhibit NF-kappaB and to thus downregulate inflammatory responses.[477] **Results**: Within 6 weeks, this patient had happily lost 10 lbs of excess weight and was able to work without pain for the first time in years. Follow-up testing showed that his previously astronomical CRP had dropped from 124 to 7—a drop of 114 points in less than one month: better than had ever been achieved even with the use of intravenous immune-suppressing drugs! This patient continues to make significant progress. Obviously this case was complex, and we needed to do more than the basic protocol. Nonetheless, the basic protocol still served as the foundation for the treatment plan. Note that vitamin D has significant anti-inflammatory benefits and can cause major reductions in inflammation measured by CRP.[478] The correction of the hormonal abnormalities and the dysbiosis, and downregulating NF-kappaB with several botanical extracts were also critical components of this successful treatment plan.[1]

## Summary and Conclusions

These examples show how the nutritional wellness protocol that I described in the September issue of *Nutritional Wellness* can be used as the foundational treatment for a wide range of health problems. In many cases, implementation of the basic protocol is all that is needed. In more complex situations, we use the basic protocol and then add more specific treatments to address dysbiosis and hormonal problems, and we can add additional nutrients as needed. However, there will never be a substitute for a healthy diet, sufficiencies of vitamin D and all five of the health-promoting fatty acids (ie, ALA, GLA, EPA, DHA, and oleic acid), and normalization of gastrointestinal flora. Without these basics, survival and the appearance of health are possible, but true health and recovery from "untreatable" illnesses is not possible. In order to attain optimal health, we have to create the conditions that allow for health to be attained[1,] and we start this process by supplying the body with the nutrients that it needs to function optimally. In the words of naturopathic physician Jared Zeff from the *Journal of Naturopathic Medicine*, *"The work of the naturopathic physician is to elicit healing by helping patients to create or recreate the conditions for health to exist within them. Health will occur where the conditions for health exist. Disease is the product of the conditions which allow for it."*[479]

Although the chiropractic profession has emphasized spinal manipulation as its primary therapeutic tool, the profession has always appreciated holistic, integrative models of therapeutic intervention, health and disease. Chiropractic was the first healthcare profession in America to

---

[475] Tak PP, Firestein GS. NF-kappaB: a key role in inflammatory diseases. *J Clin Invest*. 2001 Jan;107(1):7-11
[476] Sandoval M, et al. Peroxynitrite-induced apoptosis in epithelial (T84) and macrophage (RAW 264.7) cell lines: effect of legume-derived polyphenols (phytolens). *Nitric Oxide*. 1997;1(6):476-83
[477] **Vasquez A**. Reducing pain and inflammation naturally - Part 4: Nutritional and Botanical Inhibition of NF-kappaB, the Major Intracellular Amplifier of the Inflammatory Cascade. A Practical Clinical Strategy Exemplifying Anti-Inflammatory Nutrigenomics. *Nutritional Perspectives* 2005;July: 5-12 www.OptimalHealthResearch.com/part4
[478] Timms PM, et al. Circulating MMP9, vitamin D and variation in the TIMP-1 response with VDR genotype. *QJM*. 2002 Dec;95(12):787-96
[479] Zeff JL. The process of healing: a unifying theory of naturopathic medicine. *Journal of Naturopathic Medicine* 1997; 7: 122-5

specifically claim that the optimization of health requires attention to the spiritual (emotional, psychological), mechanical (physical, structural), and chemical (nutritional, hormonal) aspects of our lives.[1] Chiropractic's founder DD Palmer[480] wrote, "The human body represents the actions of three laws—spiritual, mechanical, and chemical—united as one triune. As long as there is perfect union of these three, there is health." Accordingly, these cornerstones are fundamental to the modern definition of the chiropractic profession recently articulated by the American Chiropractic Association[481]: *"Doctors of Chiropractic are physicians who consider man as an integrated being and give special attention to the physiological and biochemical aspects including structural, spinal, musculoskeletal, neurological, vascular, nutritional, emotional and environmental relationships."* The cases that I have described in this article demonstrate the importance of attending to the nutritional, hormonal, environmental and gastrointestinal aspects of human physiology for helping our patients attain optimal health.

## Common Oversights and Shortcomings in the Study and Implementation of Nutritional Supplementation

*Alex Vasquez, D.C., N.D.*

This article was originally published in *Naturopathy Digest*
http://www.naturopathydigest.com/archives/2007/jun/vasquez.php

### Introduction
An impressive discrepancy often exists between the low efficacy of nutritional interventions reported in the research literature and the higher efficacy achieved in the clinical practices of clinicians trained in the use of interventional nutrition (i.e., chiropractic and naturopathic physicians). This discrepancy is dangerous for at least two reasons. First, it results in an undervaluation of the efficacy of nutritional supplementation, which ultimately leaves otherwise treatable patients untreated. Second, such untreated and undertreated patients are often then forced to use dangerous and expensive pharmaceutical drugs and surgical interventions to treat conditions that could have otherwise been easily and safely treated with nutritional supplementation and diet modification. Consequently, the burden of suffering, disease, and healthcare expense in the US is higher than it would be if nutritionally-trained clinicians were more fully integrated into the healthcare system.

### Obstacles to Efficacy in the Use of Nutritional Supplementation
Below are listed some of the most common causes for the underachievement of nutritional supplementation in practice and in published research. While this list is not all-inclusive, it will serve as a review for clinicians and an introduction for chiropractic/naturopathic students. In both practice and research, the problems listed below often overlap and function synergistically to reduce the efficacy of nutritional supplementation.

---

[480] Palmer DD. *The Science, Art, and Phiosophy, of Chiropractic*. Portland, OR; Portland Printing House Company, 1910: 107
[481] American Chiropractic Association. What is Chiropractic? http://amerchiro.org/media/whatis/ Accessed January 9, 2005

1. **Inadequate dosing (quantity)**: Many clinical trials published in major journals and many doctors in clinical practice have used inadequate doses of vitamins (and other natural therapeutics) and have thus failed to achieve the results that would have easily been obtained had they implemented their protocol with the proper physiologic or supraphysiologic dose of intervention. The best example in my experience centers on vitamin D, where so many of the studies are performed with doses of 400-800 IU per day only to conclude that vitamin supplementation is ineffective for the condition being treated. The problem here is that the researchers failed to appreciate that the physiologic requirement for vitamin D3 in adults is approximately 3,000-5,000 IU per day[482] and that therefore their supplemental dose of 400-800 IU is only 10-20% of what is required. Subphysiologic doses are generally subtherapeutic. In this regard, I have had to correct journals such as *The Lancet*[483], *JAMA*[484], and *British Medical Journal*[485] from misleading their readers (many of whom are major policymakers) from concluding that nutritional supplementation is impotent; rather, their researchers and editors were not sufficiently educated in the design and review of studies using nutritional interventions. These journals should hire chiropractic and naturopathic physicians so that they have staff trained in natural treatments and who can thus provide an educated review of studies on these topics.[486]

2. **Inadequate dosing (duration)**: Often the effects of long-term nutritional deficiency are not fully reversible and/or may require a treatment period of months or years to achieve maximal clinical response. For example, full replacement of fatty acids in human brain phospholipids is an ongoing process that occurs over a period of several years; thus studies using fatty acid supplements for a period of weeks or 2-3 months generally underestimate the enhanced effectiveness that can be obtained with administration over many months or several years of treatment. Relatedly, recovery from vitamin D deficiency takes several weeks of high-dose supplementation in order to achieve tissue saturation and subsequent cellular replenishment; studies of short duration are destined to underestimate the results that could have been achieved with supplementation carried out over several months.[487]

3. **Failure to use proper forms of nutrients**: Nutrients are often available in different forms, not the least of which are "active" versus "inactive" and "natural" versus "unnatural." Most vitamin supplements, particularly high-potency B vitamins, are manufactured synthetically and are not from "natural sources" despite the marketing hype promulgated by companies that, for example, mix their synthetic vitamins with a vegetable powder and then call their vitamin supplements "natural." The simple fact is that production of high-potency supplements from purely natural sources would be prohibitively wasteful, inefficient, and expensive. Thus, while it is not necessary for vitamins to be "natural" in order to be useful, it is necessary that the vitamins are useable and preferably not "unnatural." The best example of the use of unnatural supplements is the use of synthetic DL-tocopherol in the so-called "vitamin E" studies; DL-tocopherol is by definition 50% comprised of the L-isomer of

---

[482] Heaney RP, Davies KM, Chen TC, Holick MF, Barger-Lux MJ. Human serum 25-hydroxycholecalciferol response to extended oral dosing with cholecalciferol. *Am J Clin Nutr*. 2003 Jan;77(1):204-10 http://www.ajcn.org/cgi/content/full/77/1/204

[483] **Vasquez A**. Subphysiologic Doses of Vitamin D are Subtherapeutic: Comment on the Study by The Record Trial Group. *The Lancet* 2005 Published on-line May 6  http://OptimalHealthResearch.com/lancet

[484] Muanza DN, **Vasquez A**, Cannell J, Grant WB. Isoflavones and Postmenopausal Women. [letter] *JAMA* 2004; 292: 2337

[485] **Vasquez A**, Cannell J. Calcium and vitamin D in preventing fractures: data are not sufficient to show inefficacy. [letter] *BMJ: British Medical Journal* 2005;331:108-9 http://www.optimalhealthresearch.com/reprints/vasquez-cannell-bmj-reprint.pdf

[486] **Vasquez A**. Allopathic Usurpation of Natural Medicine: The Blind Leading the Sighted. *Naturopathy Digest* 2006 February http://www.naturopathydigest.com/archives/2006/feb/vasquez.php

[487] **Vasquez A**, Manso G, Cannell J. The clinical importance of vitamin D (cholecalciferol): a paradigm shift with implications for all healthcare providers. *Altern Ther Health Med*. 2004 Sep-Oct;10(5):28-36 http://optimalhealthresearch.com/monograph04

tocopherol which is not only unusable by the human body but is actually harmful in that it interferes with normal metabolism and can exacerbate hypertension and cause symptomatic complications (e.g., headaches). Further, tocopherols exist within the body in relationship with the individual forms of the vitamin, such that supplementation with one form (e.g., alpha-tocopherol) can result in a relative deficiency of another form (e.g., gamma-tocopherol). One final example of the failure to use proper forms of nutrients is in the use of pyridoxine HCl as a form of vitamin B6; while this practice itself is not harmful, clinicians need to remember that pyridoxine HCl is ineffective until converted to the more active forms of the vitamin including pyridoxal-5-phosphate. Since this conversion requires co-nutrients such as magnesium and zinc, we can easily see that the reputed failure of B6 supplementation when administered in the form of pyridoxine HCl might actually be due to untreated insufficiencies of required co-nutrients, as discussed in the following section.

4. **Failure to ensure adequacy of co-nutrients**: Vitamins, minerals, amino acids, and fatty acids work together in an intricately choreographed and delicately orchestrated dance that culminates in the successful completion of interconnected physiologic functions. If any of the performers in this event are missing (i.e., nutritional deficiency) or if successive interconversions are impaired due to lack of enzyme function, then the show cannot go on, or—if it does go on—impaired metabolism and defective function will result. So, if we take a patient with "vitamin B6 deficiency" and give him vitamin B6 in the absence of other co-nutrients needed for the proper activation and metabolic utilization of vitamin B6, we cannot honestly expect the "nutritional supplementation" to work in this case; rather, we might see a marginal benefit or perhaps even a negative outcome as an imbalanced system is pushed into a different state of imbalance despite supplementation with the "correct" vitamin. In the case of vitamin B6, necessary co-nutrients include zinc, magnesium, and riboflavin; deficiency of any of these will result in a relative "failure" of B6 supplementation even if a patient has a B6-responsive condition. Notably, overt magnesium deficiency is alarmingly common among patients and citizens in industrialized nations[488,489,490], and this epidemic of magnesium deficiency is due not only to insufficient intake but also to excessive excretion caused by consumption of high-glycemic foods, caffeine, and a diet that promotes chronic metabolic acidosis with resultant urinary acidification.

5. **Failure to achieve urinary alkalinization**: Western/American-style diets typified by overconsumption of grains, dairy, sugar, and salt result in a state of subclinical chronic metabolic acidosis which results in urinary acidification, relative hypercortisolemia, and consequent hyperexcretion of minerals such as calcium and magnesium.[491,492] Thus, the common conundrum of magnesium replenishment requires not only magnesium

---

[488] "Altogether 43% of 113 trauma patients had low magnesium levels compared to 30% of noninjured cohorts." Frankel H, Haskell R, Lee SY, Miller D, Rotondo M, Schwab CW. Hypomagnesemia in trauma patients. *World J Surg*. 1999 Sep;23(9):966-9
[489] "There was a 20% overall prevalence of hypomagnesemia among this predominantly female, African American population." Fox CH, Ramsoomair D, Mahoney MC, Carter C, Young B, Graham R. An investigation of hypomagnesemia among ambulatory urban African Americans. *J Fam Pract*. 1999 Aug;48(8):636-9
[490] "Suboptimal levels were detected in 33.7 per cent of the population under study. These data clearly demonstrate that the Mg supply of the German population needs increased attention." Schimatschek HF, Rempis R. Prevalence of hypomagnesemia in an unselected German population of 16,000 individuals. *Magnes Res*. 2001 Dec;14(4):283-90
[491] Cordain L, Eaton SB, Sebastian A, Mann N, Lindeberg S, Watkins BA, O'Keefe JH, Brand-Miller J. Origins and evolution of the Western diet: health implications for the 21st century. *Am J Clin Nutr*. 2005 Feb;81(2):341-54
[492] Maurer M, Riesen W, Muser J, Hulter HN, Krapf R. Neutralization of Western diet inhibits bone resorption independently of K intake and reduces cortisol secretion in humans. *Am J Physiol Renal Physiol*. 2003 Jan;284(1):F32-40

supplementation but also dietary interventions to change the internal climate to one that is conducive to bodily retention and cellular uptake of magnesium.[493]

6. **Use of mislabeled supplements**: Even in the professional arena of nutritional supplement manufacturers, some companies habitually underdose their products either in an attempt to spend less in the manufacture of their products or as a consequence of poor quality control. If a product is labeled to contain 1,000 IU of vitamin D but only contains 836 IU of the nutrient, then obviously full clinical efficacy will not be achieved; this was a problem in a recent clinical trial involving vitamin D.[494] The problem for clinicians is in trusting the companies that supply nutritional supplements; some companies do "in house" testing which lacks independent review, while other companies use questionable "independent testing" which is not infrequently performed by a laboratory that is a wholly owned subsidiary of the parent nutritional company. Manufacturing regulations that are sweeping through the industry will cleanse the nutritional supplement world of poorly made products, and these same regulations will sweep some unprepared companies right out the door when they are unable to meet the regulatory requirements.

7. **Assurance of bioavailability and optimal serum/cellular levels**: Clinical trials with nutritional therapies need to monitor serum or cellular levels to ensure absorption, product bioavailability, and the attainment of optimal serum levels. This is particularly relevant in the treatment of chronic disorders such as the autoimmune diseases, wherein so many of these patients have gastrointestinal dysbiosis and often have concomitant nutrient malabsorption.[495] Simply dosing these patients with supplements is not always efficacious; often the gut must be cleared of dysbiosis so that the mucosal lining can be repaired and optimal nutrient absorption can be reestablished.

8. **Coadministration of food with nutritional supplements (sometimes right, sometimes wrong)**: Food can help or hinder the absorption of nutritional supplements. Some supplements, like coenzyme Q10, should be administered with fatty food to enhance absorption. Other supplements, like amino acids, should be administered away from protein-rich foods and are often better administered with simple carbohydrate to enhance cellular uptake; this is especially true with tryptophan.

9. **Correction of gross dietary imbalances enhances supplement effectiveness**: If the diet is grossly imbalanced, then nutritional supplementation is less likely to be effective. The best example of this is in the use of fatty acid supplements, particularly in the treatment of inflammatory disorders. If the diet is laden with dairy, beef, and other sources of arachidonate, then fatty acid supplementation with EPA, DHA, and GLA is much less likely to be effective, or much higher doses of the supplements will need to be used in order to help restore fatty acid balance. Generally speaking, the diet needs to be optimized to enhance the efficacy of nutritional supplementation.

## Conclusion

In this brief review, I have listed and discussed some of the most common impediments to the success of nutritional supplementation. I hope that chiropractic and naturopathic students, clinicians, and researchers will find these points helpful in their design of clinical treatment protocols.

---

[493] Vormann J, Worlitschek M, Goedecke T, Silver B. Supplementation with alkaline minerals reduces symptoms in patients with chronic low back pain. *J Trace Elem Med Biol*. 2001;15(2-3):179-83

[494] Heaney RP, Davies KM, Chen TC, Holick MF, Barger-Lux MJ. Human serum 25-hydroxycholecalciferol response to extended oral dosing with cholecalciferol. *Am J Clin Nutr*. 2003 Jan;77(1):204-10 http://www.ajcn.org/cgi/content/full/77/1/204

[495] **Vasquez A**. Reducing Pain and Inflammation Naturally. Part 6: Nutritional and Botanical Treatments Against "Silent Infections" and Gastrointestinal Dysbiosis, Commonly Overlooked Causes of Neuromusculoskeletal Inflammation and Chronic Health Problems. *Nutritional Perspectives* 2006; January http://www.optimalhealthresearch.com/part6

# Review of Clinical Assessments and Concepts

Topics:
- **Musculoskeletal Medicine: The Goal is *Wellness***
- **Clinical Assessments**
    - History taking & Physical examination
    - Orthopedic/musculoskeletal examination: Concepts and goals
    - Neurologic assessment: Review
    - Laboratory assessments: General considerations of commonly used tests
        i. CRP, ESR, CBC, Chemistry/metabolic panel
        ii. Complements C3 and C4
        iii. Ferritin
        iv. 25(OH)-vitamin D
        v. TSH: Thyroid stimulating hormone
        vi. ANA: Antinuclear antibodies
        vii. ANCA: Antineutrophilic cytoplasmic antibodies
        viii. RF: Rheumatoid factor
        ix. CCP: Cyclic citrullinated protein antibodies; anticitrullinated protein antibodies
        x. HLA-B27
        xi. Lactulose-mannitol assay
        xii. Comprehensive stool analysis and comprehensive parasitology
- **High-Risk Pain Patients**
- **Clinical Concepts**
    - Not all injury-related problems are injury-related problems
    - Safe patient + safe treatment = safe outcome
    - Four clues to underlying problems
    - Special considerations in the evaluation of children
    - No errors allowed: Differences between primary healthcare and spectator sports
    - "Disease treatment" is different from "patient management"
    - Clinical Practice Involves Much More than "Diagnosis and Treatment"
    - Risk Management: A Note Especially to Students and Recent Licensees
- **Musculoskeletal Emergencies**
    - Acute compartment syndrome
    - Acute red eye, including acute iritis and scleritis
    - Atlantoaxial subluxation and instability
    - Cauda equina syndrome
    - Giant cell arteritis, temporal arteritis
    - Myelopathy, spinal cord compression
    - Neuropsychiatric lupus
    - Osteomyelitis
    - Septic arthritis, acute nontraumatic monoarthritis
- **Chiropractic: Overview of History and Current Science**
    - Chiropractic training and clinical benefits
    - Spinal manipulation: mechanistic considerations
    - Wilk versus American Medical Association: Permanent anti-trust anti-conspiracy injunction order against AMA by Judge Getzendanner, 1987

> **Review**
> This review is included for students and for graduates desiring a concise overview of basic and essential clinical concepts.

## Core Competencies:
- You must know how to test and grade muscle reflexes and muscle strength.
- You must be able to explain and apply the "principle of neurologic localization" in conjunction with your comprehensive neurologic examination.
- You must know how to rapidly diagnose and effectively manage the following musculoskeletal emergencies:
    - Acute compartment syndrome
    - Acute red eye, including acute iritis and scleritis
    - Atlantoaxial subluxation and instability
    - Cauda equina syndrome
    - Giant cell arteritis, temporal arteritis
    - Myelopathy, spinal cord compression
    - Neuropsychiatric lupus
    - Osteomyelitis
    - Septic arthritis, acute nontraumatic monoarthritis
- Regarding acute monoarthritis, what are the main differential diagnoses and what (beyond routine history and physical examination) is the single most important diagnostic procedure?
- You must demonstrate competency in the correlative and differential interpretation of the following routine blood tests:
    - ANA
    - CBC
    - CCP antibodies
    - Chemistry/metabolic panel
    - CRP
    - ESR
    - Ferritin
    - Serum 25(OH)D
    - TSH

Sample questions about laboratory test interpretation:
- What is the diagnostic difference between "elevated CRP with a normal ferritin" and "elevated CRP with elevated ferritin"?
- What is the standard of care when you find that your adult asymptomatic patient has a ferritin less than 20 mcg/L?
- What is the proper management of an asymptomatic patient with a ferritin > 300 mcg/L (male) or > 200 mcg/L (female)?
- Name two common nutritional deficiencies that would be correlated with a MCV > 95 fL; also name the corresponding treatments and appropriate doses.
- What are the six most common causes of an elevated lactulose-mannitol ratio and how are these differentially diagnosed?
- Name six causes of hypercalcemia and means for assessing each.
- Describe the two components of "composite seropositivity" and describe the patient management for 1) a young patient who is asymptomatic, and 2) a middle-aged patient with peripheral polyarthropathy and recent onset of hyperreflexia, iritis, and visual changes.

*Review of Clinical Assessments and Concepts*

## Integrative Musculoskeletal Medicine: the Goal is *Wellness*

Since **approximately 1 of every 7 (14% of total) visits to a primary healthcare provider is for the treatment of musculoskeletal pain or dysfunction**[1], every healthcare provider needs to have 1) knowledge of important concepts related to musculoskeletal medicine, 2) the ability to recognize urgent and emergency conditions, 3) the ability to competently perform orthopedic examination procedures and interpret laboratory assessments, and 4) the knowledge and ability to design and implement effective treatment plans and to coordinate patient management. Written for students and experienced clinicians, this chapter introduces and reviews many new and common terms, procedures, and concepts relevant to the management of patients with musculoskeletal disorders. Especially for students, the reading of this chapter is essential to understanding the extensive material in this book and will facilitate the clinical assessment and management of patients with musculoskeletal disorders.

> **Medical iatrogenesis kills 493 Americans per day**
>
> "Recent estimates suggest that each year more than 1 million patients are injured while in the hospital and approximately 180,000 die because of these injuries. Furthermore, drug-related morbidity and mortality are common and are estimated to cost more than $136 billion a year."
>
> Holland EG, Degruy FV. Drug-induced disorders. *Am Fam Physician*. 1997;56(7):1781-8, 1791-2

Healthcare is currently in a time of significant fluctuation and is ready for changes in the balance of power and the paradigms which direct our therapeutic interventions. For nearly a century, allopathic medicine has hailed itself as "the gold standard", and other professions have either submitted to or been crushed by their ongoing political/scientific manipulations and their continual proclamation of intellectual and therapeutic superiority[2,3,4,5,6,7,8,9,10,11,12,13,14] despite 180,000-220,000 iatrogenic *medically-induced* deaths per year (500-600 iatrogenic deaths per day)[15,16] and consistent documentation that most medical/allopathic physicians are unable to provide accurate musculoskeletal diagnoses due to pervasive inadequacies in medical

---

[1] American College of Rheumatology Ad Hoc Committee on Clinical Guidelines. Guidelines for the initial evaluation of the adult patient with acute musculoskeletal symptoms. *Arthritis Rheum*. 1996 Jan;39(1):1-8 See also: **Vasquez A**. Musculoskeletal disorders and iron overload disease: comment on the American College of Rheumatology guidelines. *Arthritis Rheum* 1996;39: 1767-8
[2] Wilk CA. Medicine, Monopolies, and Malice: How the Medical Establishment Tried to Destroy Chiropractic. Garden City Park: Avery, 1996
[3] Getzendanner S. Permanent injunction order against AMA. *JAMA*. 1988 Jan 1;259(1):81-2 http://optimalhealthresearch.com/archives/wilk.html
[4] Carter JP. Racketeering in Medicine: The Suppression of Alternatives. Norfolk: Hampton Roads Pub; 1993
[5] Morley J, Rosner AL, Redwood D. A case study of misrepresentation of the scientific literature: recent reviews of chiropractic. *J Altern Complement Med*. 2001 Feb;7(1):65-78
[6] Terrett AG. Misuse of the literature by medical authors in discussing spinal manipulative therapy injury. *J Manipulative Physiol Ther*. 1995 May;18(4):203-10
[7] National Alliance of Professional Psychology Providers. AMA Seeks To Control and Restrict Psychologist's Scope of Practice. http://www.nappp.org/scope.pdf Accessed November 25, 2006
[8] "In an effort to marshal the medical community's resources against the growing threat of expanding scope of practice for allied health professionals, the AMA has formed a national partnership to confront such initiatives nationwide… The committee will use $25,000..." Daly R, American Psychiatric Association. AMA Forms Coalition to Thwart Non-M.D. Practice Expansion. *Psychiatric News* 2006 March; 41: 17 http://pn.psychiatryonline.org/cgi/content/full/41/5/17-a?eaf Accessed November 25, 2006
[9] Spivak JL. The Medical Trust Unmasked. Louis S. Siegfried Publishers; New York: 1961
[10] Trever W. In the Public Interest. Los Angeles; Scriptures Unlimited; 1972. This is probably the most authoritative documentation of the illegal actions of the AMA up to 1972; contains numerous photocopies of actual AMA documents and minutes of official meetings with overt intentionality of destroying Americans' healthcare options so that the AMA and related organizations would have a monopoly in national healthcare.
[11] Wenban AB. Inappropriate use of the title 'chiropractor' and term 'chiropractic manipulation' in the peer-reviewed biomedical literature. *Chiropr Osteopat*. 2006;14:16 http://chiroandosteo.com/content/14/1/16
[12] Orme-Johnson DW, Herron RE. An innovative approach to reducing medical care utilization and expenditures. *Am J Manag Care*. 1997 Jan;3:135-44 http://www.ajmc.com/Article.cfm?Menu=1&ID=2154
[13] van der Steen WJ, Ho VK. Drugs versus diets: disillusions with Dutch health care. *Acta Biother*. 2001;49(2):125-40
[14] Texas Medical Association. Physicians Ask Court to Protect Patients From Illegal Chiropractic Activities. http://www.texmed.org/Template.aspx?id=5259 Accessed February 20, 2007
[15] Starfield B. Is US health really the best in the world? *JAMA*. 2000 Jul 26;284(4):483-5
[16] "Recent estimates suggest that each year more than 1 million patients are injured while in the hospital and approximately 180,000 die because of these injuries. Furthermore, drug-related morbidity and mortality are common and are estimated to cost more than $136 billion a year." Holland EG, Degruy FV. Drug-induced disorders. *Am Fam Physician*. 1997;56(7):1781-8, 1791-2

training.[17,18,19,20] Increasing disenchantment with allopathic *heroic medicine* and its adverse outcomes of inefficacy, exorbitant expenses, and unnecessary death are fostering change, such that allopathic medicine has been dethroned as the leading paradigm among American patients, who spend the majority of their volitional healthcare dollars on consultations and treatments provided by "alternative" healthcare providers.[21,22] With the ever-increasing utilization of chiropractic, naturopathic, and osteopathic medical services, we must see that our paradigms and interventions keep pace with the evolving research literature and our increasing professional responsibilities so that we can deliver the highest possible quality of care.

> **Ever-increasing popularity of nonallopathic medicine**
>
> "…Americans made an estimated 425 million visits to providers of unconventional therapy. This number exceeds the number of visits to all U.S. primary care physicians (388 million)."
>
> Eisenberg DM, Kessler RC, Foster C, Norlock FE, Calkins DR, Delbanco TL. Unconventional medicine in the United States. Prevalence, costs, and patterns of use. *N Engl J Med*. 1993 Jan 28;328(4):246-52

In allopathic medicine, the goal of musculoskeletal treatment is to address the patient's injury or disorder by alleviating pain with the use of drugs, preventing further injury, and returning the patient to his/her previous status and activities. The most commonly employed interventions are 1) rest and "watchful waiting", 2) non-steroidal anti-inflammatory drugs (NSAIDS) and cyclooxygenase-2-inhibitors ("coxibs"), and 3) surgery. Chiropractic, naturopathic, and osteopathic physicians criticize this approach because, although avoidance of and "rest" from damaging activities is reasonable and valuable, too much rest without an emphasis on active preventive rehabilitation encourages patient passivity, assumption of the sick role, fails to actively promote tissue healing, and fails to address the underlying proprioceptive deficits that are common in patients with chronic musculoskeletal pain and recurrent injuries.[23,24,25] **NSAIDs are considered "first line" therapy for musculoskeletal disorders by allopaths** despite the data showing that "**There is no evidence that widely used NSAIDs have any long-term benefit on osteoarthritis.**"[26] What is worse than this lack of efficacy is the evidence showing that NSAIDs *exacerbate* musculoskeletal disease (rather than *cure* it). **NSAIDs are known to inhibit cartilage formation and to promote bone necrosis and joint degradation with long-term use**[27,28,29,30] and

> "…only about 15% of medical interventions are supported by solid scientific evidence…"
>
> Smith R. Where is the wisdom...? The poverty of medical evidence. *BMJ*. 1991 Oct 5;303:798-9

---

[17] Freedman KB, Bernstein J. The adequacy of medical school education in musculoskeletal medicine. *J Bone Joint Surg Am*. 1998;80(10):1421-7
[18] Freedman KB, Bernstein J. Educational deficiencies in musculoskeletal medicine. *J Bone Joint Surg Am*. 2002;84-A(4):604-8
[19] Matzkin E, Smith ME, Freccero CD, Richardson AB. Adequacy of education in musculoskeletal medicine. *J Bone Joint Surg Am*. 2005 Feb;87-A(2):310-4
[20] Schmale GA. More evidence of educational inadequacies in musculoskeletal medicine. *Clin Orthop Relat Res*. 2005 Aug;(437):251-9
[21] "…Americans made an estimated 425 million visits to providers of unconventional therapy. This number exceeds the number of visits to all U.S. primary care physicians (388 million)." Eisenberg DM, Kessler RC, Foster C, Norlock FE, Calkins DR, Delbanco TL. Unconventional medicine in the United States. Prevalence, costs, and patterns of use. *N Engl J Med*. 1993 Jan 28;328(4):246-52
[22] "Estimated expenditures for alternative medicine professional services increased 45.2% between 1990 and 1997 and were conservatively estimated at $21.2 billion in 1997, with at least $12.2 billion paid out-of-pocket. This exceeds the 1997 out-of-pocket expenditures for all US hospitalizations." Eisenberg DM, Davis RB, Ettner SL, Appel S, Wilkey S, Van Rompay M, Kessler RC. Trends in alternative medicine use in the United States, 1990-1997: results of a follow-up national survey. *JAMA*. 1998 Nov 11;280(18):1569-75
[23] McPartland JM, Brodeur RR, Hallgren RC. Chronic neck pain, standing balance, and suboccipital muscle atrophy--a pilot study. *J Manipulative Physiol Ther*. 1997;20(1):24-9
[24] Bullock-Saxton JE, Janda V, Bullock MI. Reflex activation of gluteal muscles in walking. An approach to restoration of muscle function for patients with low-back pain. *Spine* 1993 May;18(6):704-8
[25] Sinaki M, Brey RH, Hughes CA, Larson DR, Kaufman KR. Significant reduction in risk of falls and back pain in osteoporotic-kyphotic women through a Spinal Proprioceptive Extension Exercise Dynamic (SPEED) program. *Mayo Clin Proc*. 2005 Jul;80(7):849-55
[26] Beers MH, Berkow R (eds). The Merck Manual. 17th Edition. Whitehouse Station; Merck Research Laboratories 1999 page 451
[27] "At…concentrations comparable to those… in the synovial fluid of patients treated with the drug, several NSAIDs suppress proteoglycan synthesis… These NSAID-related effects on chondrocyte metabolism … are much more profound in osteoarthritic cartilage than in normal cartilage, due to enhanced uptake of

**NSAIDs are responsible for more than 16,000 gastrohemorrhagic deaths and 100,000 hospitalizations each year.**[31] The "coxibs" were supposed to provide anti-inflammatory benefits with an enhanced safety profile, but the gastrocentric focus of these drug developers failed to appreciate that COX-2 is necessary for the formation of prostacyclin, a prostaglandin created from arachidonic acid via COX-2 that plays an important role in vasodilation and antithrombosis; not surprisingly therefore, use of COX-2-inhibiting drugs has consistently been associated with increased risk for adverse cardiovascular effects including myocardial infarction, unstable angina, cardiac thrombus, resuscitated cardiac arrest, sudden or unexplained death, ischemic stroke, and transient ischemic attacks.[32] Additionally, the use of a COX-2 inhibiting treatment in patients who overconsume arachidonic acid (i.e., most people in America and other industrialized nations[33]) would be expected to shunt bioavailable arachidonate into the formation of leukotrienes, a group of inflammatory mediators now known to contribute directly to atherogenesis.[34] Thus, it was entirely predictable that overuse of COX-2 inhibitors would create a catastrophe of iatrogenic cardiovascular death, and this is exactly what was allowed to occur—clearly indicating independent but synergistic failures on the part of pharmaceutical companies, the FDA, and the medical profession.[35,36,37,38] According to David J. Graham, MD, MPH, (Associate Director for Science, Office of Drug Safety, FDA) **an estimated 139,000 Americans who took Vioxx suffered serious complications including stroke or myocardial infarction; between 26,000 and 55,000 Americans died as a result of their doctors' prescribing Vioxx.**[39] Furthermore, the surgical procedures employed by allopaths for the treatment of musculoskeletal pain do not consistently show evidence of efficacy, safety, or cost-effectiveness. Arthroscopic surgery for osteoarthritis of the knee, for example, costs thousands of dollars to each individual and billions of dollars to the American healthcare system but is no more effective than placebo.[40,41,42] In a review which also noted that only 15% of medical procedures are supported by literature references and that only 1% of such references are deemed scientifically valid, Rosner[43] showed that the risks of serious injury (i.e., cauda equina syndrome or vertebral artery dissection) associated with spinal manipulation are *"400 times lower* than the death rates observed from

---

NSAIDs by the osteoarthritic cartilage." Brandt KD. Effects of nonsteroidal anti-inflammatory drugs on chondrocyte metabolism in vitro and in vivo. *Am J Med.* 1987 Nov 20; 83(5A): 29-34
[28] "The case of a young healthy man, who developed avascular necrosis of head of femur after prolonged administration of indomethacin, is reported here." Prathapkumar KR, Smith I, Attara GA. Indomethacin induced avascular necrosis of head of femur. *Postgrad Med J.* 2000 Sep; 76(899): 574-5
[29] "This highly significant association between NSAID use and acetabular destruction gives cause for concern, not least because of the difficulty in achieving satisfactory hip replacements in patients with severely damaged acetabula." Newman NM, Ling RS. Acetabular bone destruction related to non-steroidal anti-inflammatory drugs. *Lancet.* 1985 Jul 6; 2(8445): 11-4
[30] Vidal y Plana RR, Bizzarri D, Rovati AL. Articular cartilage pharmacology: I. In vitro studies on glucosamine and non steroidal antiinflammatory drugs. *Pharmacol Res Commun.* 1978 Jun;10(6):557-69
[31] Singh G. Recent considerations in nonsteroidal anti-inflammatory drug gastropathy. *Am J Med.* 1998;105(1B):31S-38S
[32] Mukherjee D, Nissen SE, Topol EJ. Risk of cardiovascular events associated with selective COX-2 inhibitors. *JAMA.* 2001 Aug 22-29;286(8):954-9
[33] Seaman DR. The diet-induced proinflammatory state: a cause of chronic pain and other degenerative diseases? *J Manipulative Physiol Ther.* 2002;25(3):168-79
[34] Dwyer JH, Allayee H, Dwyer KM, Fan J, Wu H, Mar R, Lusis AJ, Mehrabian M. Arachidonate 5-lipoxygenase promoter genotype, dietary arachidonic acid, and atherosclerosis. *N Engl J Med.* 2004 Jan 1;350(1):29-37
[35] Topol EJ. Arthritis medicines and cardiovascular events--"house of coxibs". *JAMA.* 2005 Jan 19;293(3):366-8. Epub 2004 Dec 28
[36] Ray WA, Griffin MR, Stein CM. Cardiovascular toxicity of valdecoxib. *N Engl J Med.* 2004 Dec 23;351(26):2767. Epub 2004 Dec 17
[37] Topol EJ. Failing the public health--rofecoxib, Merck, and the FDA. *N Engl J Med.* 2004 Oct 21;351(17):1707-9
[38] Horton R. Vioxx, the implosion of Merck, and aftershocks at the FDA. *Lancet.* 2004 Dec 4-10;364(9450):1995-6
[39] David J. Graham, MD, MPH, (Associate Director for Science, Office of Drug Safety, US FDA) estimated that 139,000 Americans who took Vioxx suffered serious side effects; he estimated that the drug killed between 26,000 and 55,000 people. http://www.commondreams.org/views05/0223-35.htm http://www.fda.gov/cder/drug/infopage/vioxx/vioxxgraham.pdf Accessed November 25, 2006
[40] Gina Kolata. A Knee Surgery for Arthritis Is Called Sham. *The New York Times,* July 11, 2002
[41] Moseley JB, O'Malley K, Petersen NJ, Menke TJ, Brody BA, Kuykendall DH, Hollingsworth JC, Ashton CM, Wray NP. A controlled trial of arthroscopic surgery for osteoarthritis of the knee. *N Engl J Med.* 2002;347:81-8
[42] Bernstein J, Quach T. A perspective on the study of Moseley et al: questioning the value of arthroscopic knee surgery for osteoarthritis. *Cleve Clin J Med.* 2003;70(5):401, 405-6, 408-10
[43] Rosner AL. Evidence-based clinical guidelines for the management of acute low-back pain: response to the guidelines prepared for the Australian Medical Health and Research Council. *J Manipulative Physiol Ther.* 2001;24(3):214-20

gastrointestinal bleeding due to the use of nonsteroidal anti-inflammatory drugs and *700 times lower* than the overall mortality rate for spinal surgery."

In chiropractic, osteopathic, and naturopathic medicine, the goal and means of musculoskeletal treatment is to address the patient's injury or disorder by simultaneously alleviating pain with the use of natural, noninvasive, low-cost, and low-risk interventions while improving the patient's overall health, preventing future health problems, and "upgrading" the patient's overall paradigm of health maintenance and disease prevention from one that is passive and reactive to one that is empowered and pro-active. Commonly employed therapeutics include spinal manipulation[44,45,46], exercise[47] and the use of nutritional supplements and botanical medicines[48] which have been demonstrated in peer-reviewed clinical trials to be safe and effective for the treatment of musculoskeletal pain. More specifically, chiropractic and naturopathic physicians are well versed in the clinical utilization of such treatments as niacinamide[49], glucosamine and chondroitin sulfates[50], vitamin D[51], vitamin B-12[52], balanced and complete fatty acid therapy[53,54], anti-inflammatory diets[55,56,57], proteolytic/pancreatic enzymes[58], and botanical medicines such as *Boswellia*[59], *Harpagophytum*[60], *Uncaria*, and willow bark[61,62] —each of these interventions has been validated in peer-reviewed research for safety and effectiveness.[63] Furthermore, from the perspective of integrative chiropractic and naturopathic medicine, aiming for such a limited accomplishment as mere "returning the patient to previous status and activities" would be considered substandard, since the patient's overall health was neither addressed nor improved and since returning the patient to his/her previous status and activities would be a direct invitation for the problem to recur indefinitely. Chiropractic and naturopathic physicians appreciate that, especially regarding chronic health problems, any treatment plan that allows the patient to resume his/her previous lifestyle is by definition doomed to fail because a return to the patient's previous lifestyle and activities that allowed the onset of the disease/disorder in the first

---

[44] Manga P, Angus D, Papadopoulos C, et al. The Effectiveness and Cost-Effectiveness of Chiropractic Management of Low-Back Pain. Richmond Hill, Ontario: Kenilworth Publishing; 1993

[45] Meade TW, Dyer S, Browne W, Townsend J, Frank AO. Low-back pain of mechanical origin: randomised comparison of chiropractic and hospital outpatient treatment. *BMJ*. 1990;300(6737):1431-7

[46] Meade TW, Dyer S, Browne W, Frank AO. Randomised comparison of chiropractic and hospital outpatient management for low-back pain: results from extended follow up. *BMJ*. 1995;311(7001):349-5

[47] Harold Elrick, MD. Exercise is Medicine. *The Physician and Sportsmedicine* - Volume 24 - No. 2 - February 1996

[48] **Vasquez A**. Reducing pain and inflammation naturally - Part 3: Improving overall health while safely and effectively treating musculoskeletal pain. *Nutr Perspect* 2005; 28: 34-38, 40-42 http://optimalhealthresearch.com/part3

[49] Kaufman W. Niacinamide therapy for joint mobility. Therapeutic reversal of a common clinical manifestation of the "normal" aging process. *Conn State Med J* 1953;17:584-591

[50] Reginster JY, Deroisy R, Rovati LC, Lee RL, Lejeune E, Bruyere O, Giacovelli G, Henrotin Y, Dacre JE, Gossett C. Long-term effects of glucosamine sulphate on osteoarthritis progression: a randomised, placebo-controlled clinical trial. *Lancet*. 2001;357(9252):251-6

[51] **Vasquez A**, Manso G, Cannell J. The clinical importance of vitamin D: a paradigm shift with implications for all healthcare providers. *Altern Ther Health Med* 2004;10:28-36 http://optimalhealthresearch.com/monograph04

[52] Mauro GL, Martorana U, Cataldo P, Brancato G, Letizia G. Vitamin B12 in low back pain: a randomised, double-blind, placebo-controlled study. *Eur Rev Med Pharmacol Sci*. 2000 May-Jun;4(3):53-8

[53] **Vasquez A**. Reducing Pain and Inflammation Naturally. Part 1: New Insights into Fatty Acid Biochemistry and the Influence of Diet. *Nutrl Perspect* 2004; Oct: 5, 7-10,12,14

[54] **Vasquez A**. Reducing Pain and Inflammation Naturally. Part 2: New Insights into Fatty Acid Supplementation and Its Effect on Eicosanoid Production and Genetic Expression. *Nutritional Perspectives* 2005; January: 5-16 http://optimalhealthresearch.com/part2

[55] Seaman DR. The diet-induced proinflammatory state: a cause of chronic pain and other degenerative diseases? *J Manipulative Physiol Ther*. 2002 Mar-Apr;25(3):168-7

[56] **Vasquez A**. *Integrative Orthopedics*. Revised edition August 2004, Second Edition 2007

[57] **Vasquez A**. Reducing Pain and Inflammation Naturally. Part 1: New Insights into Fatty Acid Biochemistry and the Influence of Diet. *Nutritional Perspectives* 2004; October: 5, 7-10, 12, 14 http://optimalhealthresearch.com/part1

[58] Trickett P. Proteolytic enzymes in treatment of athletic injuries. *Appl Ther*. 1964;30:647-52

[59] Kimmatkar N, Thawani V, Hingorani L, Khiyani R. Efficacy and tolerability of Boswellia serrata extract in treatment of osteoarthritis of knee--a randomized double blind placebo controlled trial. *Phytomedicine*. 2003 Jan;10(1):3-7

[60] Chrubasik S, Junck H, Breitschwerdt H, Conradt C, Zappe H. Effectiveness of Harpagophytum extract WS 1531 in the treatment of exacerbation of low-back pain: a randomized, placebo-controlled, double-blind study. *Eur J Anaesthesiol* 1999 Feb;16(2):118-29

[61] Chrubasik S, Eisenberg E, Balan E, Weinberger T, Luzzati R, Conradt C. Treatment of low-back pain exacerbations with willow bark extract: a randomized double-blind study. *Am J Med*. 2000;109:9-14

[62] **Vasquez A**, Muanza DN. Comment: Evaluation of Presence of Aspirin-Related Warnings with Willow Bark. *Ann Pharmacotherapy* 2005 Oct;39(10):1763

[63] **Vasquez A**. Reducing pain and inflammation naturally. Part 3: Improving overall health while safely and effectively treating musculoskeletal pain. *Nutr Perspect* 2005;28:34-42

place will most certainly result in the perpetuation and recurrence of the illness or disorder. **Stated more directly: for *healing* to truly be effective, the comprehensive treatment plan must generally result in a permanent and profound change in the patient's lifestyle and emotional climate, which are the primary modifiable determinants of either health or disease.**

While we all readily acknowledge the importance of emergency care for emergency situations, those of us who advocate and practice a more complete approach to healthcare and life readily see the shortcomings of a limited and mechanical approach to healthcare, and we aspire to do more than simply fix problems. The implementation of *multidimensional* (i.e., *comprehensive* and *multifaceted*) treatment plans that address many aspects of pathophysiologic phenomena is a huge step forward in creating improved health and preventing future illness in the patients who seek our professional assistance. However, even complete multidimensional treatment plans still fall short of the goal of creating wellness, if for no other reasons than 1) they are still disease- and problem-oriented, rather than health-oriented, 2) they are prescribed from outside ("The doctor told me to do it.") rather than originating internally and spontaneously by the patient's own direction and affirmation ("I *do* this because I *am* this."), and, finally and most difficult to relay, 3) they are mechanistic rather than organic, they can do no better than the sum of their parts, they flow exclusively from the mind ("do") and not also from the body-soul ("am"). The art of creating wellness takes time to understand, longer to implement clinically, and even longer to apply to one's own life. Wellness is a state of being rather than a checklist of activities in a "preventive health program." The subtle differences that distinguish "wellness" from any "program" or "prescription" are the differences between *leading* versus *following* and *flowing* versus *performing*. **Wellness is multidimensional self-actualization, full integration of one's life—present, past, and future; physical, mental, emotional, spiritual, biochemical—one's shadow[64], work[65], feelings, thoughts, and goals into a cohesive living whole – "a wheel rolling from its own center."[66]**

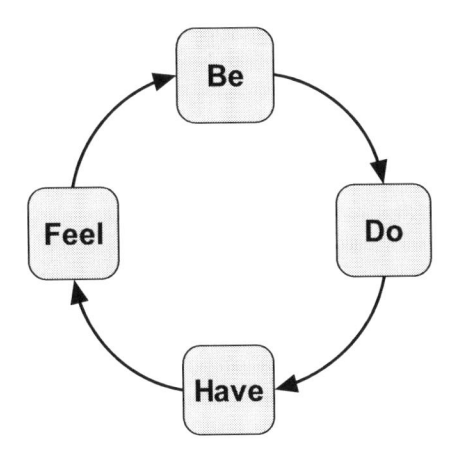

---

[64] Robert Bly. The Human Shadow. Sound Horizons, New York 1991 [ISBN: 1879323001] and Bly R. A Little Book on the Human Shadow.[ ISBN: 0062548476]
[65] Rick Jarow. Creating the Work You Love: Courage, Commitment and Career; Inner Traditions Intl Ltd; (December 1995) [ISBN: 0892815426]
[66] Walter Kaufmann (Translator), Friedrich Wilhelm Nietzsche. Thus Spoke Zarathustra. Penguin USA; 1978, page 27

# Clinical Assessments

The clinical assessments reviewed in the following sections are history-taking, orthopedic/musculoskeletal, and neurologic examinations, and commonly used laboratory tests.

**History taking is the art of conducting an *informative* and *collaborative* patient interview.**

The role of the doctor during the interview process is not merely that of a data-collecting machine, spewing out questions and receiving responses. Patient interviews can be a creative, enjoyable, comforting opportunity to build rapport and to establish meaningful connection with another human being. Patients are not simply people with health problems – they are first and foremost our fellow human beings, not so dissimilar from ourselves perhaps, and always full of complexity. Our task is not to fully understand their complexity nor to solve all of their mysteries, but rather to help orchestrate these dynamics into a coordinated if not unified direction that promotes health and healing.

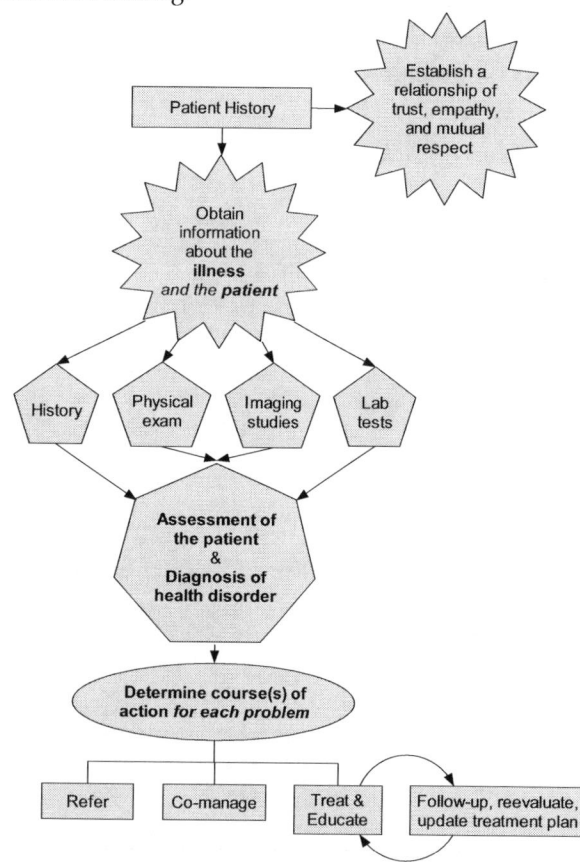

## History & Assessment

**History of the primary complaint**: "D.O.P.P. Q.R.S.T."
- Description/location
- Onset
- Provocation: exacerbates
- Palliation: alleviates
- Quality
- Radiation of pain
- Severity
- Timing

**Associated complaints**
- Additional manifestations
- Concomitant diseases

**Review of systems**
- Head-to-toe inventory of health status, associated health problems, and complications

**Past health history**
- Surgeries
- Hospitalizations
- Traumas
- Vaccinations and medications
- Successful and failed treatments for the current complaint(s)

**Family health history**
- Genotropic illnesses and predispositions
- Lifestyle patterns
- Emotional expectations about health

**Social history**
- Hobbies, work, exposures
- Relationships and emotional experiences
- Interpersonal support
- Malpractice litigation

**Health Habits**
- Diet: appropriate intake of protein, fruits, vegetables, fats, sugars
- Sleep
- Stress management
- Exercise / Sedentary Lifestyle
- Spirituality / Centeredness
- Caffeine and tobacco
- Ethanol and recreational drugs

**Medication and supplements**
- Reason, doses, duration, cost
- Side-effects
- Interactions

**Responsibility and Compliance**
- Ability and willingness to comply with prescribed treatment plan and to incorporate the necessary diet-exercise-relationship-emotional-lifestyle modifications
- *Internal* versus *external* locus of control

[Flowchart: Patient History → Establish a relationship of trust, empathy, and mutual respect; Obtain information about the illness *and the patient* → History, Physical exam, Imaging studies, Lab tests → Assessment of the patient & Diagnosis of health disorder → Determine course(s) of action *for each problem* → Refer, Co-manage, Treat & Educate → Follow-up, reevaluate, update treatment plan]

## Components of a Complete Patient History: "D.O.P.P. Q.R.S.T."

| Category | Application and considerations |
|---|---|
| **Description, Location:** Always start with open-ended questions | • What is it like for you?<br>• What do you experience?<br>• What are you feeling?<br>• Where is the pain/sensation/problem?<br>• Ask about specifics: **Pain, numbness, weakness, tingling**, fatigue, recent or chronic infections, burning, aching, dull, sharp, cramping, stretching, pins and needles, weakness, changes in function (i.e., bowel and bladder continence). |
| **Onset** | • When did it begin? Have you ever had anything like this before?<br>• Was there a specific event associated with the onset of the problem, such as an injury or an illness, or did the problem start gradually or insidiously?<br>• How has it changed over time?<br>• Prior injuries to site?<br>• Why are you seeking care for this now (rather than last week or last month)?<br>• What has changed? How is the pain/problem developing over time—getting worse or getting better? |
| **Palliation** | • How have you tried treating it? Does anything make it go away?<br>• What makes it better? What relieves the pain?<br>• Ask about prior and current treatments, radiographs, medications, supplements (herbs, vitamins, minerals), injections, surgery, massage, manipulation, counseling.<br>• Knowing response/resistance to previous treatments can provide clinical insight. |
| **Provocation** | • Are your symptoms constant, or does the problem come and go?<br>• What makes it worse? What makes the pain worse?<br>• When during the day/week/month/year are your symptoms the worst? |
| **Quality** | • Can you describe the pain to me?<br>• What does it feel like?<br>• What do you experience?<br>• Get a clear understanding of the type of sensation(s): stabbing, shooting pain, pins and needles, sharp pain, electric sensation, numbness, burning, aching, throbbing, weakness, tingling, gel phenomenon, dizziness, confusion, fatigue, shortness of breath. |
| **Radiation** | • Does the pain stay localized or does it move to your arm/leg/head/face?<br>• Do you feel pain in other areas of your body? |
| **Severity** | • How bad is it? How would you rate it on a scale of one to ten if one were almost no pain and ten was the worst pain you could imagine? Use the validated VAS—visual analog scale—to quantify the level of pain and impairment.<br>• Does this problem prevent you from engaging in your daily activities, such as work, exercise, or hobbies? This is a very important question for determining functional impairment and internal consistency; if the patient is "too injured to work" yet is still able to fully participate in recreational activities that are physically challenging, then malingering needs to be strongly considered. |
| **Timing** | • When do you notice this problem?<br>• Is it constant, or does it come and go? Where are you when you notice it the most?<br>• Is it worse in the morning, or worse in the evening?<br>• Does anyone else in your [home/office/worksite] have this same problem?<br>• What times of the day or what days of the week is it the worst? |

# Components of a Complete Patient History—*continued*

| Category | Application and considerations |
|---|---|
| **Associated manifestations and constitutional symptoms** | • *Have you noticed any other problems associated with this problem?*<br>• *Fatigue?*<br>• *Fever?*<br>• *Weight loss? Weight gain?*<br>• *Night sweats?*<br>• *Diarrhea? Constipation?*<br>• *Weakness?*<br>• *Nausea?*<br>• *Bowel or bladder difficulties or changes? Difficulty with sexual function?* These could be related to hormonal imbalances, drug side-effects, relationship problems, nutritional deficiencies, nerve compression, and/or depression<br>• *Change in sensation near your anus/genitals?* Cauda equina syndrome is an important consideration in patients with low-back pain<br>• *Loss of appetite?*<br>• *Difficulty sleeping?*<br>• *Skin rash or change in pigmentation?* |
| **ROS: review of systems** | • <u>General constitution</u>: fatigue, malaise, fever, chills, weight gain/loss…<br>• *"Now we are going to conduct a head-to-toe inventory just to make sure that we have covered everything."*<br>• <u>Head</u>: headaches, head pain, pressure inside head, difficulty concentrating, difficulty remembering, mental function<br>• <u>Ears</u>: ringing in ears, dizziness, hearing loss, hypersensitivity to noise, ear pain, discharge from ear, pressure in ears<br>• <u>Eyes</u>: eye pain, loss of vision or decreased vision or ability to focus, redness or irritation, seeing flashing lights or spots, double vision<br>• <u>Nose</u>: sinus problems, chronically stuffy nose, difficulty smelling things, nose bleeds, change or decrease in sense of smell or taste<br>• <u>Mouth</u>, teeth, TMJ, pain or sores in mouth, difficulty chewing, sensitive teeth, bleeding gums, pain in jaw joint, change or decrease in sense of taste<br>• <u>Neck</u>: pain at the base of skull, pain in neck, stiffness<br>• <u>Throat</u>: difficulty swallowing, pain in throat, feeling like things get stuck in throat, change in voice, difficulty getting air or food in or out<br>• <u>Chest and breasts</u>: any chest pain, difficult breathing, wheezing, coughing, pain, lumps, or discharge from nipple<br>• <u>Shoulders</u>: pain or aching in your shoulders, restricted motion or stiffness<br>• <u>Arms, elbows, hands</u>: pain or problems with your arms, elbows, hands, …in the joints or the muscles…, numbness, tingling, weakness, swelling, changes in fingernails, cold hands?<br>• <u>Stomach, abdomen, pelvis, genitals, urinary tract, rectum,</u> : pain in stomach or abdomen, difficulty with digestion, gas, bloating, regurgitation, ulcer, any problems lower down in your abdomen—near your lower intestines? Pain, lumps, swelling, difficulty passing stool, pain or itching near your anus, genitalia; any genital pain, burning, discharge, redness, irritation, sexual dysfunction or impotence, loss of bowel or bladder control? Diarrhea or constipation? How often do you have a bowel movement?<br>• <u>Hips, legs, knees, ankles, feet</u>: numbness, weakness, pain or tingling in the hips, knees, ankles, or feet; pain in calves with walking, swelling of ankles, cold feet<br>• *Is there anything else that you think I should know in order to help you?* |

## Components of a Complete Patient History—*continued*

| Category | Application and considerations |
|---|---|
| **Medical history** | - *Are you taking any **medications**? What medications have you taken in the past few years? Finding out that your new patient recently discontinued his 20-year regimen of valproic acid, lithium, and risperidone may significantly change your interpretation of the clinical interview*<br>- *Have you been **treated for any medical conditions** or health problems?*<br>- *Have you ever been **hospitalized**?*<br>- *Have you ever had **surgery**?*<br>- *Have you ever been **diagnosed with any health problems** such as high blood pressure or diabetes?*<br>- Investigate for specific problems in the past health history that would be a major oversight to miss:<br>    o Current or past diseases: Cancer, Diabetes, Mental illness<br>    o Hypertension or high cholesterol<br>    o Medications, especially corticosteroids<br>    o Surgeries & Hospitalizations<br>    o Infections, Immune disorders<br>    o Trauma or previous injuries |
| **Social history** | - **Work**—*What do you do for work? Are you exposed to chemicals or fumes at your workplace?*<br>- **Hobbies**—*What do you do for recreation or hobbies? Are you exposed to chemicals or fumes at home or with your hobbies (e.g., painting, gardening)?*<br>- **Eat**—*Tell me about your breakfast, lunch, dinner, snacks… Do you consume foods or drinks that contain NutraSweet/aspartame* (linked to increased incidence of brain tumors[67]) *or carrageenan* (possibly linked to increased risk of breast cancer and inflammatory bowel disease[68,69])*?*<br>- **Exercise**—*What do you do for exercise or physical activity?*<br>- **Drink**—*Do you **drink alcohol**? Coffee/caffeine? Water?*<br>- **Drugs**—*Do you use recreational **drugs**? **Now or in the past?***<br>- **Smoke**—*Do you **smoke**?*<br>- **Sex**—*Are you **sexually active**? If so, do you practice safer sex practices? For all women: Is there any chance you could be pregnant right now?*<br>- **Emotional support**<br>- **Family contact and relationships** |
| **Family health history** | - *Does anyone in your family have any health problems, especially your parents and siblings?*<br>- *Do you have any children? Do they have any health problems?*<br>- *Do any diseases "run in the family" such as cancer, diabetes, arthritis, heart disease?* |
| **Additional questions** | - *Do you have any other information for me? Is there anything that I did not ask?*<br>- *What is your opinion as to why you are having this health problem?*<br>- *Are you in litigation for your illness or injuries?* |

---

[67] "In the past two decades brain tumor rates have risen in several industrialized countries, including the United States... Compared to other environmental factors putatively linked to brain tumors, the artificial sweetener aspartame is a promising candidate to explain the recent increase in incidence and degree of malignancy of brain tumors." Olney JW, Farber NB, Spitznagel E, Robins LN. Increasing brain tumor rates: is there a link to aspartame? *J Neuropathol Exp Neurol* 1996 Nov;55(11):1115-23
[68] Tobacman JK. Review of harmful gastrointestinal effects of carrageenan in animal experiments. *Environ Health Perspect.* 2001 Oct;109(10):983-94
[69] "However, the gum carrageenan which is comprised of linked, sulfated galactose residues has potent biological activity and undergoes acid hydrolysis to poligeenan, an acknowledged carcinogen." Tobacman JK, Wallace RB, Zimmerman MB. Consumption of carrageenan and other water-soluble polymers used as food additives and incidence of mammary carcinoma. *Med Hypotheses.* 2001 May;56(5):589-98

## Physical Examination

<u>Goals and purpose of the orthopedic/musculoskeletal examination</u>:
1. **To establish an accurate diagnosis (or diagnoses)**
2. **To assess the patient's functional status**
3. **To assess for concomitant and/or underlying and preexisting problems**
4. **To rule out emergency situations**
- *Example*: If your patient presents with low back and leg pain, and you determine that his fall off a horse resulted in ischial bursitis, have you also excluded a lumbar compression fracture? You can send the patient home with anti-inflammatory treatments and icepacks for the bursitis; but if you missed the spinal fracture, your patient could suffer neurologic injury resultant from your "failure to diagnose." **Don't assume that the patient has only one problem until you have proven with your history and examination that other likely problems do not exist.**

**Functional assessment**: When working with patients with acute injuries and systemic diseases, **take a wider view of the patient than simply diagnosing the problem.**
- *Will she be able to return to work?*
- *Will he be able to drive home safely?*
- *Will she need help with activities of daily living?*
- *Is there an occult disease, infection, malignancy, or toxic exposure that is causing these problems?*

**Neurologic examination**: One of the most important areas to assess when a patient presents with a musculoskeletal complaint is the neurologic system, especially if the complaint is related to a recent traumatic injury. Blood circulation is essential for life; but lack of circulation is only a major consideration in a small number of injuries, and it is usually readily apparent when severe because the problem will become acute quickly. Nerve injuries, however, can be subtle and insidious. All patients with spine (neck, thoracic, low back) pain must be questioned thoroughly for evidence of neurologic compromise. Nerve injuries can be painless, can progress rapidly, and can lead to permanent functional disability from muscle weakness or paralysis. **Every patient with pain, weakness, or recent trauma must be evaluated for neurologic deficits before the patient is treated and released from care.** Neurologic examinations are briefly reviewed in the pages that follow; citations can be used for sources of additional information.

<u>Resources for neurologic assessment</u>:
- Goldberg S. The Four-Minute Neurologic Exam. Medmaster http://www.medmaster.net/
- http://www.neuroexam.com Information and free on-line videos of a neurologic exam
- http://rad.usuhs.mil/rad/eye_simulator/eyesimulator.html Excellent interactive simulation of assessment of extraocular muscles in a neurologic examination; important for visualizing the combination of lesions and the subtlety of clinical presentation
- http://www.pennhealth.com/health_info/animationplayer/ Many health-related animations
- http://www.emedicine.com/neuro/topic632.htm This is an excellent review, noteworthy for its description of a "+5" level of reflex grading that denotes sustained clonus; most textbooks use a 0-4 scale

# Orthopedic Musculoskeletal Examination: Concepts and Goals

Orthopedic tests are detailed or reviewed in each respective chapter of *Integrative Orthopedics*[70] (i.e., shoulder exams are in the chapter on shoulders, knee exams in the chapter on knees). This section reviews the concepts and goals that provide the rationale for performing these tests. **Orthopedic tests are designed to place particular types of stress on specific body tissues.** Types of stress include tension/distraction, compression/pressure, shear force, vibration, friction, and percussion. Each type of stress is applied to elicit specific information about the exact tissue or structure that is being tested. **If you understand the reason for the type of stress that you are applying, and you are aware of the tissue/structure that you are testing, then you will find it much easier to perform the dozens of tests that are required in clinical practice.** If you understand the "how" and the "why" then you won't be overwhelmed with named tests that otherwise appear illogical or superfluous. Except for certain tests that all doctors need to know, illogical and superfluous tests have intentionally been omitted from this text. The tests that are described here meet at least one of the following two criteria: 1) it is a common test that all doctors know and which you will need to know for the sake of communication and for passing your academic and licensing examinations, or 2) it is going to be a useful test in your clinical practice.

Always remember that abnormalities found during the physical examination—particularly the neurologic examination—are often indicative of an underlying *nonmusculoskeletal* problem that must be identified or—at the very least—considered and then excluded by additional testing. For example, a patient **shoulder pain** and neurologic deficits found during the neuromusculoskeletal portion of your examination could have a **herniated cervical disc** as the underlying cause; but the cause could also be **syringomyelia**, or an **apical lung tumor** that is invading local bone and destroying the nerves of the brachial plexus.[71] As a clinician, the successful management and treatment of your patients depends in large part on the following: ❶ **knowledge**: your ability to conceptualize broadly and to consider many *functional* and *pathologic* causes of your patient's complaints, ❷ **tact**: the efficiency and accuracy with which you assess, accept, and exclude the various differential diagnoses into your final working diagnosis from which your treatment, management, referral, and co-management decisions are made, ❸ **art**: your ability to create the changes in your patient's outlook, lifestyle, biochemistry, biomechanics/anatomy, and physiology to effect the desired outcome.

| Type of stress | General application |
|---|---|
| Tension, traction | To provoke pain from injured/compromised tissues: tendons, muscles, ligaments, and nerves |
| Compression, pressure | To provoke pain from inflamed tissues; also used to assess for swelling and fluid accumulation in subcutaneous tissue, bursa, and joint spaces such as the knee |
| Shearing force | To test the integrity of ligaments and intervertebral discs |
| Vibration | To assess vibration sense (neurologic: peripheral nerves and dorsal columns) and screen for broken bones (orthopedic) |
| Friction, grinding | To elicit pain from injured tissues (cross-fiber friction) and articular surfaces (grinding tests) |
| Percussion, over bone and discs | To assess for bone fractures, bone infections, and acute disc injuries |
| Percussion, over peripheral nerves | To assess hypesthesia/tingling suggesting reduced threshold for depolarization secondary to nerve irritation or compression, i.e., Tinel's sign |
| Fulcrum tests | To assess for bone fractures: commonly the doctor's arm or a firm object is placed centrally under the bone in question and increasingly firm downward stress is applied to both ends of the bone to test for occult fracture |
| Torque, twisting | To test joint integrity (restriction or laxity) or for occult bone fracture (particularly of the digits) |

---

[70] **Vasquez A.** Integrative Orthopedics: Concepts, Algorithms, and Therapeutics. www.OptimalHealthResearch.com
[71] "Pancoast tumor has long been implicated as a cause of brachial plexopathy...The possibility of Pancoast lesion should be considered not only in the presence of brachial plexopathy, but also when C8 or T1 radiculopathy is found." Vargo MM, Flood KM. Pancoast tumor presenting as cervical radiculopathy. *Arch Phys Med Rehabil*. 1990 Jul;71(8):606-9

# Neurologic Assessment

Clinical neurology is a complex area of study. However, for most doctors, knowledge of clinical neurology hinges on answering three questions:
- **Is this patient's presentation normal or abnormal?**
- **If it is abnormal, does it indicate a specific disease or lesion?**
- **Does this condition require referral to a specialist or emergency care?**

Every clinician needs thorough training in anatomy and clinical neurology to be competent in the management of patients, because even common problems such as "pain" and "fatigue" and "headache" may herald devastating neurologic illness that must be assessed accurately and managed skillfully. While a complete review of clinical neurology is beyond the scope of this text, the following section provides a basic review of the clinical essentials. Clinicians needing an efficient refresher course in clinical neurology are encouraged to read the concise review texts by Goldberg.[72,73]

**Reliable indicators of organic neurologic disease**: These cannot be feigned and must be assumed to reveal organic neurologic illness that **must be evaluated by a neurologist**:
- **Significant asymmetry of pupillary light reflex**
- **Ocular divergence**
- **Papilledema**
- **Marked nystagmus**
- **Muscle atrophy and fasciculation**
- **Muscle weakness with neurologic deficit**; upper motor neuron lesions (UMNL) indicate a CNS lesion and need to be fully evaluated, probably by a neurologist; the need for referral is less necessary in cases of chronic neuropathy of known cause

**Purpose of Neurologic Examination and *Principle of Neurologic Localization*:**
The purpose of the neurologic examination is to qualify ("yes" or "no") the presence of a neurologic deficit, and—if present—to localize the lesion so that it can be further assessed with the proper laboratory, imaging, electrodiagnostic, or biopsy techniques. The following 9-point summary of localized lesions does not supplant independent studies of neurology and neuroanatomy but is useful for a quick clinically-relevant review.
1. **Cerebral cortex and internal capsule**: Neurologic deficit depends on location of lesion but is typically a combination of sensory/motor deficit and impaired higher neurologic function such as comprehension (superior temporal gyrus) or socially appropriate behavior (frontal lobe, ventral frontal gyri)
2. **Basal ganglia and striatal system**: Athetosis (lentiform nucleus: putamen and globus pallidus), (hemi)ballism (subthalamic nucleus), chorea (putamen), akinesia, bradykinesia, hypokinesia (lack of nigrostriatal dopamine)
3. **Cerebellum**: Ataxia, awkward clumsy execution of *intentional* motions; may have nystagmus, hypotonia
4. **Brainstem**: Cranial nerve deficit(s) with contralateral distal sensory and/or UMN motor deficits

---
[72] Goldberg S. Clinical Neuroanatomy Made Ridiculously Simple. Miami, Medimaster, Inc, 1990. Now in a third edition with interactive CD.
[73] Goldberg S. The Four-Minute Neurologic Exam. Miami, Medimaster, Inc, 1992

5. **Spinal cord**: Cranial nerves and higher cortical functions are intact; lesion can be a combination of sensory and motor (UMN and LMN) deficits and the pattern distal to lesion may be a complete or incomplete pattern of sensory and motor deficits on one or both sides of body depending on area of spinal cord affected
6. **Nerve root**: Segmental unilateral motor deficit; dermatomal distribution pain or sensory disturbance
7. **Peripheral nerve**: Localized combination of sensory and motor deficits; may be bilateral or unilateral
8. **Neurmuscular junction**: Painless weakness and "fatigable weakness": weakness that *worsens* with repeated testing; typically involves cranial nerves first in myasthenia gravis; also consider Eaton-Lambert Syndrome (ELS: autoimmune neuromuscular junction disorder associated with occult malignancy; contrasts with myasthenia gravis in that ELS strength *increases* with repeated testing)
9. **Muscle disease**: Painless weakness, typically involving proximal hip/shoulder muscles first; elevated serum aldolase and (phospho)creatine kinase

| *Cortex* | *Cerebellum* |
|---|---|
| <ul><li>Orientation: Person, place, time, situation.</li><li>Mood and cooperation</li><li>Level of consciousness: Alert, lethargic, stupor, coma (indirect assessment of reticular system in brainstem)</li><li>Memory: Remember objects or numbers; *recent* memory is most commonly affected by brain lesions: *What day of the month is it? How did you get here?*</li><li>Mentation: *Count backward from 100 by 7's.*</li><li>Spelling: *Spell the word "hand" backwards.*</li><li>Stereognosis: Identify by touch a familiar object such as a key or coin.</li><li>Hoffman's reflex: Doctor rapidly extends DIP of patient's middle finger and watches for patient's hand to perform grasp reflex; this test is performed for motor tract lesions involving the cerebral cortex, cerebellum, and upper motor neurons of the spinal cord.</li><li>Pronator drift: Supinated hands and arms outstretched forward for 30 seconds; doctor taps on palms; falling of hands and arms into pronation suggests UMNL.</li><li>Babinski reflex: Scraping the bottom of the foot results in splaying and flexing of the toes and extension (dorsiflexion) of the big toe; normal in infants.</li></ul> | <ul><li>Gait (lesion: ataxia)</li><li>Heel-to-toe walk</li><li>Tandem gait</li><li>Hand flip, foot tap (lesion: dysdiadochokinesia)</li><li>Finger-to-nose: Patient reaches out to doctor's finger, then patient touches patient nose, then back to new location of doctor's finger.</li><li>Heel-to-shin: Slide heel along shin.</li><li>Walk in circle around chair</li><li>Move eyes in a rapid "figure 8": Technique for provoking latent nystagmus</li><li>Rhomberg's test: Patient stands with feet close together and eyes closed; tests proprioception (peripheral nerves, dorsal columns, spinocerebellar tracts); vision (eyes open tests optic righting reflex) and coordinated motor activity (cerebellum).</li></ul> |

Several of the above '"cerebral" deficits may also result from intoxicative, nutritional, or metabolic disorders rather than an organic irreversible physical lesion. Likewise "cerebellar" deficits may also result from lesion of the brainstem tracts/nuclei and cerebellar peduncles, rather than the cerebellum itself.

Deep tendon reflexes are summarized below and on the following page. Hyperreflexia is noted with upper motor neuron lesions (UMNL) in the cortex, subcortical nuclei, brainstem, or corticospinal tracts of the spinal cord, whereas hyporeflexia can result from lesions of lower motor neurons (LMNL) in spinal cord, peripheral nerves, as well as from sensory/afferent defects including diabetic neuropathy, vitamin B-12 deficiency, and Guillain-Barre disorder. Muscle strength should always be "five over five" to be considered normal, whereas in the testing of reflexes, symmetry/asymmetry is generally more important than the grade of response (except with sustained clonus). **Asymmetry of reflex or strength (especially when seen together) is never normal and requires clinical correlation and investigation.**

| *Deep tendon reflexes* | *Muscle strength* |
|---|---|
| +5 Hyperreflexia *with sustained clonus*: Sustained clonus strongly suggests UMNL and requires investigation; most textbooks use a 0-4 scale, yet this 0-5 scale facilitates clear communication of observed lesions.[74] | 5/5 Normal: Full strength: able to withstand gravity and full resistance. |
| +4 Marked hyperreflexia: Up to 4 beats of *unsustained* clonus may be normal[75]; suggests UMNL but may be caused by medications, electrolyte disturbances, etc. | 4/5 Partial strength: Able to withstand gravity and partial resistance. |
| +3 Hyperreflexia: More than normal. | 3/5 Partial strength: Only able to resist gravity. |
| **+2 *Normal*: Neither hyporeflexia nor hyperreflexia.** | 2/5 Partial strength: Able to contract muscle but unable to resist gravity. |
| +1 Hyporeflexia: Less than normal | 1/5 Slight flicker of muscle contraction: Does not result in joint movement. |
| 0 No reflex: Requires clinical correlation for lesion of sensory receptors, peripheral nerve, spinal cord, anterior horn, or neuromuscular junction; this is a common finding in normal individuals. | 0/5 No clinically detectable contraction: Correlate with lesion of peripheral nerve, cord, cerebrum, anterior horn, or neuromuscular junction. |

---

[74] Oommen K, edited by Berman SA, et al. Neurological History and Physical Examination. Last Updated: October 4, 2006. *eMedicine* http://www.emedicine.com/neuro/topic632.htm

[75] "…three to four beats of clonus can be elicited at the ankles in some normal individuals." Waxman SG. Clinical Neuroanatomy 25th Edition. McGraw Hill Medical, New York, 2003, p 325

# Review of Clinical Assessments and Concepts

| Brainstem and Cranial Nerves | Spinal Cord, Roots, Nerves |
|---|---|

**Brainstem and Cranial Nerves**

1. Olfactory: **smell**
   - Smell: Test with strong and common odors such as coffee; do not use ammonia or other irritants which are perceived via trigeminal nerve (cranial nerve 5)
   - This is a worthwhile test in patients with recent head trauma (direct or indirect) such as from motor vehicle accidents (MVA); any violent motion of the head may result in injury to the olfactory fibers passing through the cribiform plate; patients may have associated anosmia or altered sense of flavor; frontal lobe disorders such as altered social behavior may be noted in lesioned patients
2. Ophthalmic: **reading, peripheral vision, fundoscopic**
   - Snellen chart for far vision, Rosenbaum card for near vision
   - Peripheral vision
   - Fundoscopic examination
3. Oculomotor: **move eyes and constrict pupils**
   - Eye motion in cardinal fields of gaze
   - Pupil contraction to light
   - Pupil contraction to accommodation
4. Trochlear: **motor to superior oblique**
   - Look "down and in" toward nose
5. Trigeminal: **bite, sensory to face and eyes**
   - Bite (motor to muscles of mastication)
   - Feel (sensory to face, eyes, and tongue)
6. Abducens: **motor to lateral rectus**
   - Looks laterally to the ear
7. Facial: **face muscles and taste to anterior tongue**
   - Furrow forehead, close eyes forcefully, smile and frown
   - Taste to anterior tongue
8. Vestibulocochlear: **hearing and balance**
   - Hearing, Rinne-Weber tests[76]
   - Balance: observe gait and Romberg test
9. Glossopharyngeal: **swallowing, and gag reflex**
   - Swallow
   - Gag reflex (sensory component)
10. Vagus: **motor to palate**
    - Say "ahh" to raise uvula
    - Gag reflex (motor component)
11. Spinal accessory: **motor to SCM and trapezius**
    - Raise your shoulders (against resistance)
    - Turn your head (against resistance)
12. Hypoglossal: **motor to tongue**
    - Stick out tongue to front

**Spinal Cord, Roots, Nerves**

Motor and reflex
- Strength: Specific muscles are tested and rated 0-5
- Plantar (Babinski) reflex: Signifies UMNL
- Abdominal reflexes: "Present" or "absent" (not rated 0-4); superficial reflexes are lost (rather than hyperactive) with UMNL
  - Upper abdominal: T8-10
  - Lower abdominal: T10-12
- Anal reflex: Cauda equina and sacral nerve roots
- Reflexes: Rate 0-4; asymmetric reflexes are more significant than finding absent or hyperactive (+3) reflexes; +4 reflex with sustained clonus is almost always pathologic and requires neurologist referral. Deep tendon reflexes with main spinal root levels are as follows:
  - Biceps: C5
  - Brachioradialis: C6
  - Triceps: C7
  - Patellar: L3-L4
  - Hamstring: L5
  - Achilles: S1

Sensory
- Light touch
- Two-point discrimination
- Vibration (use 128 Hz tuning fork)
- Joint position sense and proprioception (eyes closed, locate position of joint)
- Sharp and dull
- Hot and cold
- Sensory loss mapping (if deficits are found)
- Romberg (peripheral nerves, dorsal columns, vestibular, cerebellar)
- Nerve root tension tests such as straight leg raising
- *Subjective pain and discomfort can be indicated on pain diagrams and VAS (visual analog scale) as shown on the following page*

---

[76] "The Rinne and Weber tuning fork tests are the most important tools in distinguishing between conductive and sensorineural hearing loss." Ruckenstein MJ. Hearing loss. A plan for individualized management. *Postgrad Med.* 1995 Oct;98(4):197-200, 203, 206

**Patients can be asked to localize and describe their pain/discomfort on drawings such as these.** *Examples of descriptions*:

- Numb
- Hypersensitive
- Tingling
- Shooting pain
- Electrical pain
- Stabbing pain
- Burning pain
- Dull ache
- Muscle weakness

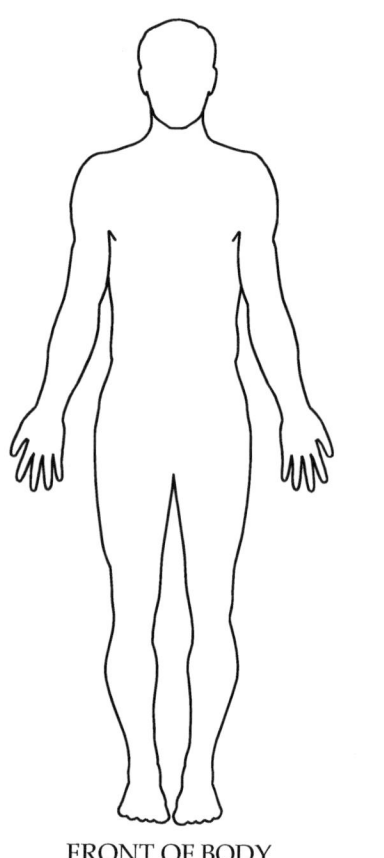

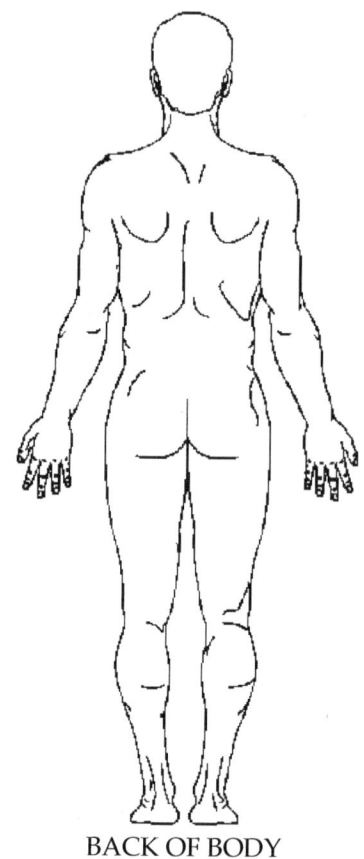

FRONT OF BODY                BACK OF BODY

On the lines below, indicate which pain/discomfort you are referring to and then quantify it by placing an "X" on the line.

Location of pain:_____

|—————————————————————————|
No pain at all                                             Worst pain imaginable

Location of pain:_____

|—————————————————————————|
No pain at all                                             Worst pain imaginable

# Laboratory Assessments: General Considerations of Commonly Used Tests

"The laboratory evaluation of patients with rheumatic disease is often informative but rarely definitive."[77]

Laboratory tests are immensely important in evaluating patients with musculoskeletal pain, as these tests allow you to 1) assess for infection (e.g., subacute osteomyelitis), 2) quantify the degree of inflammation (i.e., with CRP or ESR), 3) assess or exclude other disease processes that may be the cause of pain or dysfunction, and 4) assess for concomitant diseases (e.g., septic arthritis complicating rheumatoid arthritis). Additionally, 5) these tests open the door to more complete patient care and holistic management of the whole person because they allow for a more comprehensive and complete understanding of the patient's underlying physiology. **The recommended routine is to use the following panel of tests when assessing patients with musculoskeletal pain: 1) CBC, 2) CRP, 3) chemistry/metabolic panel, and preferably also 4) ferritin, 5) 25(OH)-vitamin D, and 6) thyroid assessment, minimally including TSH** and optimally including free T4 and anti-thyroid antibodies. The use of this screening evaluation on a routine basis helps identify patients with occult diseases and also allows for more comprehensive management of the patient's overall health. Other tests are indicated in specific situations. *Orthopedics* relies heavily upon physical examination and imaging, whereas *Rheumatology* relies more heavily upon laboratory analysis. In Orthopedics, laboratory tests are used mainly for the purposes of discovering or excluding rheumatic and systemic diseases. In Rheumatolgy, lab tests are used to specifically identify the type of illness, quantify the severity of the condition, and to assess for concomitant illnesses and complications.

**Essential Tests: These Tests are <u>Required</u> for <u>Basic</u> Patient Assessment**

| Test | Purpose | Clinical application |
|---|---|---|
| CRP (or ESR) | Screening for **infection**, **inflammation**, and possibly **cancer**; if inflammation is present, then these tests allow for a generalized quantification of severity. | **Useful in all new patients** for helping to differentiate systemic/inflammatory disorders from those which are noninflammatory and mechanical. Also very helpful as a general "barometer" of health since higher values correlate with increased risk for diabetes mellitus and cardiovascular disease; thus this test helps bridge the gap between acute care and wellness promotion. |
| CBC | Screening for **anemia**, **infection**, certain cancers (namely **leukemia**). | Useful in any patient with **nontraumatic musculoskeletal pain** or **systemic manifestations**, especially **fever or weight loss**; commonly detects occult B-12 and folate deficiencies. |
| Chemistry panel | Screening for **diabetes**, **liver disease, kidney failure**, bone lesions (alkaline phosphatase), **electrolyte disturbances**, adrenal insufficiency (hyponatremia with hyperkalemia), **hyperparathyroidism, hypercalcemia.** | Any patient with **nontraumatic musculoskeletal pain** or **systemic manifestations**; all patients with **hypertension, diabetes**, or who use **medications** that cause **hepatotoxicity, nephrotoxicity**, etc. |

---

[77] Klippel JH (ed). *Primer on the Rheumatic Diseases.* 11th Edition. Atlanta: Arthritis Foundation. 1997 page 94

## Overview of Important Tests: Common Components of Routine Evaluation

| Test | Purpose | Clinical Application |
|---|---|---|
| **Ferritin** | Important for assessing for **iron overload** (e.g., hemochromatoic polyarthropathy), and **iron deficiency** (e.g., low back pain due to colon cancer metastasis). Ferritin values less than 20 in adults (e.g., iron deficiency) or greater than 200 in women and 300 in men (e.g., iron overload) necessitate evaluation and effective treatment. | Ferritin is the ideal test for both iron overload and iron deficiency. All patients should be screened for hemochromatosis and other hereditary forms of iron overload regardless of age, gender, or ethnicity.[78] Iron deficiency—particularly in adults—may be the first clue to gastric/colon cancer and generally necessitates referral to gastroenterologist. |
| **Serum 25-hydroxy-vitamin D, 25(OH)D** | **Vitamin D deficiency is a common cause of musculoskeletal pain and inflammation**[79,80], and vitamin D deficiency is a significant risk factor for cancer and other serious health problems.[81,82,83] | Measurement of serum 25(OH) vitamin D (or empiric treatment with 2,000 – 4,000 IU vitamin D3 per day for adults) is indicated in patients with chronic musculoskeletal pain.[84,85] Optimal vitamin D status correlates with serum 25(OH)D levels of 50 – 100 ng/mL.[86] |
| **Thyroid stimulating hormone (TSH)** | Hypothyroidism is a common problem and is an often overlooked cause of musculoskeletal pain.[87] | This is a reasonable test for any patient with fatigue, cold extremities, depression, "arthritis", muscle pain, hypercholesterolemia, or other manifestations of hypothyroidism. |
| **Antinuclear antibodies (ANA)** | Sensitive (but not specific) for the detection of several autoimmune diseases, especially systemic lupus erythematosus (SLE). | This test is particularly valuable for assessing patients with polyarthropathy, facial rash, and/or fatigue. |
| **Rheumatoid factor (RF)** | The primary value of this test is in supporting a diagnosis of rheumatoid arthritis; specificity is low. | RF may be positive in normal health, iron overload, chronic infections, hepatitis, sarcoidosis, and bacterial endocarditis. |
| **Cyclic citrullinated protein (CCP) antibodies** | Cyclic citrullinated protein (CCP) antibodies are currently the single best laboratory test for rheumatoid arthritis (RA). | Citrullinated protein antibodies are rapidly becoming *the test* for diagnosing and confirming RA; used with RF for highly specific "conjugate seropositivity." |
| **Lactulose-mannitol assay** | Assesses for malabsorption and excess intestinal permeability—"leaky gut." | Diagnostic test for intestinal damage; excellent screening test for pathology or pathophysiology |
| **Comprehensive parasitology, stool analysis** | Identification and quantification of intestinal yeast, bacteria, and other microbes. | Extremely valuable test when working with patients with chronic fatigue syndromes, fibromyalgia, or autoimmunity; see chapter 4 of *Integrative Rheumatology*. |

[78] Vasquez A. Musculoskeletal disorders and iron overload disease: comment on the American College of Rheumatology guidelines for the initial evaluation of the adult patient with acute musculoskeletal symptoms. *Arthritis Rheum* 1996;39: 1767-8
[79] Masood H, Narang AP, Bhat IA, Shah GN. Persistent limb pain and raised serum alkaline phosphatase the earliest markers of subclinical hypovitaminosis D in Kashmir. *Indian J Physiol Pharmacol*. 1989 Oct-Dec;33(4):259-61
[80] Al Faraj S, Al Mutairi K. Vitamin D deficiency and chronic low back pain in Saudi Arabia. *Spine*. 2003 Jan 15;28(2):177-9
[81] Grant WB. An estimate of premature cancer mortality in the U.S. due to inadequate doses of solar ultraviolet-B radiation. *Cancer*. 2002 Mar 15;94(6):1867-75
[82] Zittermannn A. Vitamin D in preventive medicine: are we ignoring the evidence? *Br J Nutr*. 2003 May;89(5):552-72
[83] Holick MF. Vitamin D: importance in the prevention of cancers, type 1 diabetes, heart disease, and osteoporosis. *Am J Clin Nutr*. 2004;79(3):362-71
[84] Plotnikoff GA, Quigley JM. Prevalence of severe hypovitaminosis D in patients with persistent, nonspecific musculoskeletal pain. *Mayo Clin Proc*. 2003 Dec;78(12):1463-70
[85] Al Faraj S, Al Mutairi K. Vitamin D deficiency and chronic low back pain in Saudi Arabia. *Spine*. 2003 Jan 15;28(2):177-9
[86] Vasquez A, Manso G, Cannell J. The Clinical Importance of Vitamin D (Cholecalciferol): A Paradigm Shift with Implications for All Healthcare Providers. *Alternative Therapies in Health and Medicine* 2004; 10: 28-37. Also published in *Integrative Medicine: A Clinician's Journal* 2004; 3: 44-54. See www.optimalhealthresearch.com/monograph04
[87] "Hypothyroidism is frequently accompanied by musculoskeletal manifestations ranging from myalgias and arthralgias to true myopathy and arthritis." McLean RM, Podell DN. Bone and joint manifestations of hypothyroidism. *Semin Arthritis Rheum*. 1995 Feb;24(4):282-90

## Review of Clinical Assessments and Concepts

| CRP: C-reactive protein | |
|---|---|
| *Overview and interpretation:* | - CRP is a protein made by the liver in response to the immunologic activation characteristic of infectious and inflammatory conditions. Generally, any tissue injury or inflammatory process especially that involves the immune system's increased production of IL-6 will result in increased production of CRP.[88] High sensitivity CRP (hsCRP) is preferred over normal CRP due to its greater sensitivity and use in assessing cardiovascular risk.<br>- Elevated values are seen with:<br>  - <u>Infections</u>: Bacterial, fungal, parasitic, viral diseases; some patients with dysbiosis[89] will have mildly-moderately elevated CRP<br>  - <u>Inflammatory bowel disease</u>: Crohn's disease and ulcerative colitis (higher in CD than UC)<br>  - <u>Autoimmune disease</u>: Rheumatoid arthritis, polymyalgia rheumatica, giant cell arteritis, polyarteritis nodosa, (not always SLE)<br>  - <u>Acute myocardial infarction or other tissue ischemia</u><br>  - <u>Organ transplant rejection</u>: Renal, (NOT cardiac)<br>  - <u>Trauma</u>: Burns, surgery<br>  - <u>Obesity</u>: Leads to modest elevations in CRP |
| *Advantages:* | - This is an excellent screening test for differentiating "serious problems" (e.g., inflammatory and infectious arthropathy) from "benign problems" such as osteoarthritis.<br>- Since higher values of CRP are a well-recognized risk factor for cardiovascular disease, screening "musculoskeletal patients" with hsCRP provides data for cardiovascular risk assessment and a more comprehensive and holistic treatment approach, thus bridging the gap between acute care and preventive care. |
| *Limitations:* | - Elevations in CRP are completely nonspecific, requiring clinical investigation to determine the underlying cause of the immune activation.<br>- CRP may be normal in some patients with severe systemic diseases (such as lupus or cancer), and therefore a normal CRP does not entirely exclude the presence of significant illness. |
| *Comments:* | - Writing in *The New England Journal of Medicine*, authors Gabay and Kushner[90] note that measurements of plasma or serum **C-reactive protein can help differentiate inflammatory from non-inflammatory conditions and are useful in managing the patient's disease, since "the concentration often reflects the response to and the need for therapeutic intervention."** Additionally, they note, "Most normal subjects have plasma C-reactive protein concentrations of 2 mg per liter or less, but some have concentrations as high as 10 mg per liter." Deodhar[91] noted that **"Any clinical disease characterized by tissue injury and/or inflammation is accompanied by significant elevation of serum CRP..."** and that **CRP should replace ESR as a method of laboratory evaluation.** Deodhar also noted that **some patients with severe SLE will have normal CRP levels.** |

---

[88] Deodhar SD. C-reactive protein: the best laboratory indicator available for monitoring disease activity. *Cleve Clin J Med* 1989 Mar-Apr;56(2):126-30
[89] See chapter 4 of *Integrative Rheumatology* and Vasquez A. Reducing Pain and Inflammation Naturally. Part 6: Nutritional and Botanical Treatments Against "Silent Infections" and Gastrointestinal Dysbiosis, Commonly Overlooked Causes of Neuromusculoskeletal Inflammation and Chronic Health Problems. *Nutr Perspect* 2006; Jan http://optimalhealthresearch.com/part6
[90] Gabay C, Kushner I. Acute-phase proteins and other systemic responses to inflammation. *N Engl J Med*. 1999 Feb 11;340(6):448-54
[91] Deodhar SD. C-reactive protein: the best laboratory indicator available for monitoring disease activity. *Cleve Clin J Med* 1989 Mar-Apr;56(2):126-30

| ESR: erythrocyte sedimentation rate | |
|---|---|
| *Overview and interpretation:* | - Values may be elevated even when no pathology is present because ESR increases with anemia and with age.
- Much more sensitive than WBC count when screening for infection.[92]
- May be normal in about 10% of patients who have pathology such as **giant cell arteritis** and **polymyalgia rheumatica** (conditions where it is generally the only lab abnormality); may also be normal in several other diseases.
- **May be normal in patients with septic arthritis and patients with crystal-induced arthritis: joint aspiration for synovial fluid analysis is indicated if septic arthritis is suspected.**[93]
- Increased with age, anemia, inflammation; higher in women than men. Age-adjusted normal ranges: any value over 25 is considered high in young people, or 40 in elderly women.
- Age-related adjustments for men and women are as follows:
    - MEN: age divided by 2
    - WOMEN: (age + 10) divided by 2 |
| *Advantages:* | - Inexpensive and easy to perform—use the same lavender-topped tube that you use for CBC.
- Provides a quick screen for infection, inflammation, and multiple myeloma—the most common primary bone tumor in adults.
- In patients with elevated levels, ESR can be used to monitor progression of disease and response to treatment.[94] However, a negative/normal test result does not exclude the presence of significant disease; some noteworthy examples include the following: 1) elderly—due to diminished ability to mount an inflammatory response, 2) patients taking anti-inflammatory drugs and immunosuppressants, 3) a significant proportion of patients with lupus will have normal ESR despite aggressive disease, and 4) many cancer patients with clinically significant tumor burden will not show signs of systemic inflammation.
- **ESR may be more reliable than CRP for multiple myeloma.**[95] |
| *Limitations:* | - ESR may be normal in a subset of patients with clinically significant infection or inflammation.
- Values are elevated in the elderly and patients with anemia and are thus not necessarily indicative of disease in these populations. |
| *Comments:* | - **This test is generally considered *outdated* and has been replaced in most circumstances by CRP for the evaluation of inflammation and infection.**
- **The only time I use this test clinically is when I am highly suspicious of inflammation and the CRP is normal. Further, this test may be preferred when assessing for temporal arteritis and for multiple myeloma, two conditions which are classically associated with elevated ESR.** |

---

[92] Shaw BA, Gerardi JA, Hennrikus WL. How to avoid orthopedic pitfalls in children. *Patient Care* 1999; Feb 28: 95-116
[93] Klippel JH (ed). Primer on the Rheumatic Diseases. 11th Edition. Atlanta: Arthritis Foundation. 1997 page 94
[94] Shojania K. Rheumatology: 2. What laboratory tests are needed? *CMAJ*. 2000 Apr 18;162(8):1157-63 http://www.cmaj.ca/cgi/content/full/162/8/1157
[95] "We conclude that ESR, a simple and easily performed marker, was found to be an independent prognostic factor for survival in patients with multiple myeloma." Alexandrakis MG, Passam FH, Ganotakis ES, Sfiridaki K, Xilouri I, Perisinakis K, Kyriakou DS. The clinical and prognostic significance of erythrocyte sedimentation rate (ESR), serum interleukin-6 (IL-6) and acute phase protein levels in multiple myeloma. *Clin Lab Haematol*. 2003 Feb;25(1):41-6

*Review of Clinical Assessments and Concepts*

| | |
|---|---|
| **CBC: complete blood count** | |
| *Overview and interpretation:* | This test measures numbers and indices of white and red blood cells and platelets:<br>- WBC (white blood cells): The primary value of the WBC count in patients with musculoskeletal pain is that it allows screening assessment for 1) infection and 2) hematologic malignancies such as leukemia. **However, relying on the WBC count for the assessment of infection is potentially problematic since it is elevated in less than 50% of patients with acute and chronic musculoskeletal infections. "Therefore, it is helpful when it is high, but potentially misleading when it is normal."**[96] Be alert to the possibility of gaining additional information by assessing quantitative WBC indices of neutrophils, lymphocytes, and eosinophils, elevations of which may suggest bacterial infections, viral infections, or allergic or parasitic conditions, respectively.<br>- RBC (red blood cells and associated indices): In most clinical situations you are looking for anemia, which may be related to:<br>   o Nutritional deficiency of B-12 or folate: My approach is to critique the mean corpuscular volume (MCV) and to interpret MCV values greater than 90 with an increased suspicion for folate and/or B-12 deficiency. Clinical experience has shown that MCV values greater than 95 correlate with increased homocysteine levels, and a clinical response (improvement in mood, energy, and a reduction in MCV) is commonly seen following three months of nutritional supplementation. Deficiency of vitamin B-12 can easily be treated with oral administration of 2,000 mcg per day of vitamin B-12.[97] I generally use 5 mg (occasionally up to 20 mg) per day of oral folate for the treatment of probable or documented folic acid deficiency; this is safe for most patients, excluding those on antiepileptic drugs.[98] B-12 and folic acid *function together* and should be *administered together*.<br>   o Iron deficiency (confirmed with assessment of serum ferritin): While inadequate intake, malabsorption, or menstrual bleeding may cause iron deficiency, **adult patients with iron deficiency are at higher probability for gastrointestinal pathology and should therefore be evaluated with endoscopy or other comprehensive assessment** beyond fecal occult-blood testing to rule out gastrointestinal disease.[99,100] **The standard of care for all healthcare professionals is that adult patients with iron deficiency are referred for gastroenterological evaluation to evaluate for occult gastric or colon cancer.**<br>   o The anemia of chronic disease: Generally associated with a corresponding disease history such as long-term RA or renal insufficiency and often associated with increased ESR/CRP and ferritin. **Do not assume that an anemic patient has iron deficiency until proven with measurement of serum ferritin.** |
| *Advantages:* | - Inexpensive and easy to perform. Allows a quick screen for anemia, leukemia, infection, and for provisional evidence of B-12/folate and iron deficiencies; can also identify more complex conditions such as pancytopenia. |
| *Limitations:* | - WBC count may be normal even in patients with serious infections.<br>- RBC indices may be normal in people with clinically significant nutritional deficiencies. Ferritin should be used to confirm iron deficiency—*I have seen many patients with no evidence of anemia on the CBC, yet they have ferritin values less than 6 mcg/L.* |
| *Comments:* | - This test is part of a routine assessment for all new patients. |

---

[96] Shaw BA, Gerardi JA, Hennrikus WL. How to avoid orthopedic pitfalls in children. *Patient Care* 1999; Feb 28: 95-116
[97] "In cobalamin deficiency, 2 mg of cyanocobalamin administered orally on a daily basis was as effective as 1 mg administered intramuscularly on a monthly basis and may be superior." Kuzminski AM, Del Giacco EJ, Allen RH, Stabler SP, Lindenbaum J. Effective treatment of cobalamin deficiency with oral cobalamin. *Blood* 1998 Aug 15;92(4):1191-8 http://www.bloodjournal.org/cgi/content/full/92/4/1191
[98] "PGA administered in doses up to 1,000 mg orally a day… The folate was well absorbed, as reflected by marked increases in the serum and erythrocyte folate concentrations… There was no evidence of clinical or laboratory toxicity at these high doses of folate." Boss GR, Ragsdale RA, Zettner A, Seegmiller JE. Failure of folic acid (pteroylglutamic acid) to affect hyperuricemia. *J Lab Clin Med* 1980 Nov;96(5):783-9
[99] Rockey DC, Cello JP. Evaluation of the gastrointestinal tract in patients with iron-deficiency anemia. *N Engl J Med.* 1993;329(23):1691-5
[100] "Endoscopy revealed a clinically important lesion in 23 (12%) of 186 patients. … CONCLUSIONS: Endoscopy yields important findings in premenopausal women with iron deficiency anemia, which should not be attributed solely to menstrual blood loss." Bini EJ, Micale PL, Weinshel EH. Evaluation of the gastrointestinal tract in premenopausal women with iron deficiency anemia. *Am J Med.* 1998 Oct;105(4):281-6

| Chemistry/metabolic panel | |
|---|---|
| *Overview and interpretation:* | <ul><li>Measures glucose, electrolytes, markers for kidney and liver function, and other parameters.</li><li>Requires knowledge and pattern-recognition by the doctor to translate numbers into differential diagnoses that are correlated with the clinical presentation, examination and imaging findings to arrive at probable diagnoses.</li></ul> |
| *Advantages:* | <ul><li>Inexpensive and easy to perform—use serum separator tube.</li><li>Provides a quick screen for diabetes, hepatitis, renal insufficiency, alcohol abuse, hyperparathyroidism, and other problems.</li></ul> |
| *Limitation and considerations:* | <ul><li><u>Liver enzymes</u>: may be normal in patients with chronic viral hepatitis, hemochromatosis, or other cause of ongoing liver damage.</li><li><u>Hypercalcemia</u>: some of the more common causes in clinical practice are:<ol><li><u>Calcium-sparing diuretics</u>: Such as hydrochlorothiazide</li><li><u>Hyperparathyroidism</u>: Assess by measuring parathyroid hormone</li><li><u>Sarcoidosis</u>: Begin investigation with lab evaluation and chest radiograph</li><li><u>Vitamin D excess</u>: Measure 25-OH-vitamin D</li><li><u>Multiple myeloma</u>: ESR and serum electrophoresis</li><li><u>Lymphoma or cancer</u>: Assess with imaging, lab tests, clinical correlation, referral</li></ol></li><li><u>BUN and creatinine</u>: may be normal in patients with early kidney failure—always assess with urinalysis if renal insufficiency is suspected, such as in diabetic or hypertensive patients. Conversely, BUN and creatinine may be significantly elevated—mimicking renal failure—simply by dehydration.</li></ul> |
| *Comments:* | <ul><li>Abnormalities need to be pursued—repeat test within 2-4 weeks as part of routine follow-up along with additional investigation.</li><li>Many ill patients (such as those with chronic fatigue syndrome, fibromyalgia, etc) will have normal results with the metabolic panel. Therefore, normal results do not ensure that the patient is healthy.</li></ul> |


| Complement C3 and C4 | |
|---|---|
| *Overview and interpretation:* | <ul><li>Complement proteins are consumed in the complement cascades (typically activated by immune complexes) and thus low levels of complement proteins provide indirect evidence of extensive consumption due to immune complex-mediated inflammation. **Low levels of complement are seen with immune complex disorders (such as SLE, vasculitis, mixed cryoglobulinemia, rheumatoid vasculitis, glomerulonephritis) and inherited complement deficiencies.**</li><li>10%–15% of Caucasian patients with SLE have an inherited complement deficiency.[101]</li></ul> |
| *Advantages:* | <ul><li>Low complement levels provide indirect evidence of immune complex-mediated inflammation.</li><li>Elevated levels of complement are seen in conditions of infection or inflammation.</li></ul> |
| *Limitations:* | <ul><li>Some patients have a hereditary absence of complement proteins and thus their levels are always abnormally low; obviously the test cannot be used in these patients for monitoring inflammatory disease.</li></ul> |

---

[101] Shojania K. Rheumatology: 2. What laboratory tests are needed? *CMAJ*. 2000 Apr 18;162(8):1157-63 http://www.cmaj.ca/cgi/content/full/162/8/1157

## Review of Clinical Assessments and Concepts

| **Ferritin** | |
|---|---|
| *Overview and interpretation:* | - Ferritin levels are directly proportional to body iron stores, except in patients with inflammation, infection, hepatitis, or cancer. Therefore, **measuring ferritin allows assessment for iron deficiency (as a cause of fatigue, or early manifestation of colon cancer) and allows for assessment of iron overload (as a cause of joint pain and arthropathy).** This test should be performed in all African Americans[102,103], white men over age 30 years[104], diabetics[105], and patients with peripheral arthropathy[106] (i.e., pain in one or more joints, such as the hands, wrists, knees, hips, shoulders, shoulders, elbows, ankles, or feet), and exercise-associated joint pain[107,108] The research also justifies testing children[109], women[110], young adults[111] and the general asymptomatic public.[112]<br>- Low ferritin = iron deficiency<br>- High ferritin = iron overload, cancer, inflammation, infection, and/or hepatitis (viral, alcoholic, or toxic) |
| *Advantages:* | - Reliable screening test for iron overload when used in conjunction with patient assessment and evidence (e.g., normal CRP) of no infection or acute phase response.<br>- This is the blood test of choice for iron deficiency *and* iron overload. |
| *Limitations:* | - Iron-deficient patients with an acute phase response may have a falsely normal level of ferritin since ferritin is an acute phase reactant and will be elevated *disproportionate to iron status* during inflammation.<br>- Elevations of ferritin (i.e., >200 mcg/L in women and >300 mcg/L in men) need to be retested along with CRP (to rule out false elevation due to excessive inflammation) before making the presumptive diagnosis of iron overload. **In the absence of significant inflammation, ferritin values >200 mcg/L in women and >300 mcg/L in men indicate iron overload and the need for treatment regardless of the absence of symptoms or end-stage complications.**[113] |
| *Comments:* | - Note that since ferritin is an acute-phase reactant, a high level of serum ferritin by itself does not allow differentiation between iron overload, infection, and the inflammation associated with tissue injury or metastatic disease. Ferritin must be evaluated within the context of the patient's clinical condition and the assessment of at least one other marker for inflammation such as CRP. If the patient is not acutely ill or has not recently suffered tissue injury (e.g., myocardial infarction) and the CRP is normal, then an elevated ferritin value indicates iron overload until proven otherwise with diagnostic phlebotomy, which is safer and less expensive than liver biopsy or MRI. Transferrin saturation can also be measured when the interpretation of ferritin is unclear. By itself, serum iron is unreliable. |

---

[102] Barton JC, Edwards CQ, Bertoli LF, Shroyer TW, Hudson SL. Iron overload in African Americans. *Am J Med.* 1995 Dec;99(6):616-23
[103] Wurapa RK, Gordeuk VR, Brittenham GM, Khiyami A, Schechter GP, Edwards CQ. Primary iron overload in African Americans. *Am J Med.* 1996;101(1):9-18
[104] Baer DM, Simons JL, Staples RL, Rumore GJ, Morton CJ. Hemochromatosis screening in asymptomatic ambulatory men 30 years of age and older. *Am J Med.* 1995 May;98(5):464-8
[105] Phelps G, Chapman I, Hall P, Braund W, Mackinnon M. Prevalence of genetic haemochromatosis among diabetic patients. *Lancet* 1989; 2: 233-4
[106] Olynyk J, Hall P, Ahern M, KwiatekR, MackinnonM. Screening for hemochromatosis in a rheumatology clinic. *Aust NZ J Med* 1994; 24: 22-5
[107] McCurdie I, Perry JD. Haemochromatosis and exercise related joint pains. *BMJ.* 1999 Feb 13;318(7181):449-5
[108] "RESULTS: Our findings indicate a high prevalence of HFE gene mutations in this population (49.2%) compared with sedentary controls (33.5%). No association was detected in the athletes between mutations and blood iron markers. CONCLUSIONS: The findings support the need to assess regularly iron stores in elite endurance athletes." Chicharro JL, Hoyos J, Gomez-Gallego F, Villa JG, Bandres F, Celaya P, Jimenez F, Alonso JM, Cordova A, Lucia A. Mutations in the hereditary haemochromatosis gene HFE in professional endurance athletes. *Br J Sports Med.* 2004 Aug;38(4):418-21. Erratum in: *Br J Sports Med.* 2004 Dec;38(6):793 http://bjsm.bmjjournals.com/cgi/content/full/38/4/418 Accessed September 12, 2005
[109] Kaikov Y, Wadsworth LD, Hassall E, Dimmick JE, Rogers PCJ. Primary hemochromatosis in children: report of three newly diagnosed cases and review of the pediatric literature. *Pediatrics* 1992; 90: 37-42
[110] Edwards CQ, Kushner JP. Screening for hemochromatosis. *N Engl J Med* 1993; 328: 1616-20
[111] Gushusrt TP, Triest WE. Diagnosis and management of precirrhotic hemochromatosis. *W Virginia Med J* 1990; 86: 91-5
[112] Balan V, Baldus W, Fairbanks V, et al. Screening for hemochromatosis: a cost-effectiveness study based on 12, 258 patients. *Gastroenterology* 1994; 107: 453-9
[113] Barton JC, McDonnell SM, Adams PC, Brissot P, Powell LW, Edwards CQ, Cook JD, Kowdley KV. Management of hemochromatosis. Hemochromatosis Management Working Group. *Ann Intern Med.* 1998 Dec 1;129(11):932-9

**Ferritin**—*Interpretation of serum levels*

| Serum levels | Categorization and management |
|---|---|
| ≥ 800 mcg/L | **Practically diagnostic of iron overload**[114,115]: Repeat tests; rule out inflammation or occult pathology. Initiate phlebotomy and consider liver biopsy or MRI |
| ≥ 300 mcg/L | **Probable iron overload**[116]: Repeat tests; rule out inflammation or occult pathology. In men, initiate phlebotomy and consider liver biopsy or MRI[117] |
| ≥ 200 mcg/L | *In women*: **Suggestive of iron overload**[118]: Repeat tests, rule out inflammation or occult pathology. In women, initiate phlebotomy and consider liver biopsy or MRI[119] <br><br> *In men*: **High-normal *unhealthy* iron status with increased risk of myocardial infarction**[120]: Rule out inflammation or occult pathology. No follow-up is mandated, yet blood donation and/or abstention from dietary iron are recommended preventative healthcare measures |
| ≥ 160 mcg/L | *In women*: **Abnormal iron status**[121]: Repeat tests, rule out inflammation or occult pathology. Consider phlebotomy and liver biopsy or MRI |
| ≥80-120 mcg/L | **High-normal unhealthy iron status**[122,123]: No follow-up is mandated; blood donation and abstention from dietary iron are suggested preventative healthcare measures |
| 40-70 mcg/L | **Optimal iron status**[124,125] |
| < 20 mcg/L | **Iron deficiency:** Search for occult gastrointestinal blood loss with endoscopy or imaging assessments in adults; refer to gastroenterologist[126,127] |

Ferritin is an acute-phase reactant, which means that its production is increased during the acute phase of inflammatory and/or infectious disorders. Therefore the numeric value and hence its clinical meaning can be interpreted only within a context that also includes assessment of the patient's inflammatory status, which is best assessed with either ESR or CRP. If CRP/ESR is high, then the physician might assume that the ferritin value is "falsely elevated"—disproportionately elevated with respect to body iron stores. *Common clinical examples requiring use and skillful interpretation of ferritin*:

- **Elderly or arthritic patient with iron deficiency despite normal serum ferritin**: An elderly patient with normal ferritin and elevated CRP/ESR is probably iron deficient; retesting of ferritin and measurement of transferrin saturation and CBC should be performed promptly. If iron deficiency is confirmed or cannot be excluded, referral for endoscopic examination must be implemented. In a patient with known inflammatory arthropathy, the ferritin may appear normal even though the patient is iron deficient and in need of supplementation and endoscopy.
- **Non-anemic iron deficiency**: A middle-aged patient (commonly a premenopausal woman) presents with fatigue and during the course of evaluation is found to have a normal CBC. **Do not let the normal CBC prevent you from assessing ferritin; many of these patients are completely iron deficient with ferritin values of 2-6 mcg/L and are in need of iron replacement and gastrointestinal evaluation.**

---

[114] Milman N, Albeck MJ. Distinction between homozygous and heterozygous subjects with hemochromatosis using iron status markers and receiver operating characteristic (ROC) analysis. *Eur J Clin Biochem* 1995; 33: 95-8
[115] MilmanN. Iron status markers in hereditary hemochromatosis:distinction between individuals beinghomozygous and heterozygous for the hemochromatosis allele.*EurJHaematol*1991;47:292-8
[116] Olynyk JK, Bacon BR. Hereditary hemochromatosis: detecting and correcting iron overload. *Postgrad Med* 1994;96: 151-65
[117] "Therapeutic phlebotomy is used to remove excess iron and maintain low normal body iron stores, ... initiated in men with serum ferritin levels of 300 microg/L or more and in women with serum ferritin levels of 200 microg/L or more, regardless of the presence or absence of symptoms." Barton JC, McDonnell SM, Adams PC, Brissot P, Powell LW, Edwards CQ, Cook JD, Kowdley KV. Management of hemochromatosis. Hemochromatosis Management Working Group. *Ann Intern Med.* 1998 Dec 1;129(11):932-9
[118] Barton JC, Edwards CQ, Bertoli LF, Shroyer TW, Hudson SL. Iron overload in African Americans. *Am J Med* 1995; 99: 616-23
[119] Barton JC, McDonnell SM, Adams PC, Brissot P, Powell LW, Edwards CQ, Cook JD, Kowdley KV. Management of hemochromatosis. Hemochromatosis Management Working Group. *Ann Intern Med.* 1998 Dec 1;129(11):932-9
[120] Salonen JT, Nyyssonen K, Korpela H, Tuomilehto J, Seppanen R, Salonen R. High stored iron levels are associated with excess risk of myocardial infarction in eastern Finnish men. *Circulation* 1992; 86: 803-11
[121] Nicoll D. Therapeutic drug monitoring and laboratory reference ranges. In: Tierney LM, McPhee SJ, Papadakis MA. Current Medical Diagnosis and Treatment 1996 (35th Edition). Stamford: Appleton and Lange, 1996: 1442
[122] Lauffer, RB. Iron and Your Heart. New York: St. Martin's Press, 1991: 79-8, 83-88, 162
[123] Sullivan JL. Iron and the sex difference in heart disease risk. *Lancet.* 1981 Jun 13;1(8233):1293-4
[124] Lauffer, RB. Iron and Your Heart. New York: St. Martin's Press, 1991: 79-8, 83-88, 162
[125] Vasquez A. High body iron stores: causes, effects, diagnosis, and treatment. *Nutritional Perspectives* 1994; 17: 13, 15-7, 19, 21, 28 and Vasquez A. Men's Health: Iron in men: why men store this nutrient in their bodies and the harm that it does. *MEN Magazine* 1997; January: 11, 21-23 http://www.vix.com/menmag/alexiron.htm
[126] Rockey DC, Cello JP. Evaluation of the gastrointestinal tract in patients with iron-deficiency anemia. *N Engl J Med.* 1993;329(23):1691-5
[127] "Endoscopy revealed a clinically important lesion in 23 (12%) of 186 patients. ... CONCLUSIONS: Endoscopy yields important findings in premenopausal women with iron deficiency anemia, which should not be attributed solely to menstrual blood loss." Bini EJ, Micale PL, Weinshel EH. Evaluation of the gastrointestinal tract in premenopausal women with iron deficiency anemia. *Am J Med.* 1998 Oct;105(4):281-6

*Review of Clinical Assessments and Concepts*

## Algorithm for the Comprehensive Assessment of Iron Status

- **Screen asymptomatic patients.**
- **Follow-up abnormal laboratory results.** (high serum iron, elevated liver enzymes, high blood glucose, etc.)
- **Screen high-risk and symptomatic patients.**

↓

**Assess iron status with transferrin saturation and serum ferritin. Use fasting morning specimen.**

**IRON-DEFICIENCY**
serum ferritin: <10-15 in women, <20 in men, transferrin saturation: <16%

→ In adults with no obvious cause of blood loss: Assume pathologic gastrointestinal bleeding until proven otherwise. Simply testing for occult blood in the stool is insufficient. **Refer for complete (endoscopic) evaluation.**

**"HEALTHY IRON STATUS"**
transferrin saturation: 25-30%
serum ferritin: 30-70

→ Periodically assess iron status as part of routine health assessment. Consider assessment for impending iron deficiency. Consider periodic blood donation and low-iron diet to maintain healthy iron status.

**"MODERATE IRON OVERLOAD"**
transferrin saturation: >33-45%
serum ferritin: 80-160

→ No treatment is mandatory. Periodically assess iron status as part of routine health assessment. Consider low-iron diet and regular blood donation to reduce risk of cancer and myocardial infarction.

**POSSIBLE SEVERE IRON OVERLOAD**
transferrin saturation: >40% and/or
serum ferritin: >160 in women; >200 in men

→ Repeat tests with fasting morning specimen. Consider other causes of elevated transferrin saturation or elevated serum ferritin.*

→ Second assessment suggests "healthy iron status" or "moderate iron overload": Average results and/or reassess within 1 month, or periodically assess iron status as part of routine health assessment.

**PROBABLE SEVERE IRON OVERLOAD**
Ferritin >200 in women, or Ferritin >300 in men.
**Confirm with diagnostic phlebotomy, or liver biopsy, or MRI.**

→ Refer as needed (usually gastroenterologist, hematologist, or internist) for **phlebotomy therapy** and/or deferoxamine chelation.

**\*Factors that alter iron assessment tests**:
**False elevations of transferrin saturation**: cancer, liver disease, inflammation, infection, excess alcohol consumption, non-fasting specimens.
**False elevations of ferritin**: inflammation, infection, cancer, excess alcohol consumption, liver disease, early pregnancy, hyperthyroidism, tissue necrosis, hyperferremia-cataract syndrome and other rare genetic/congenital syndromes.

**Basic treatment of severe iron overload:**
- **Iron-removal therapy is mandatory:** Phlebotomy therapy is generally performed weekly or twice-weekly; deferoxamine chelation is reserved for patients who do not withstand phlebotomy (due to cardiomyopathy, severe anemia, or hypoproteinemia) or may be used concurrently with phlebotomy in some patients. Periodically assess hematologic and iron indexes. Continue with weekly iron removal therapy until patient reaches mild iron-deficiency anemia, then decrease frequency and continue phlebotomy as needed (e.g., 4 times per year).
- **Laboratory tests and physical examination:** Assess general physical condition and hepatic, cardiac, endocrine, and general health status.
- **Confirm diagnosis:** Liver biopsy ("gold standard") or diagnostic phlebotomy; perhaps MRI.
- **Assess liver status:** Liver biopsy ("gold standard") or perhaps MRI. Cirrhosis indicates increased risk of hepatocellular carcinoma and reduced life expectancy. Consider liver ultrasound, serum liver enzyme measurement, and serum alpha-fetoprotein to screen for hepatocellular carcinoma every 6 months. Hepatoma surveillance is mandatory in cirrhotic patients.
- **Implement dietary modifications and nutritional therapies:** Avoid iron supplements, multivitamin supplements with iron, iron-fortified foods, liver, beef, pork, alcohol, and excess vitamin C. Ensure adequate protein intake to replace protein lost during phlebotomy. Diet modifications are not substitutes for iron removal therapy. Consider antioxidant therapy.
- **Screen all blood relatives of patients with primary iron overload**. *Mandatory!*
- **Monitor patient condition, and compliance** with lifelong phlebotomy therapy
- **Assess and address psychoemotional issues/concerns**

| | |
|---|---|
| **25(OH)D: serum 25(OH) vitamin D** | |
| *Overview and interpretation:* | • **Vitamin D deficiency is a common cause of musculoskeletal pain**[128,129,130], and vitamin D deficiency is a significant risk factor for cancer and other serious health problems.[131,132,133]<br>• Measurement of serum 25(OH) vitamin D (or empiric treatment with 2,000 – 10,000 IU vitamin D3 per day for adults) is indicated in patients with chronic musculoskeletal pain, particularly low-back pain.[134] Optimal vitamin D status correlates with serum 25(OH)D levels of 50 – 100 ng/mL (125 - 250 nmol/L)—see our review article for more details[135]; levels greater than 100 ng/mL are unnecessary and increase the risk of hypercalcemia.<br><br>**Excess vitamin D**<br>> 100 ng/mL (250 nmol/L) with hypercalcemia<br><br>**Optimal range**<br>50 - 100 ng/mL (125 - 250 nmol/L)<br><br>**Insufficiency range**<br>< 20- 40 ng/mL (50 - 100 nmol/L)<br><br>**Deficiency**<br>< 20 ng/mL (50 nmol/L)<br><br><u>Interpretation of serum 25(OH) vitamin D levels</u>. Modified from Vasquez et al, *Alternative Therapies in Health and Medicine* 2004 and Vasquez A. *Musculoskeletal Pain: Expanded Clinical Strategies* (Institute for Functional Medicine) 2008. |
| *Advantages:* | • Accurate assessment of vitamin D status. |
| *Limitations:* | • Patients with certain granulomatous conditions such as sarcoidosis or Crohn's disease and patients taking certain drugs such as thiazide diuretics (hydrochlorothiazide) can develop hypercalcemia due to "vitamin D hypersensitivity" or drug side effects—these patients require frequent monitoring of serum calcium while taking vitamin D supplements. |
| *Comments:* | • **Routine measurement and/or empiric treatment with vitamin D3 needs to become a routine component of patient care.**[136]<br>• Periodic assessment of 25(OH)D and serum calcium are required to ensure effectiveness and safety of treatment, respectively. |

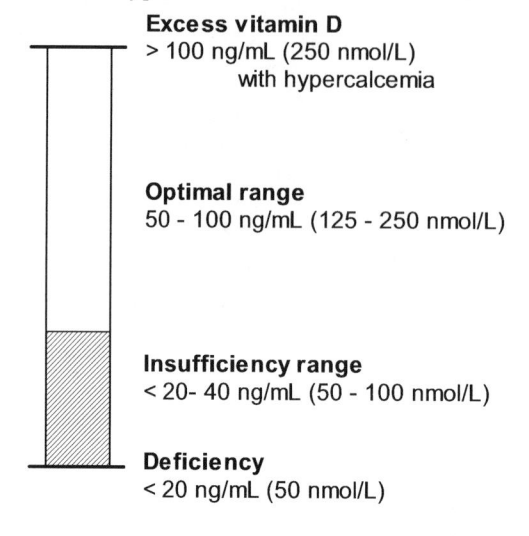

---

[128] Masood H, Narang AP, Bhat IA, Shah GN. Persistent limb pain and raised serum alkaline phosphatase the earliest markers of subclinical hypovitaminosis D in Kashmir. *Indian J Physiol Pharmacol*. 1989 Oct-Dec;33(4):259-61

[129] Al Faraj S, Al Mutairi K. Vitamin D deficiency and chronic low back pain in Saudi Arabia. *Spine*. 2003 Jan 15;28(2):177-9

[130] Plotnikoff GA, Quigley JM. Prevalence of severe hypovitaminosis D in patients with persistent, nonspecific musculoskeletal pain. *Mayo Clin Proc*. 2003 Dec;78(12):1463-70

[131] Grant WB. An estimate of premature cancer mortality in the U.S. due to inadequate doses of solar ultraviolet-B radiation. *Cancer*. 2002 Mar 15;94(6):1867-75

[132] Zittermannn A. Vitamin D in preventive medicine: are we ignoring the evidence? *Br J Nutr*. 2003 May;89(5):552-72

[133] Holick MF. Vitamin D: importance in the prevention of cancers, type 1 diabetes, heart disease, and osteoporosis. *Am J Clin Nutr*. 2004;79(3):362-71

[134] Al Faraj S, Al Mutairi K. Vitamin D deficiency and chronic low back pain in Saudi Arabia. *Spine*. 2003 Jan 15;28(2):177-9

[135] **Vasquez A, Manso G, Cannell J. The Clinical Importance of Vitamin D (Cholecalciferol): A Paradigm Shift with Implications for All Healthcare Providers.** *Alternative Therapies in Health and Medicine* **2004; 10: 28-37.** www.optimalhealthresearch.com/monograph04

[136] Heaney RP. Vitamin D, nutritional deficiency, and the medical paradigm. *J Clin Endocrinol Metab*. 2003 Nov;88(11):5107-8 http://jcem.endojournals.org/cgi/content/full/88/11/5107

## TSH: thyroid stimulating hormone

**Overview and interpretation:**

- TSH is produced by the anterior pituitary to stimulate the thyroid gland to produce T4 and T3. If the thyroid gland begins to fail, then TSH levels increase as the body attempts to stimulate production of thyroid hormones from a failing gland. Thyroid hormones have many different functions in the body, and their chief effect is contributing to the control of the basal metabolic rate, or the "speed" of reactions and the "temperature" of the body. For reasons that are not entirely clear, some people do not make enough thyroid hormone to function optimally.[137] Williams[138] noted that "a wide variation in thyroid activity exists among 'normal' human beings."

- TSH values greater than 2 represent a disturbance of the thyroid-pituitary axis and an increased risk for future thyroid problems[139], and the American Association of Clinical Endocrinologists encourages doctors to consider treatment for patients who test outside the boundaries of a narrower margin based on a target TSH level of 0.3 to 3.0.[140] It appears reasonable to implement a therapeutic trial of thyroid hormone treatment in patients who are clinically hypothyroid even if they are biochemically euthyroid provided that treatment is implemented cautiously, in appropriately selected patients, and patients are appropriately informed.[141,142]

- This is a routine test for general health assessment in asymptomatic patients, especially women and those with clinical manifestations of hypothyroidism which can include: fatigue, depression, dry skin, constipation, menstrual irregularities, infertility, PMS, uterine fibroids, excess menstrual bleeding, low body temperature, cold hands and feet, weak fingernails, increased need for sleep (hypersomnia), slow heart rate (bradycardia), overweight, gain weight easily, difficulty loosing weight, high cholesterol, slow healing, decreased memory and concentration, muscle weakness or myopathy, sleep apnea, frog-like husky voice, low libido, recurrent infections, high blood pressure, poor digestion, acid reflux, and delayed Achilles return.

**Advantages:**

- A quick and inexpensive screening test for overt primary hypothyroidism.

**Limitations:**

- Some patients will have a completely normal TSH value but a low free T4 or low free T3. Thus, even a properly interpreted TSH test may overlook problems of T4 production or conversion to active T3. Additionally, in some patients, all of these tests are normal but they may have thyroid autoimmunity (i.e., thyroid peroxidase antibodies, anti-TPO) and should receive treatment with thyroid hormone[143] or some other corrective treatment (e.g., selenium supplementation[144,145] and a gluten-free diet[146]) to normalize thyroid status.

**Comments:**

- The combination of T3 and T4 (as in the prescription Liotrix/Thyrolar or Armour thyroid) appears to have similar safety to T4 alone (Levothyroxine, Synthroid) and may result in greater improvements in mood and neuropsychological function.[147]

- Glandular thyroid supplements and Armour thyroid should *not* be used in patients with thyroid autoimmunity or Hashimoto's Thyroiditis because the bovine/porcine antigens will exacerbate the anti-thyroid immune response as evidenced by increased anti-TPO antibodies.

---

[137] Broda Barnes MD, Lawrence Galton, Hypothyroidism: The Unsuspected Illness. Ty Crowell Co; 1976
[138] Williams RJ. Biochemical Individuality : The Basis for the Genetotrophic Concept. Austin and London: University of Texas Press, 1956 page 82
[139] Weetman AP. Fortnightly review: Hypothyroidism: screening and subclinical disease. *BMJ: British Medical Journal* 1997;314: 1175
[140] American Association of Clinical Endocrinologists: "Until November 2002, doctors had relied on a normal TSH level ranging from 0.5 to 5.0 to diagnose and treat patients with a thyroid disorder who tested outside the boundaries of that range . Now AACE encourages doctors to consider treatment for patients who test outside the boundaries of a narrower margin based on a target TSH level of 0.3 to 3.04. AACE believes the new range will result in proper diagnosis for millions of Americans who suffer from a mild thyroid disorder, but have gone untreated until now." Available at http://www.aace.com/pub/tam2003/press.php on January 2004. For more current information, see "The target TSH level should be between 0.3 and 3.0 µIU/mL." American Association of Clinical Endocrinologists Medical Guidelines for Clinical Practice for the Evaluation and Treatment of Hyperthyroidism and Hypothyroidism. http://www.aace.com/pub/pdf/guidelines/hypo_hyper.pdf December 20,2005
[141] Skinner GR, Thomas R, Taylor M, Sellarajah M, Bolt S, Krett S, Wright A. Thyroxine should be tried in clinically hypothyroid but biochemically euthyroid patients. *BMJ: British Medical Journal* 1997 Jun 14; 314(7096): 1764
[142] McLaren EH, Kelly CJ, Pollack MA. Trial of thyroxine treatment for biochemically euthyroid patients has been approved. *BMJ* 1997 Nov 29; 315(7120): 1463
[143] Beers MH, Berkow R (eds). The Merck Manual. 17th Edition. Whitehouse Station; Merck Research Laboratories 1999 page 96
[144] Duntas LH, Mantzou E, Koutras DA. Effects of a six month treatment with selenomethionine in patients with autoimmune thyroiditis. *Eur J Endocrinol*. 2003 Apr;148(4):389-93 http://eje-online.org/cgi/reprint/148/4/389
[145] "We recently conducted a prospective, placebo-controlled clinical study, where we could demonstrate, that a substitution of 200 wg sodium selenite for three months in patients with autoimmune thyroiditis reduced thyroid peroxidase antibody (TPO-Ab) concentrations significantly." Gartner R, Gasnier BC. Selenium in the treatment of autoimmune thyroiditis. *Biofactors*. 2003;19(3-4):165-70
[146] Sategna-Guidetti C, Volta U, Ciacci C, Usai P, Carlino A, De Franceschi L, Camera A, Pelli A, Brossa C. Prevalence of thyroid disorders in untreated adult celiac disease patients and effect of gluten withdrawal: an Italian multicenter study. *Am J Gastroenterol*. 2001 Mar;96(3):751-7
[147] "CONCLUSIONS: In patients with hypothyroidism, partial substitution of triiodothyronine for thyroxine may improve mood and neuropsychological function; this finding suggests a specific effect of the triiodothyronine normally secreted by the thyroid gland." Bunevicius R, Kazanavicius G, Zalinkevicius R, Prange AJ Jr. Effects of thyroxine as compared with thyroxine plus triiodothyronine in patients with hypothyroidism. *N Engl J Med*. 1999 Feb 11;340(6):424-9

| Antinuclear antibody: ANA | |
|---|---|
| *Overview and interpretation:* | - **Good screening test for autoimmune conditions**: SLE, Sjogren's syndrome, and various other connective tissue diseases.<br>- Good and "highly sensitive" for initial assessment of SLE; positive in 95-98% of SLE patients; negative result strongly suggests against diagnosis of SLE.[148] Only 2% of patients with SLE have a negative ANA test—these patients may be identified by testing with anti-RO antibodies and CH50 (complement levels).<br>- This test measures for the presence of antibodies that react to nucleoproteins. Some labs report titers of 1:20 or 1:40 as "positive"; however, low levels of ANA are common (5-15%) in the general population. Thus, ANA is not specific for any one disease; may be positive in SLE, RA, scleroderma, Sjogren's, also seen with elderly, infected patients, cancer, and certain medications. Titers less than 1:160 should be interpreted cautiously as they may not indicate the presence of *clinical* autoimmunity.[149] Titers greater than 1:320 are considered indicative of clinically significant autoimmunity.<br>Methodologies (indirect immunofluorescence is most popular), subtypes, and patterns reported for ANA results may be irrelevant or clinically meaningful; the most common descriptors are provided in the table below. |

| *ANA patterns and descriptions*[150,151] | *Clinical correlation* |
|---|---|
| **Homogeneous**, diffuse nuclear staining | Nonspecific |
| **Speckled** | Least specific |
| **Rim** or peripheral staining | Suggests SLE and warrants assessment for anti-dsDNA, which is specific for lupus |
| **Anti-centromere**: selective staining of the centromeres of nuclei in metaphase | Highly specific for the limited scleroderma subtype associated with CREST syndrome |
| **Nucleolar** | Correlated with diffuse scleroderma (systemic sclerosis) |
| **FANA**: fluorescent ANA | The standard ANA test in the US |
| **Anti-Sm**: anti-Smith[152] | Virtually diagnostic of SLE: Highly specific for SLE; insensitive: positive in 20-30% of SLE patients |
| **Anti-dsDNA**: anti-double stranded DNA | Virtually diagnostic of SLE: Highly specific for SLE and indicative of an increased likelihood of poor prognosis with major organ involvement[153] especially active renal disease |
| **Anti-Ro (anti-SS-A)** | Correlates with SLE, Sjögren's syndrome, and neonatal SLE |
| **Anti-La (anti-SS-B)** | Sjögren's syndrome or low risk of SLE nephritis |
| **Anti-RNP** | SLE and/or mixed connective tissue disease (MCTD) |
| **Anti-Jo-1** | Specific but not sensitive for polymyositis/dermatomyositis |
| **Antihistone** | SLE and especially drug-induced SLE |
| **Antitopoisomerase (Scl-70)** | Correlates with diffuse scleroderma, especially with interstitial lung disease |

---

[148] Shojania K. Rheumatology: 2. What laboratory tests are needed? *CMAJ*. 2000 Apr 18;162(8):1157-63 http://www.cmaj.ca/cgi/content/full/162/8/1157
[149] Hardin JG, Waterman J, Labson LH. Rheumatic disease: Which diagnostic tests are useful? *Patient Care* 1999; March 15: 83-102
[150] Shojania K. Rheumatology: 2. What laboratory tests are needed? *CMAJ*. 2000 Apr 18;162(8):1157-63 http://www.cmaj.ca/cgi/content/full/162/8/1157
[151] Ward MM. Laboratory testing for systemic rheumatic diseases. *Postgrad Med*. 1998 Feb;103(2):93-100.
[152] Lane SK, Gravel JW Jr. Clinical utility of common serum rheumatologic tests. *Am Fam Physician*. 2002;65:1073-80 http://www.aafp.org/afp/20020315/1073.html
[153] Shojania K. Rheumatology: 2. What laboratory tests are needed? *CMAJ*. 2000 Apr 18;162(8):1157-63 http://www.cmaj.ca/cgi/content/full/162/8/1157

| **Antinuclear antibody: ANA**—*continued* | |
|---|---|
| *Advantages:* | • ANA has 98% sensitivity and 90% specificity for SLE in an unselected population.<br>• The negative predictive value in an unselected population is greater than 99%. ANA is therefore an excellent test for *excluding* the diagnosis of SLE. |
| *Limitations:* | • The positive predictive value in an unselected population is about 30%; **only 30% of unselected people with a positive result will have SLE**—this fact underscores the importance of patient selection and judicious interpretation of this test.<br>• Positive ANA is seen in patients with conditions other than SLE, including rheumatoid arthritis, Sjogren's syndrome, scleroderma, polymyositis, vasculitis, juvenile rheumatoid arthritis (JRA), and infectious diseases. |
| *Comments:* | • ANA is most often used to support the diagnosis of SLE in a patient with multisystemic illness and a clinical picture compatible with SLE. Nearly all patients with SLE will have positive ANA. **A positive ANA does not mean that the patient necessarily has SLE; be weary of paraneoplastic syndromes and viral hepatitis as underlying causative processes in patients with an unclear clinical picture.**<br>• I view any "positive ANA" as an indicator of poor health in general and immune dysfunction in particular. The goal, then, is to restore health. I have seen ANA show a trend toward normalization or completely normalize with effective health restoration as detailed in *Integrative Rheumatology* (chapter 4). I realize that my experience in this regard contrasts sharply with the allopathic view that serial measurements of ANA are worthless because the result never normalizes once a patient is ANA-positive[154]; I consider this evidence of the effectiveness of my naturopathic approach and the comparable failure of the allopathic approach. |

| **Antineutrophilic cytoplasmic antibodies: ANCA** | |
|---|---|
| *Overview:* | • ANCA are autoantibodies to the cytoplasmic constituents of granulocytes and are characteristically found in vasculitic syndromes and also in (Chinese) patients with inflammatory bowel disease[155] and nearly all patients with hepatic amebiasis due to *Entamoeba histolytica*.[156]<br>Two types:<br>• Cytoplasmic ANCA (C-ANCA): classically seen in **Wegener's granulomatosis**; also seen in some types of glomerulonephritis and vasculitis; this test is highly sensitive and specific for these conditions. In fact, a positive C-ANCA result can replace biopsy in a patient with a clinical picture of **Wegener's granulomatosis**.[157]<br>• Perinuclear ANCA (P-ANCA): considered a nonspecific finding[158] that correlates with SLE, drug induced lupus, and some types of glomerulonephritis and vasculitis. Shojania[159] stated that this test must be confirmed with antimyeloperoxidase antibodies to evaluate for Churg–Strauss syndrome, crescentic glomerulonephritis, and microscopic polyarteritis. |
| *Advantages, limitations, and comments* | • Obviates biopsy in a patient with clinical Wegener's granulomatosis.<br>• Not to be used as a screening test, except in patients with idiopathic vasculitis or glomerulonephritis.<br>• The fact that hepatic amebiasis due to *Entamoeba histolytica* induces production of C-ANCA antibodies in nearly 100% of infected patients may support the hypothesis that autoimmunity can be induced or exacerbated by parasitic infections. |

---

[154] Shojania K. Rheumatology: 2. What laboratory tests are needed? *CMAJ*. 2000 Apr 18;162(8):1157-63 http://www.cmaj.ca/cgi/content/full/162/8/1157
[155] "Fourteen patients (73.5%) were positive, of which six (31.5%) showed a perinuclear staining pattern and eight (42%) demonstrated a cytoplasmic pattern." Sung JY, Chan KL, Hsu R, Liew CT, Lawton JW. Ulcerative colitis and antineutrophil cytoplasmic antibodies in Hong Kong Chinese. *Am J Gastroenterol*. 1993 Jun;88(6):864-9
[156] "ANCA was detected in 97.4% of amoebic sera; the pattern of staining was cytoplasmic, homogeneous, without central accentuation (C-ANCA)." Pudifin DJ, Duursma J, Gathiram V, Jackson TF. Invasive amoebiasis is associated with the development of anti-neutrophil cytoplasmic antibody. *Clin Exp Immunol*. 1994 Jul;97(1):48-5
[157] Shojania K. Rheumatology: 2. What laboratory tests are needed? *CMAJ*. 2000 Apr 18;162(8):1157-63 http://www.cmaj.ca/cgi/content/full/162/8/1157
[158] Shojania K. Rheumatology: 2. What laboratory tests are needed? *CMAJ*. 2000 Apr 18;162(8):1157-63 http://www.cmaj.ca/cgi/content/full/162/8/1157
[159] Shojania K. Rheumatology: 2. What laboratory tests are needed? *CMAJ*. 2000 Apr 18;162(8):1157-63 http://www.cmaj.ca/cgi/content/full/162/8/1157

| RF: Rheumatoid Factor | |
|---|---|
| *Overview and application:* | - Rheumatoid factor—"anti-IgG antibodies"—are antibodies directed to the Fc portion of the patient's own IgG. Rheumatoid factors are anti-immunoglobulin antibodies, classically anti-IgG IgM. RF are found in low levels in most patients, and despite the "rheumatoid" name, RF is not specific for rheumatoid arthritis.[160] Current tests (latex fixation or nephelometry) detect IgM anti-immunoglobulin antibodies; however IgA-RF appears to have clinical superiority over other forms of RF because it correlates more strongly with clinical status.[161]
- This test is most commonly used to support the diagnosis of rheumatoid arthritis in a patient with a compelling clinical picture: peripheral polyarthritis lasting >6 weeks.[162] A negative result with a compelling clinical presentation of RA is termed "seronegative rheumatoid arthritis" by allopathic textbooks whereas a more appropriate term might be oligoarthritis, a condition described as "idiopathic" by allopathic text books despite the clear evidence that the majority of patients have one or more subsets of multifocal dysbiosis.[163]
- **Titers (latex fixation) of 1:160 are considered clinically significant, favoring the diagnosis of RA.**[164] However the positive predictive value is low—only 20-34% of people in an unselected population with a positive test result actually have RA.[165,166] |
| *Advantages:* | - Supports the diagnosis of rheumatoid arthritis: about 60-85% positive/sensitive in patients with rheumatoid arthritis (RA).[167,168] Quantitative titers of RF correlate with prognosis: a very high RF value portends a poor prognosis.[169] |
| *Limitations:* | - **Positive findings are common in the following conditions: rheumatoid arthritis, viral hepatitis, Sjögren's syndrome, endocarditis, scleroderma, mycobacteria diseases, polymyositis and dermatomyositis, syphilis, systemic lupus erythematosus, old age, mixed connective tissue disease, sarcoidosis**; positive results may also been noted in: **cryoglobulinemia, parasitic infection, interstitial lung disease, asymptomatic relatives of people with autoimmune diseases.**
- Febrile patients with arthralgia are more likely to have endocarditis than RA.[170]
- Patients with iron overload present with a similar clinical picture (i.e., polyarthropathy with systemic complaints) and may have a positive RF. Thus, patients with positive RF and polyarthropathy should be tested for iron overload; use serum ferritin.[171,172] |
| *Comments:* | - This test should only be used to confirm the diagnosis of rheumatoid arthritis in patients with a compelling clinical picture of the disease: inflammatory peripheral polyarthropathy with systemic complaints for > 6 weeks. A negative result does not mean that the patient *does not* have rheumatoid arthritis; a positive result does not mean that the patient *does* have rheumatoid arthritis.[173]
- **CCP (cyclic citrullinated protein) antibodies appear to be more specific and sensitive for RA and is becoming the test of choice for RA as described on the following page.** |

---

[160] Shojania K. Rheumatology: 2. What laboratory tests are needed? *CMAJ*. 2000 Apr 18;162(8):1157-63 http://www.cmaj.ca/cgi/content/full/162/8/1157
[161] Jonsson T, Valdimarsson H. What about IgA rheumatoid factor in rheumatoid arthritis? *Ann Rheum Dis*. 1998 Jan;57(1):63-4 http://ard.bmjjournals.com/cgi/content/full/57/1/63
[162] Shojania K. Rheumatology: 2. What laboratory tests are needed? *CMAJ*. 2000 Apr 18;162(8):1157-63 http://www.cmaj.ca/cgi/content/full/162/8/1157
[163] See chapter 4 of *Integrative Rheumatology* and Vasquez A. Reducing Pain and Inflammation Naturally. Part 6: Nutritional and Botanical Treatments Against "Silent Infections" and Gastrointestinal Dysbiosis, Commonly Overlooked Causes of Neuromusculoskeletal Inflammation and Chronic Health Problems. *Nutr Perspect* 2006; Jan http://optimalhealthresearch.com/part6
[164] Beers MH, Berkow R (eds). The Merck Manual. Seventeenth Edition. Whitehouse Station; Merck Research Laboratories 1999 Page 417
[165] Ward MM. Laboratory testing for systemic rheumatic diseases. *Postgrad Med*. 1998 Feb;103(2):93-100.
[166] Shojania K. Rheumatology: 2. What laboratory tests are needed? *CMAJ*. 2000 Apr 18;162(8):1157-63 http://www.cmaj.ca/cgi/content/full/162/8/1157
[167] Tierney ML. McPhee SJ, Papadakis MA (eds). Current Medical Diagnosis and Treatment 2002, 41st Edition. New York: Lange Medical Books, 2002 Page 854
[168] Shojania K. Rheumatology: 2. What laboratory tests are needed? *CMAJ*. 2000 Apr 18;162(8):1157-63 http://www.cmaj.ca/cgi/content/full/162/8/1157
[169] Shojania K. Rheumatology: 2. What laboratory tests are needed? *CMAJ*. 2000 Apr 18;162(8):1157-63 http://www.cmaj.ca/cgi/content/full/162/8/1157
[170] Klippel JH (ed). Primer on the Rheumatic Diseases. 11th Edition. Atlanta: Arthritis Foundation. 1997 page 96
[171] Bensen WG, Laskin CA, Little HA, Fam AG. Hemochromatoic arthropathy mimicking rheumatoid arthritis. A case with subcutaneous nodules, tenosynovitis, and bursitis. *Arthritis Rheum* 1978; 21: 844-8
[172] **Vasquez A**. Musculoskeletal disorders and iron overload disease: comment on the American College of Rheumatology guidelines for the initial evaluation of the adult patient with acute musculoskeletal symptoms. *Arthritis Rheum* 1996;39: 1767-8
[173] Shojania K. Rheumatology: 2. What laboratory tests are needed? *CMAJ*. 2000 Apr 18;162(8):1157-63 http://www.cmaj.ca/cgi/content/full/162/8/1157

## CCP: Cyclic citrullinated protein antibody; Citrullinated protein antibodies (CPA); anti-CCP antibodies: anticyclic citrullinated peptide antibody

| | |
|---|---|
| *Overview and use:* | - CCP—cyclic citrullinated protein antibodies; anticitrullinated protein antibodies: this is a relatively new auto-antibody marker that shows great promise and specificity for the early diagnosis of rheumatoid arthritis (RA). The test often becomes positive/present in asymptomatic patients years before the onset of clinical manifestations of RA.
- As of the first inclusion of this information in my books in December 2006, the information on anti-CCP antibodies is so new that it is not even included in most 2006-edition medical and rheumatology reference textbooks; nonetheless, doctors nationwide are already starting to use this test for the early diagnosis of RA. This may be particularly important because some research has shown that *early* and *aggressive* treatment of RA has an important impact on long-term prognosis[174]; however, the importance of early intervention is debatable.[175]
- Anti-CCP antibodies are directed toward several native proteins (e.g., filaggrin, fibrinogen, and vimentin) that have become posttranslationally modified by a uncharged citrulline in contrast to the normal positively charged arginine. This "citrullination" is catalyzed by a calcium-dependent enzyme, **peptidylarginine deiminase (PAD)**. These changes in protein charge and sequence make the native protein a target of auto-antibody attack by IgG antibodies in RA.[176] However, this does not necessarily imply that citrullination of native proteins is "the cause" of RA because citrullination of native proteins can also occur *de novo* in inflamed joints, which are then further targeted for inflammatory destruction. Until more information is available, we should withhold final judgment as to the ultimate role and origin of anti-CCP antibodies and in the meanwhile view them as a very strong and sensitive association with RA that facilitates the early diagnosis of this disease. |
| *Advantages:* | - Anti-CCP antibodies have 98% specificity for RA[177] and is likely to become the future laboratory standard in the diagnosis and prognosis of RA.[178]
- Anti-CCP antibodies with a positive rheumatoid factor (RF) is termed "composite seropositivity" and appears to be more specific than isolated anti-CCP antibodies or RF.[179] |
| *Limitations:* | - **The best current data indicates that anti-CCP antibodies are sensitive and specific for RA[180], and clinicians should use this test to diagnose and confirm RA**; however, continue to monitor research on this test as its value is verified or questioned in future reports. |
| *Comments:* | - Healthy people do not generally have anti-CCP antibodies. Asymptomatic patients with anti-CCP antibodies are at increased risk for clinical RA and are probably *en route* to the manifestation of clinical autoimmunity—RA, Sjogren's disease, or SLE. *Holistically intervene.*
- I hypothesize that PAD may become upregulated in synovial joints exposed to allergens, xenobiotics, bacterial debris/toxins/lipopolysaccharides and that the subsequent citrullination of joint proteins may lead to an autoimmune arthropathy that persists, perhaps despite removal of the inciting immunogen. More obviously, given that PAD is calcium-dependent, it may be upregulated secondary to intracellular hypercalcinosis secondary to vitamin D deficiency, magnesium deficiency, or fatty acid imbalance.[181] |

---

[174] "CONCLUSION: An initial 6-month cycle of intensive combination treatment that includes high-dose corticosteroids results in sustained suppression of the rate of radiologic progression in patients with early RA, independent of subsequent antirheumatic therapy." Landewe RB, Boers M, Verhoeven AC, Westhovens R, van de Laar MA, Markusse HM, van Denderen JC, Westedt ML, Peeters AJ, Dijkmans BA, Jacobs P, Boonen A, van der Heijde DM, van der Linden S. COBRA combination therapy in patients with early rheumatoid arthritis: long-term structural benefits of a brief intervention. *Arthritis Rheum.* 2002 Feb;46(2):347-56

[175] "By 5 years patients receiving early DMARDs had similar disease activity and comparable health assessment questionnaire scores to patients who received DMARDs later in their disease course." Scott DL. Evidence for early disease-modifying drugs in rheumatoid arthritis. *Arthritis Res Ther.* 2004;6(1):15-18 http://arthritis-research.com/content/6/1/15

[176] Hill J, Cairns E, Bell DA. The joy of citrulline: new insights into the diagnosis, pathogenesis, and treatment of rheumatoid arthritis. *J Rheumatol.* 2004 Aug;31(8):1471-3 http://www.jrheum.com/subscribers/04/08/1471.html

[177] Hill J, Cairns E, Bell DA. The joy of citrulline: new insights into the diagnosis, pathogenesis, and treatment of rheumatoid arthritis. *J Rheumatol.* 2004 Aug;31(8):1471-3

[178] "We conclude that, at present, the antibody response directed to citrullinated antigens has the most valuable diagnostic and prognostic potential for RA." van Boekel MA, Vossenaar ER, van den Hoogen FH, van Venrooij WJ. Autoantibody systems in rheumatoid arthritis: specificity, sensitivity and diagnostic value. *Arthritis Res.* 2002;4(2):87-93 http://arthritis-research.com/content/4/2/87

[179] "...our findings suggest that a positive anti-CCP antibody result does not necessarily exclude SLE in African American patients presenting with inflammatory arthritis. In such patients, the additional assessment of IgA-RF or IgM-RF isotypes may be of added value since composite seropositivity appears to be nearly exclusive to patients with RA." Mikuls TR, Holers VM, Parrish L, Kuhn KA, Conn DL, Gilkeson G, Smith EA, Kamen DL, Jonas BL, Callahan LF, Alarcon GS, Howard G, Moreland LW, Bridges SL Jr. Anti-cyclic citrullinated peptide antibody and rheumatoid factor isotypes in African Americans with early rheumatoid arthritis. *Arthritis Rheum.* 2006 Sep;54(9):3057-9

[180] "Serum antibodies reactive with citrullinated proteins/peptides are a very sensitive and specific marker for rheumatoid arthritis." Migliorini P, Pratesi F, Tommasi C, Anzilotti C. The immune response to citrullinated antigens in autoimmune diseases. *Autoimmun Rev.* 2005 Nov;4(8):561-4

[181] See http://optimalhealthresearch.com/archives/intracellular-hypercalcinosis and www.naturopathydigest.com/archives/2006/sep/vasquez.php for additional discussion

| HLA-B27: Human leukocyte antigen B-27 | |
|---|---|
| Overview and interpretation: | <ul><li>A common (5-10% of general population) genetic marker strongly associated with seronegative* spondyloarthropathy (all of which occur more commonly in men[182]):<ul><li>Ankylosing spondylitis (90-95% of 'whites' and 50% of 'blacks')[183]</li><li>Reiter's syndrome (85%)</li><li>Enteropathic spondyloarthropathy</li><li>Psoriatic spondylitis (<60%)</li></ul></li></ul> * Recall that "seronegative" in this context implies that the *rheumatoid factor is negative*, even though *the HLA-B27 may be positive.* |
| Advantages: Limitations: Comments: | <ul><li>*From a diagnostic perspective*: The clinical application and significance of this test is of limited value. All of the above-listed conditions are better assessed with the combination of clinical assessment and radiographs. In a patient with early and mild disease, this test may add evidence either supporting or refuting the diagnosis; but the test itself is not diagnostic of anything other than a genetic/histologic marker associated with various types of infection-induced arthropathy and autoimmunity (dysbiotic arthropathy[184]).</li><li>*From an integrative/functional medicine perspective*: This test can be of some value if the result is positive and the patient has evidence of a systemic inflammatory/autoimmune disorder since it therefore more strongly suggests that a dysbiotic locus is the cause of disease.[185]<ul><li>A consistent theme in the rheumatology literature is that of "molecular mimicry"—the phenomenon by which structural similarities between human and microbial structures lead to targeting of human tissues by immune responses aimed at microbial antigens. This topic is explored in considerable detail in the section on multifocal dysbiosis in *Integrative Rheumatology*. The important link between microbe-induced autoimmunity and HLA-B27 is that many dysbiotic bacteria produce an HLA-B27-like molecule that appears to trigger an immune response which then erroneously affects human tissues, leading to the clinical picture of autoimmune inflammation. Many of these HLA-B27-producing bacteria colonize the gastrointestinal and genitourinary tracts, promoting musculoskeletal inflammation via molecular mimicry and other mechanisms.[186,187] A strong and growing body of research shows that HLA-B27 is a risk factor for microbe-induced autoimmunity. "Autoimmune" patients positive for HLA-B27 are presumed to have an occult infection—especially gastrointestinal, genitourinary, or sinorespiratory—until proven otherwise.</li></ul></li><li>**<u>Keep in mind that HLA-B27 itself is not a disease</u>** and therefore a "positive" result merely means that the patient has this particular human leukocyte antigen; this test is not and will never be diagnostic of a specific disease—it simply correlates with increased propensity toward dysbiotic arthropathy and suggests the need for dysbiosis testing and the (re)establishment of eubiosis.[188]</li></ul> |

---

[182] "The major diseases associated with HLA-B27 (Reiter's disease, ankylosing spondylitis, acute anterior uveitis, and psoriatic arthritis) all occur much more commonly in men." James WH. Sex ratios and hormones in HLA related rheumatic diseases. *Ann Rheum Dis.* 1991 Jun;50(6):401-4

[183] Shojania K. Rheumatology: 2. What laboratory tests are needed? *CMAJ.* 2000 Apr 18;162(8):1157-63 http://www.cmaj.ca/cgi/content/full/162/8/1157

[184] See chapter 4 of *Integrative Rheumatology* and **Vasquez A**. Reducing Pain and Inflammation Naturally. Part 6: Nutritional and Botanical Treatments Against "Silent Infections" and Gastrointestinal Dysbiosis, Commonly Overlooked Causes of Neuromusculoskeletal Inflammation and Chronic Health Problems. *Nutr Perspect* 2006; Jan http://optimalhealthresearch.com/part6

[185] "The association between HLA-B27 and reactive arthritis (ReA) has also been well established… In a similar way, microbiological and immunological studies have revealed an association between Klebsiella pneumoniae in AS and Proteus mirabilis in RA." Ebringer A, Wilson C. HLA molecules, bacteria and autoimmunity. *J Med Microbiol.* 2000 Apr;49(4):305-11

[186] **Inman RD. Antigens, the gastrointestinal tract, and arthritis.** *Rheum Dis Clin North Am.* 1991 May;17(2):309-21

[187] **Hunter JO. Food allergy--or enterometabolic disorder?** *Lancet.* 1991 Aug 24;338(8765):495-6

[188] Dysbiotic arthropathy—joint inflammation and destruction as a result of a neuroimmune inflammatory response to microorganisms. Phrase coined by Alex Vasquez on December 15, 2005. No matching term on Medline or Google search. See chapter 4 of *Integrative Rheumatology* and **Vasquez A**. Reducing Pain and Inflammation Naturally. Part 6: Nutritional and Botanical Treatments Against "Silent Infections" and Gastrointestinal Dysbiosis, Commonly Overlooked Causes of Neuromusculoskeletal Inflammation and Chronic Health Problems. *Nutr Perspect* 2006; Jan http://optimalhealthresearch.com/part6

# Review of Clinical Assessments and Concepts

| | **Lactulose-mannitol assay: assessment for intestinal hyperpermeability and malabsorption** |
|---|---|
| *Overview and interpretation:* | - The lactulose-mannitol assay is a highly validated assessment for the accurate determination of small intestine permeability. This test is used to diagnose "leaky gut", which is a common problem and contributor to systemic inflammation in patients with inflammation and immune dysfunction—see chapter 4 of *Integrative Rheumatology*. Intestinal hyperpermeability reflects inflammation of and damage to the small intestine mucosa and is seen in patients with parasite infections, food allergies, celiac disease, malnutrition, bacterial infections, systemic ischemia or inflammation, ankylosing spondylitis, Crohn's disease, eczema, psoriasis, and those who consume enterotoxins such as NSAIDs and excess ethanol.[189]<br>- Elevations of **lactulose** indicate increased **paracellular** permeability caused by intestinal damage and are diagnostic of "leaky gut." *Clinical pearl*: remember that the "L" in *lactulose* rhymes with *leaky*.<br>- Decrements in **mannitol** suggest impaired **transcellular** absorption and suggest malabsorption in general and villous atrophy in particular. *Clinical pearl*: remember that the "M" in *mannitol* rhymes with *malabsorption*.<br>- Classically, in patients with damaged intestinal mucosa, we generally see a combined *increase in paracellular permeability* (measured with lactulose) and a *reduction in transcellular transport* (measured with mannitol); these divergent effects result in an increased lactulose-to-mannitol ratio. |
| *Advantages:* | - **This test is safe and affordable for the assessment of small intestine mucosal integrity. Abnormal results—"leaky gut" and/or malabsorption—generally indicate one or more of following:**<br>- <u>Malnutrition</u>**: may be due to poor intake, catabolism, or malabsorption.**<br>- <u>Enterotoxins</u>**: generally NSAIDs or ethanol**<br>- <u>Food allergies</u>**: including celiac disease**<br>- <u>"Parasites"</u>**: including yeast, bacteria, protozoa, amebas, worms, etc.**[190]<br>- <u>Systemic inflammation</u>**: tissue hypoxia, trauma, recent surgery, etc.**<br>- <u>Genetic predisposition toward enteropathy</u>**: check family history for IBD** |
| *Limitations:* | - Abnormalities and the identification of "leaky gut" are nonspecific and do not point to a specific or single diagnosis or treatment. |
| *Comments:* | - The value of this test is two-fold: 1) as a screening test for the above-mentioned disorders, and 2) as a method for determining the efficacy of treatment once the cause of the problem has been putatively identified and treated.<br>- This test can be used to promote compliance and to encourage the use of additional testing in patients who are otherwise prone to noncompliance or who resist other tests, such as stool testing. In other words, the clinician can gain an advantage by showing the patient an objective abnormality which then validates the need for treatment and additional testing.<br>- I only use this test on rare occasions because I more commonly either assume that a patient has leaky gut if he/she has one of the aforementioned conditions or we move directly to stool testing and comprehensive parasitology—clearly one of the most valuable tests in the management and treatment of systemic inflammation and immune dysfunction—otherwise known as "autoimmunity" and "allergy." |

---

[189] Miller AL. The Pathogenesis, Clinical Implications, and Treatment of Intestinal Hyperpermeability. *Alt Med Rev* 1997:2(5):330-345 http://www.thorne.com/pdf/journal/2-5/intestinalhyperpermiability.pdf

[190] See chapter 4 of *Integrative Rheumatology* and **Vasquez A**. Reducing Pain and Inflammation Naturally. Part 6: Nutritional and Botanical Treatments Against "Silent Infections" and Gastrointestinal Dysbiosis, Commonly Overlooked Causes of Neuromusculoskeletal Inflammation and Chronic Health Problems. *Nutr Perspect* 2006; Jan http://optimalhealthresearch.com/part6

| | |
|---|---|
| **Comprehensive stool analysis and comprehensive parasitology** | |
| *Overview and interpretation:* | - This is clearly one of the most valuable tests in clinical practice when working with patients with chronic fatigue, systemic inflammation, and autoimmunity. Second only to routine laboratory assessments such as CBC, chemistry panel, and CRP, the importance of stool testing and comprehensive parasitology assessments must be appreciated by progressive clinicians of all disciplines.
- Stool testing must be performed by a specialty laboratory because the quality of testing provided by most standard "medical labs" and hospitals is completely inadequate. Initial samples should be collected on three separate occasions by the patient and each sample should be analyzed separately by the laboratory.
- Important qualitative and quantitative markers include the following:
   - **Beneficial bacteria (" probiotics")**: Microbiological testing should quantify and identify various beneficial bacteria, which should be present at "+4" levels on a 0-4 scale.
   - **Harmful and potentially harmful bacteria, protozoans, amebas, etc.**: Questionable or harmful microbes should be eradicated even if they are not identified as true pathogens in the paleo-classic Pasteurian/Kochian sense.[191]
   - **Yeast and mycology**: At least two tests must be performed for a complete assessment: 1) yeast culture, and 2) microscopic examination for yeast elements. Both tests are necessary because some patients—perhaps those with the most severe symptomatology and the most favorable response to anti-yeast treatment—will have a negative yeast culture and positive findings on the microscopic examination. In other words, these patients have intestinal yeast that contributes to their disease/symptomatology but which does not grow on culture despite being clearly visible with microscopy; a similar pattern (using a swab of the rectal mucosa rather than microscopy) is referred to as "negative culture with positive smear."[192]
   - **Microbial sensitivity testing**: An important component to parasitology testing is the determination of which anti-microbial agents (natural and synthetic) the microbe is sensitive to. This helps to guide and enhance the effectiveness of anti-microbial therapy.
   - **Secretory IgA**: SIgA levels are elevated in patients who are having an immune response to either food or microbial antigens.[193] Thus, in a patient with minimal dysbiosis, say for example with *Candida albicans*, an elevated sIgA can indicate that the patient is having a hypersensitivity reaction to an otherwise benign microbe—in this case, eradication of the microbe is warranted and may result in a positive clinical response. Low sIgA |

---

[191] **Vasquez A. Reducing Pain and Inflammation Naturally. Part 6: Nutritional and Botanical Treatments Against "Silent Infections" and Gastrointestinal Dysbiosis, Commonly Overlooked Causes of Neuromusculoskeletal Inflammation and Chronic Health Problems.** *Nutr Perspect* 2006; Jan http://optimalhealthresearch.com/part6

[192] "According to Galland, the best predictor of who will respond to anticandida medication is a negative stool culture combined with a positive smear of the rectal mucosa (for the identification of intracellular hyphal forms of the organism); however, even that test is not 100% reliable." Gaby AR. Before you order that lab test: part 2. *Townsend Letter for Doctors and Patients*. 2004; January http://www.findarticles.com/p/articles/mi_m0ISW/is_246/ai_112728028

[193] Quig DW, Higley M. Noninvasive assessment of intestinal inflammation: inflammatory bowel disease vs. irritable bowel syndrome. *Townsend Letter for Doctors and Patients* 2006;Jan:74-5

suggests either primary or secondary immune defect such as selective sIgA deficiency[194] or malnutrition, stress, prednisone/corticosteroids, or possibly mycotoxicosis (immunosuppression due to fungal immunotoxins). In addition to addressing any systemic causative factors, a low sIgA may be addressed with the administration of bovine colostrum, glutamine, vitamin A, and *Saccharomyces boulardii*; the following doses may be considered for use in adults with proportionately smaller doses for children:

- Bovine colostrum: 2.4 – 3.6 grams per day in divided doses for adults. No drug interactions are known. Side effects may include increased energy, insomnia, and stimulation. One study in particular used very large doses of 10 grams per day for four days in children and found no adverse effects[195]; another case report of a child involved the use of 50 grams per day for at least two weeks and showed no adverse effects.[196]
- Glutamine: 6 grams 3 times per day (18 grams per day) is a common dosage with significant literature support.
- Vitamin A: Correction of subclinical vitamin A deficiency improves mucosal integrity and increases sIgA production in humans.[197] Common doses used by integrative clinicians are in the range of 200,000 IU to 300,000 for a limited amount of time, generally 1-4 weeks; thereafter the dose is tapered. Patients are educated as to manifestations of toxicity (see the chapter on *Therapeutics* toward the end of this book) and the importance of limited duration of treatment.
- *Saccharomyces boulardii*: Common dose for adults is 250 mg thrice daily; ability of this treatment to increase sIgA levels and its anti-infective efficacy have been documented in human and animal studies.

o **Short-chain fatty acids**: These are produced by intestinal bacteria. Quantitative excess indicates bacterial overgrowth of the intestines, while insufficiency indicates a lack of probiotics or an insufficiency of dietary substrate, i.e., soluble fiber. Abnormal patterns of individual short-chain fatty acids indicate qualitative/quantitative abnormalities in gastrointestinal microflora, particularly anaerobic bacteria that cannot be identified with routine bacterial cultures.

---

[194] "Selective IgA deficiency is the most common form of immunodeficiency. Certain select populations, including allergic individuals, patients with autoimmune and gastrointestinal tract disease and patients with recurrent upper respiratory tract illnesses, have an increased incidence of this disorder." Burks AW Jr, Steele RW. Selective IgA deficiency. *Ann Allergy*. 1986;57:3-13

[195] "In this double blind placebo-controlled trial, 80 children with rotavirus diarrhea were randomly assigned to receive orally either 10 g of IIBC (containing 3.6 g of antirotavirus antibodies) daily for 4 days or the same amount of a placebo preparation." Sarker SA, Casswall TH, Mahalanabis D, Alam NH, Albert MJ, Brussow H, Fuchs GJ, Hammerstrom L. Successful treatment of rotavirus diarrhea in children with immunoglobulin from immunized bovine colostrum. *Pediatr Infect Dis J*. 1998 Dec;17(12):1149-54

[196] Lactobin-R is a commercial hyperimmune bovine colostrum with some specificity for cryptosporidiosis; administration to a 4 year old child with AIDS and severe diarrhea resulted in significant clinical improvement in the diarrhea and "permanent elimination of the parasite from the gut as assessed through serial jejunal biopsy and stool specimens." Shield J, Melville C, Novelli V, Anderson G, Scheimberg I, Gibb D, Milla P. Bovine colostrum immunoglobulin concentrate for cryptosporidiosis in AIDS. *Arch Dis Child*. 1993 Oct;69(4):451-3

[197] "It can increase resistance to infection by increasing mucosal integrity, increasing surface immunoglobulin A (sIgA) and enhancing adequate neutrophil function. If infection occurs, vitamin A can act as an immune enhancer, increasing the adequacy of natural killer (NK) cells and increasing antibody production." Faisel H, Pittrof R. Vitamin A and causes of maternal mortality: association and biological plausibility. *Public Health Nutr*. 2000 Sep;3(3):321-7

[198] Parker RJ, Hirom PC, Millburn P. Enterohepatic recycling of phenolphthalein, morphine, lysergic acid diethylamide (LSD) and diphenylacetic acid in the rat. Hydrolysis of glucuronic acid conjugates in the gut lumen. *Xenobiotica*. 1980 Sep;10(9):689-70

|  |  |  |
|---|---|---|
| | | o **Beta-glucuronidase**: This is an enzyme produced by several different intestinal bacteria. High levels of beta-glucuronidase in the intestinal lumen serve to nullify the benefits of detoxification (specifically glucuronidation) by cleaving the toxicant from its glucuronide conjugate. This can result in re-absorption of the toxicant through the intestinal mucosa which then re-exposes the patient to the toxin that was previously detoxified ("enterohepatic recirculation" or "enterohepatic recycling"[198]). This is an exemplary aspect of "auto-intoxication" that results in chronic fatigue and upregulation of Phase 1 detoxification systems (chapter 4 of *Integrative Rheumatology*).<br>o **Lactoferrin**: The iron-binding glycoprotein lactoferrin is an inflammatory marker that helps distinguish functional disorders (i.e., IBS) from more serious diseases (i.e., IBD). Approximate values are as follows:<br>    ▪ <u>Healthy and IBS</u>: 2 mcg/ml<br>    ▪ <u>Severe dysbiosis</u>: up to 120 mcg/ml<br>    ▪ <u>Inactive IBD</u>: 60-250 mcg/ml<br>    ▪ <u>Active IBD</u>: > 400 mcg/ml.<br>o **Lysozyme**: Elevated in proportion to intestinal inflammation in dysbiosis and IBD.<br>o **Other markers**: Other markers of digestion, inflammation, and absorption are reported with the more comprehensive panels performed on stool samples. These tests are not always necessary, but such additional information is always helpful when working with complex patients. These markers are relatively self-explanatory and/or are described on the results of the test by the laboratory. |
| *Advantages:* | | ▪ **Stool analysis in general and parasitology assessments in particular provide supremely valuable information in the comprehensive assessment and treatment of patients with complex illnesses such as chronic fatigue, irritable bowel syndrome, fibromyalgia, and all of the autoimmune/rheumatic diseases.** |
| *Limitations:* | | ▪ Tests vary in price from about $250-$400.<br>▪ Anaerobic bacteria are difficult to culture.<br>▪ Specialty examinations, such as for *Helicobacter pylori* antigen and enterohemorrhagic *E. coli* cytotoxin, must be requested specifically at additional cost. |
| *Comments:* | | ▪ I have found stool testing to be the single most powerful diagnostic tool for helping chronically ill patients to attain improved health. Insights from stool/parasitology testing can be used to implement powerfully effective treatments. The value of this test in the treatment of patients with rheumatic disease must be appreciated and is extensively detailed in chapter 4 of *Integrative Rheumatology*. |

## High-risk Pain Patients:

When a patient has musculoskeletal pain and any of the following characteristics, radiographs should be considered as an appropriate component of comprehensive evaluation. These considerations are particularly—though not exclusively—relevant for spine and low-back pain.[199]

1. **More than 50 years of age**
2. **Physical trauma** (accident, fall, etc.)
3. **Pain at night**
4. **Back pain not relieved by lying supine**
5. **Neurologic deficits** (motor or sensory)
6. **Unexplained weight loss**
7. **Documentation or suspicion of inflammatory arthropathy**[200]
   - Ankylosing spondylitis
   - Lupus
   - Rheumatoid arthritis
   - Juvenile rheumatoid arthritis
   - Psoriatic arthritis
8. **Drug or alcohol abuse** (increased risk of infection, nutritional deficiencies, anesthesia)
9. **History of cancer**
10. **Intravenous drug use**
11. **Immunosuppression, due to illness (e.g., HIV) or medications (e.g., steroids or cyclosporine)**
12. **History of corticosteroid use** (causes osteoporosis and increased risk for infection)
13. **Fever above 100° F or suspicion of septic arthritis or osteomyelitis**
14. **Diabetes** (increased risk of infection, nutritional deficiencies, anesthesia)
15. **Hypertension** (abdominal aneurysm: low back pain, nausea, pulsatile abdominal mass)
16. **Recent visit for same problem and not improved**
17. **Patient seeking compensation for pain/ injury** (increased need for documentation)
18. **Skin lesion** (psoriasis, melanoma, dermatomyositis, the butterfly rash of lupus, scars from previous surgery, accident, etc....)
19. **Deformity or immobility**
20. **Lymphadenopathy** (suggests cancer or infection)
21. **Elevated ESR/CRP** (cancer, infection, inflammatory disorder)
22. **Elevated WBC count**
23. **Elevated alkaline phosphatase** (bone lesions, metabolic bone disease, hepatopathy)
24. **Elevated acid phosphatase** (occasionally used to monitor prostate cancer)
25. **Positive rheumatoid factor and/or CCP—cyclic citrullinated protein antibodies**
26. **Positive HLA-B27** (propensity for inflammatory arthropathies)
27. **Serum gammopathy** (multiple myeloma is the most common primary bone tumor)
28. **"High-risk for disease"** *examples*:
    - Long-term heavy smoking of cigarettes
    - Long-term exposure to radiation
    - Obesity
29. **Strong family history of inflammatory, musculoskeletal, or malignant disease**
30. **Others:** _____

---

[199] Remember that metastasis often travel first from the primary site to bone, therefore bone pain may be an early manifestation of occult cancer. Most of the above are from "Table 1: The high-risk patient: clinical indications for radiography in low back pain patients." J Taylor, DC, DACBR, D Resnick, MD. Imaging decisions in the management of low back pain. Advances in Chiropractic. Mosby Year Book. 1994; 1-28

[200] Radiographs are often essential for diagnosis or to rule out complications of the disease. For example, in patients with inflammatory arthropathies such as these, spontaneous rupture of the transverse ligament (at the odontoid process) has been reported; although rare, this complication could be life-threatening if mismanaged or undiagnosed.

# Concept: Not all "Injury-related Problems" are "Injury-related Problems"

In the case of most acute injuries, the underlying problem is often the injury itself. However, the physician must conduct a thorough history and examination to assess for possible underlying pathologies that cause or contribute to the problem that "appears" to be injury-related. Congenital anomalies, underlying pathology, previous injury, occult infections, and psychoemotional disorders may have been present *before* the "injury." Just because the patient reports a problem such as pain following an injury does not mean that the injury is the *sole* cause of the pain. *Do not let a biased history lead you down the wrong path.*

> "**Pediatric infections and neoplasms are notorious for masquerading as sport injuries.** …Take the relevant history directly from the patient, and keep tumors and infections high on your list of differential diagnoses… For example, about 15% of children with leukemia present with musculoskeletal complaints..."
>
> Shaw BA, Gerardi JA, Hennrikus WL. How to avoid orthopedic pitfalls in children. *Patient Care* 1999; Feb 28: 95-116

**In children and young adults, 5% of "sports-related" injuries are associated with preexisting infection, anomalies, or other conditions.** In adult women, "…between 9% and 20% of women with breast cancer attribute their symptoms to previous trauma to the breast. In these cases, the association of the breast mass with a traumatic event resulted in a delay in diagnosis ranging from four months to one year."[201]

When treating children, be very careful to get an accurate history—this is difficult since your two sources of information are not very reliable: parents often think that they already have the problem figured out, and so their history will be biased toward convincing you of what they think is the problem and solution; children are often not good historians and can form illogical relationships between events that can be misleading.

A group of German physicians describe a man who presented with a soft-tissue pain following a soccer game; he was later diagnosed with a malignant tumor—synovial sarcoma.[202] Similarly, Wakeshima and

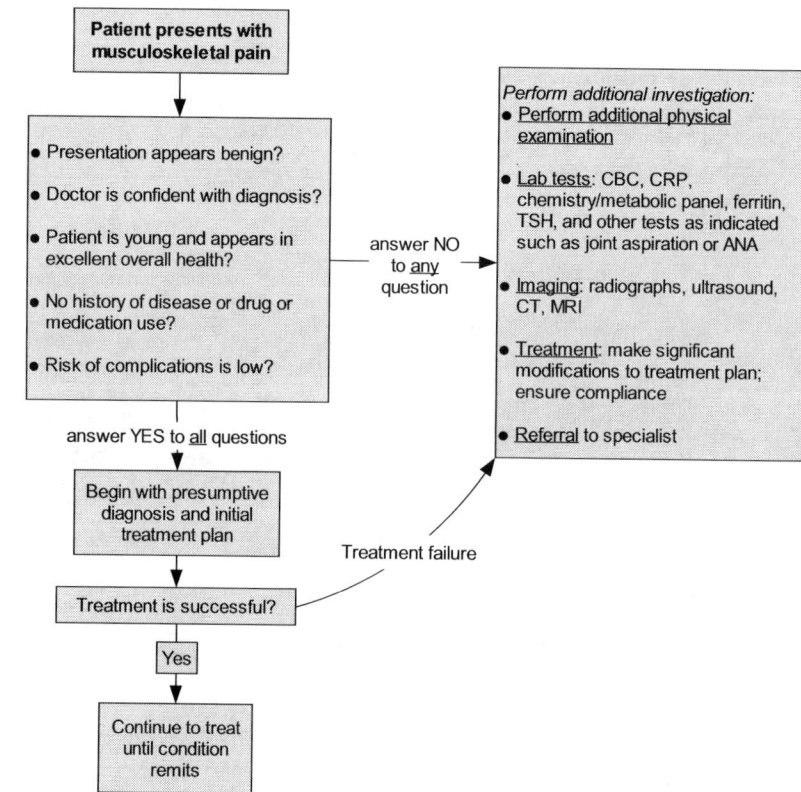

---

[201] Seifert S. Medical Illness Simulating Trauma (MIST) syndrome: case reports and discussion of syndrome. *Fam Med* 1993 Apr;25(4):273-6
[202] Engel C, Kelm J, Olinger A. Blunt trauma in soccer. The initial manifestation of synovial sarcoma. [Article in German] *Zentralbl Chir* 2001 Jan;126(1):68-71

# Review of Clinical Assessments and Concepts

Ellen[203] describe a young athletic woman who presented with chronic hip pain. The woman's history was significant for ulcerative colitis, but otherwise her radiographs were normal and her history and examination lead to a diagnosis of trochanteric bursitis. However, the patient's condition did not respond to routine treatment, and additional investigation over several months lead to a diagnosis of giant cell carcinoma. The authors concluded, "This case shows **the importance of repeat radiographic studies in patients whose joint pain does not respond or responds slowly to conservative therapy, despite initial normal findings.**"

What you expect to find and hear when taking a trauma-related history is that **1) a healthy patient** with no previous health concerns was **2) exposed to a traumatic event**, the history and consequences of which perfectly coincide with the injury you are assessing in your office, and that **3) your physical examination findings are all consistent** and lead to a specific diagnosis, which then **4) responds to your treatment**. If you find discrepancies between the history of the injury and your physical examination findings (e.g., fever after a "sports-related" injury), if the patient appears unhealthy in disproportion to the presenting complaint, or if the patient does not respond to your treatment, then you must consider the possibility of preexisting or concomitant disease.

Astute doctors search for and rule out preexisting and underlying pathology before ascribing the problem to the "obvious cause."

Always assess for consistency between the history, examination findings, and response to treatment—inconsistencies suggest the need for additional investigation.

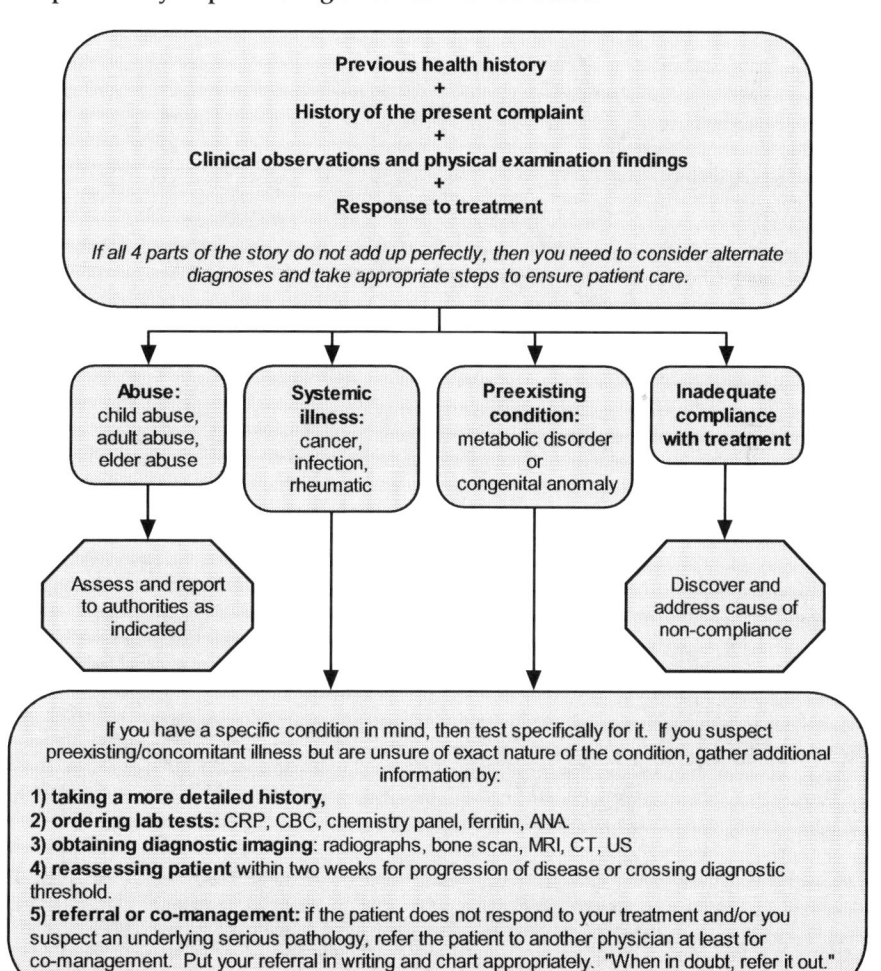

**Previous health history**
+
**History of the present complaint**
+
**Clinical observations and physical examination findings**
+
**Response to treatment**

*If all 4 parts of the story do not add up perfectly, then you need to consider alternate diagnoses and take appropriate steps to ensure patient care.*

- **Abuse:** child abuse, adult abuse, elder abuse
- **Systemic illness:** cancer, infection, rheumatic
- **Preexisting condition:** metabolic disorder or congenital anomaly
- **Inadequate compliance with treatment**

Assess and report to authorities as indicated

Discover and address cause of non-compliance

If you have a specific condition in mind, then test specifically for it. If you suspect preexisting/concomitant illness but are unsure of exact nature of the condition, gather additional information by:
1) **taking a more detailed history,**
2) **ordering lab tests:** CRP, CBC, chemistry panel, ferritin, ANA.
3) **obtaining diagnostic imaging:** radiographs, bone scan, MRI, CT, US
4) **reassessing patient** within two weeks for progression of disease or crossing diagnostic threshold.
5) **referral or co-management:** if the patient does not respond to your treatment and/or you suspect an underlying serious pathology, refer the patient to another physician at least for co-management. Put your referral in writing and chart appropriately. "When in doubt, refer it out."

---

[203] Wakeshima Y, Ellen MI. Atypical hip pain origin in a young athletic woman: a case report of giant cell carcinoma. *Arch Phys Med Rehabil* 2001 Oct;82(10):1472-5

# Concept: Safe Patient + Safe Treatment = Safe Outcome

The purpose of performing the history and physical examination on a new *or established* patient is to determine their current health status—including their mental and emotional health and their physical health, particularly as this relates to important and life-threatening possibilities such as cancer, infections, fractures, systemic diseases, and neurologic compromise. The questions that lead this investigation are: "**What is this patient's current status?**" "**Does this patient have a serious disease, neurologic injury, or are they at high risk for developing a serious complication in the near future that can be prevented with appropriate care *now*?**"

*"Is this patient safe?"*
- The question to ask yourself is, "Is this patient's health problem or current complaint/exacerbation a manifestation of an underlying condition that could result in a negative outcome?
- If a patient comes to you with a headache, and you neglect to find that their blood pressure is 230/130, then you missed the opportunity to help them avoid the stroke that they could have after leaving your office.
- If a patient comes to you with a complaint of low back pain, and you neglect to perform a neurologic examination to find that *the patient already has a neurologic deficit even before you treated them*, then you have lost the opportunity to defend yourself in court when the patient later claims that *your* treatment and *your* management of their case is the reason that they now have a permanent neurologic deficit.

**Is your treatment safe?**: Have you been perfectly clear with the patient about the risks and benefits of your treatment plan? **Have you obtained informed consent**? Have you charted **"PAR-B"** to indicate that you have discussed the **P**rocedures, **A**lternatives, **R**isks, and **B**enefits of your treatment plan? Have you been clear about the duration of treatment and the need for appropriate follow-up? If you are prescribing nutrition or botanical medicines, have you informed the patient about the duration of treatment? **Have you looked for contraindications to your otherwise brilliant treatment plan**? What about the fact that this patient was on corticosteroids for the past 15 years and only discontinued prednisone 2 months before arriving at your office? *The patient may have steroid-induced osteoporosis even though he is no longer on prednisone.* When you recommend that your patient take 100,000 IU of vitamin A to treat her throat infection, what happens when she presents to your office 8 months later with signs of vitamin A toxicity because she continued her treatment plan indefinitely rather than using it only for 7 days as you had intended? *Be sure to put a time limit on your treatment plans.* Every treatment plan should be 1) given to the patient in legible print and clear statements, 2) be copied for the chart, 3) include "what to do if things get worse" in the event of adverse treatment effect or exacerbation of problem, and 4) include patient's responsibility for returning to office/clinic for follow-up and reassessment.

> Double-check to ensure that your patient is safe (no forthcoming complications or predictable emergencies) and that your treatment is safe (appropriate, effective, clearly communicated, and time-limited with instructions to return for office visit).

**Informed consent**: From a legal standpoint, doctors can only treat a patient after the patient has given *consent to treatment*. Patients can only authoritatively consent to treatment after they have been fully educated about the treatment—thus they can provide *informed consent*. Full disclosure about the treatment plan includes informing the patient of the Procedures—what will take place; Alternatives—what options are available; Risks—what risks are involved, and (optionally) Benefits—what benefits can be expected. This is commonly charted as **"PAR—no questions"** or **"PAR—questions answered"** once the patient gives consent to treatment.

## Concept: Four Clues to Discovering Underlying Problems

When I taught Orthopedics at Bastyr University I encouraged students to search for specific **sets of clues** when evaluating patients. These clues—often insignificant in isolation but meaningful in combination—were often the "red flags" that could help make the difference between an accurate diagnosis and a missed diagnosis. These four categories can be recalled with the mnemonic "*S.C.I.N.*" or "*S.C.I.M.*" These four areas of assessment/safety emphasis differ from the "vindicates" mnemonic which is used for differential diagnosis.

| | Vindicates: a popular mnemonic for differential diagnosis |
|---|---|
| V | Vascular / Visceral referral |
| I | Infectious / Inflammatory / Immunologic |
| N | Neurologic / Nutritional / New growth: neoplasia or pregnancy |
| D | Deficiency / Degenerative |
| I | Iatrogenic (drug related) / Intoxication / Idiosyncratic |
| C | Congenital / Cardiac or circulatory |
| A | Allergy / Autoimmune / Abuse: drugs, alcohol, physical |
| T | Trauma / Toxicity |
| E | Endocrine / Exposure |
| S | Subluxation / Somatic dysfunction / Structural / Stress / Secondary gain |

- <u>**Systemic** symptoms and signs</u>: Ask about systemic signs and symptoms such as fever, weight loss, lymphadenopathy, or skin rash in patients who present with pain because these "whole body" manifestations might indicate an underlying or concomitant disease that deserves attention, either independently from the musculoskeletal pain, or as a cause of the musculoskeletal pain. For example, "headache" may appear benign, whereas "headache with fever and skin rash" suggests meningitis—a medical emergency. "Low-back pain" is a common occurrence; yet "low-back pain with weight loss and fever" might suggest occult malignancy, osteomyelitis, or other systemic disease.

- <u>**Complications**</u>: We ask about and look for already existing complications, such as "numbness, weakness, tingling in the arms or hands, legs or feet" to rapidly screen for neurologic deficits and we follow this up with screening assessments such as "squat and rise", toe walk, heel walk, and reflexes for spinal cord and lower extremity neuromuscular integrity. Additionally, when dealing with patients with spine-related complaints or injuries, we also ask about changes or loss of function in bowel and bladder control and numbness near the anus or genitals, which may be the *only* clinical clues to cauda equina syndrome—a medical emergency. Ask about effects of the condition on ADL (activities of daily living) to attain a more comprehensive view of the condition and to ensure that the patient's story is consistent.

- <u>**Indicators** from the history</u>: We look for specific "red flags" and "yellow flags" such as trauma, risk factors (such as smoking, prednisone, alcohol), or a positive history of chronic infections or cancer. Nonmechanical musculoskeletal pain in a patient with a history of or high risk for cancer is highly suspicious and mandates thorough investigation.

> Keeping these four assessment categories in mind can serve as a useful "checkpoint" to ensure that your patient is safe, and that your treatment is appropriate and therefore safe, too.

- <u>**Non-Mechanical** pain</u>: Non-mechanical pain suggests a pathologic etiology rather than simple joint dysfunction. Pain at night, pain that occurs without an inciting injury, pain that is not strongly affected by motion and is not powerfully provoked by your physical examination assessments suggests the possibility of underlying disorder such as cancer, neuropathy, or infection. However, the ability to elicit an exacerbation of pain with "mechanical" maneuvers does not indicate that the pain is "mechanical" and therefore "non-pathologic." Mechanical pain can still be pathologic pain, such as the exquisite pain felt by patients with spinal fractures—they may be neurologically intact, they do have pain worse with motion, but they are not safe to manipulate, and they require appropriate treatment and referral on an urgent basis.

# Concept: Special Considerations in the Evaluation of Children

> "Pediatric infections and neoplasms are notorious for masquerading as sport injuries. … There is only one way to avoid this trap: Take the relevant history directly from the patient, and keep tumors and infections high on your list of differential diagnoses."[204]

- **Consider the possibility of child abuse when a child presents with an injury:** As a non-naïve physician, you always have to consider the possibility of child abuse when a child presents with an injury. Be detailed in your history taking, and be sure to search for discrepancies between 1) the child's version of the incident, 2) the adult's version of the incident, and 3) what is realistic (based on your practical life experience and clinical training). As a primary care physician, you are obligated to report your *suspicion* of child abuse to law enforcement agencies and/or child protective services.
- **Children heal quickly:** This rapid healing is good as long as tissues are approximated. But if a fractured bone is displaced and not correctly replaced, then problematic malunion deformities may result *within **days***.
- **Children are more susceptible to rapidly progressing infections than are adults:** Soft tissue, joint, and bone infections need to be diagnosed expeditiously and treated aggressively.
- **Children are radiographically different from adults:** Make sure that your radiographs are interpreted by a competent radiologist with experience in the interpretation of *pediatric radiographs*. Radiographic considerations specific to children include:
    - **Epiphyseal growth plates**
    - **Secondary ossification centers**
    - **Variants in trabecular patterns and bone densities**
    - **Specific conditions that happen only in children, such as slipped capital femoral epiphysis**
    - **Congenital anomalies**
    - **Difficulty following directions with positioning** (applies to some adults, too!)
    - **Bone scans can be difficult to interpret in children:** Bone scans derive their value from the demonstration of a focal increase in uptake of radioactive isotopes, which demonstrates and localizes an area of increased metabolic activity. In adults, this increased and localized activity generally indicates pathology, especially malignant disease in bone (primary or metastatic) and recent fracture. In children, however, since their bones are already highly metabolically active due to the normal growth process, bone scans are difficult to interpret and are not highly reliable for the demonstration of focal lesions.

> Always consider the possibility of abuse, cancer, infection, or congenital anomaly as a cause of musculoskeletal pain in children, even if the injury appears to be related to injury or trauma. Strongly consider lab tests, as well as radiographs (interpreted by a pediatric radiologist). When in doubt, refer for second opinion. If you suspect abuse, you have a legal and ethical obligation to report your <u>*suspicion*</u>.

---

[204] Shaw BA, Gerardi JA, Hennrikus WL. How to avoid orthopedic pitfalls in children. *Patient Care* 1999; Feb 28: 95-116

## Concept: Differences between Primary Healthcare and Spectator Sports

In baseball, "errors" have been defined as "a defensive mistake that allows a batter to stay at the plate or reach first base, or that advances a base runner."[205] In baseball, a few errors can make the difference between winning and losing a particular game or season. However, a few errors in a game are to be expected, and ultimately the team can start over at the next game or season and try to do better.

Healthcare, however, is not a game, and even relatively minor errors such as the doctor's forgetting to ask a particular question or perform a specific test can result in a patient's catastrophic injury or death. In healthcare, when we are dealing with serious injuries and illnesses, even a single "error" is not allowed. "Failure to diagnose" is one of the biggest reasons for malpractice claims against doctors;

> While your compassion for human suffering and your love of nutrition and exercise may have directed you into healthcare, your professional success and survival will depend in large part on your ability to manage the technical and defensive aspects of clinical practice.
>
> Neuromusculoskeletal disorders and autoimmune diseases are "big league" clinical problems, and they need to be taken seriously.

such judgments often result in loss of licensure and awards of hundreds of thousands of dollars. "Failure to treat" results when the patient is injured because the doctor failed to effectively treat the patient or when the doctor failed to provide the appropriate referral to a specialist in a timely manner. Such failures are not only capable of destroying a physician's career and forcing the liquidation of his/her possessions, but such cases can also greatly damage the integrity of whole professions, especially the naturopathic and chiropractic professions which are generally guilty until proven innocent due to the double standards imposed by those adherent to the "always right" dogma of the medical paradigm.[206] Stated differently, **if the doctor does not ask the right questions and perform the right tests, then the doctor may miss an emergency diagnosis. Missing an emergency diagnosis can result in patient death. Patient death may result in litigation, loss of license for the doctor, and irreparable harm to the profession.** The upcoming section on **Musculoskeletal Emergencies** represents *core competencies* that every clinician must keep present in his/her mind during each interaction with a patient with musculoskeletal complaints, especially patients who are elderly, on medications such as prednisone, and those with known autoimmune or immunosuppressive disorders.

## Concept: "Disease Treatment" is Different from "Patient Management"

> "The key to successful intervention for orthopedic problems in a primary care practice is to know what conditions to refer and when and to whom to refer the refractory patient."[207]

Treating a problem is one thing, managing a patient is something different. "Problems" such as "low back pain" are abstract concepts, and we automatically form mental lists of treatments for problems that are irrespective of the patient who has the condition. However this list may be of only very limited applicability to the individual patient with whom you are working. Management of patients includes ❶ assessing and reassessing the differential diagnoses, ❷ monitoring compliance with treatments, including the treatments of other healthcare providers, ❸ co-treating with other healthcare providers, ❹ assessing for contraindications, ❺ monitoring patient status and effectiveness of treatments, and also ❻ the office-related tasks of charting, documentation, billing, and

---

[205] http://www.nocryinginbaseball.com/glossary/glossary.html Accessed November 11, 2006
[206] Micozzi MS. Double standards and double jeopardy for CAM research. *J Altern Complement Med*. 2001 Feb;7(1):13-4
[207] Brier S. Primary Care Orthopedics. St. Louis: Mosby, 1999 page ix

correspondence. The management of emergency conditions often involves transport to the nearest hospital. In some situations, the patient will be able to drive himself/herself without difficulty. In other situations, the patient should be driven by friend, family, or taxi. In the most extreme, the patient should be transported by ambulance. When in doubt about the mode of transport, do not hesitate to call 911 for an ambulance. If the taxi driver gets lost on the way to the hospital, or your patient goes into shock while being driven by a friend, the liability will come back to haunt the *doctor*, not the *friend* or the *taxi driver*.

## Concept: Clinical Practice Involves Much More than "Diagnosis and Treatment"

Emergency room and hospital-based physicians are appropriately able to focus solely on diagnosis and treatment as their primary spheres of activity and interaction with patients. However, those of us in private practice learn that *healthcare* involves much more than simply being a "good doctor." From an integrative perspective we have to go beyond diagnosis and treatment *for each health disorder* with each patient. Beyond *diagnosis* and *treatment* are *understanding* and *integration*. Orchestrating all of this into a treatment plan that the patient can actually implement requires creativity, resourcefulness, and the ability to enroll patients in the process of *redesigning*—often *rebuilding*—their lives.

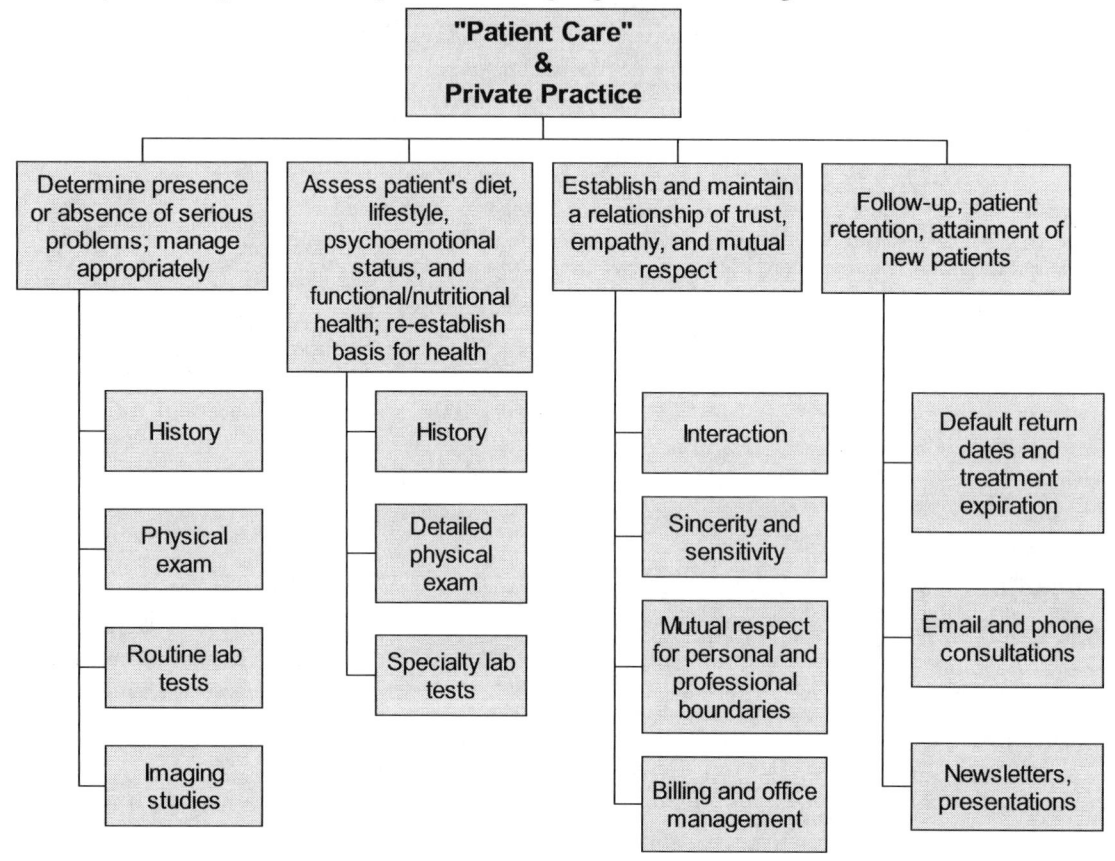

```
                        "Patient Care"
                              &
                        Private Practice
    ┌──────────────┬──────────────┬──────────────┬──────────────┐
  Determine      Assess patient's  Establish and   Follow-up, patient
  presence or    diet, lifestyle,  maintain a      retention,
  absence of     psychoemotional   relationship    attainment of
  serious        status, and       of trust,       new patients
  problems;      functional/       empathy, and
  manage         nutritional       mutual respect
  appropriately  health;
                 re-establish
                 basis for health

  History        History           Interaction     Default return
                                                   dates and
                                                   treatment
                                                   expiration

  Physical       Detailed          Sincerity and
  exam           physical exam     sensitivity

                                   Mutual respect  Email and phone
  Routine lab    Specialty lab     for personal    consultations
  tests          tests             and professional
                                   boundaries

  Imaging                          Billing and     Newsletters,
  studies                          office          presentations
                                   management
```

Recall that **28% of malpractice claims involve mistakes made by medical office staff**; this includes unreturned phone calls which can culminate in malpractice by way of "patient abandonment." Similarly, inability to get a timely consultation may result in sufficient "sense of harm" that a patient may decide to sue; this is a factor in 10% of malpractice cases.[208]

---

[208] James R. Hall, Ph.D., L.Psych., FABMP, FGICPP. Departments of Internal Medicine and Psychology, UNT Health Science Center at Fort Worth. "Communication and Medico-Legal Issues." October 19, 2006

# Risk Management: A Note Especially to Students and Recent Licensees

Even if you are a board-certified rheumatologist and an assertive and astute clinician with years of experience, the consideration of these guidelines may help protect **you** from malpractice liability and **your patient** from harm. Practicing "good medicine" is inherently defensive and in the best interests of the patient and the doctor.

1. **Document the specifics of your treatment plan and the rationale behind it.**
2. **Do not tell your patient to discontinue their anti-rheumatic drugs unless these drugs are in your scope of practice** *and* **discontinuing such drugs is therapeutically appropriate.**
3. **Give your patient written instructions, and specifically delineate time parameters for the next visit to monitor for therapeutic effectiveness, adverse effects, and disease progression/regression.**
4. **Always have an internist or rheumatologist (or appropriate specialist) on-board as part of the clinical team in case the patient experiences an exacerbation and needs to be hospitalized or acutely immunosuppressed.**
5. **When working with patients that have potentially serious diseases such as most of the autoimmune diseases, you should have a back-up plan integrated into your treatment plan from day one.** You might consider having patients sign a consent form that includes language consistent with the following:
   - *"Due to the uniqueness of each disease and each individual, including his or her willingness and ability to implement the treatment plan, no guarantees of successful treatment can be offered."*
   - *"Dr.___ may not be available on a 24-hour basis at all times. If you have a serious health problem that requires immediate attention, you should call your other doctors(s), call 911, or have someone take you to the nearest hospital emergency room. If you notice an adverse effect from one of the components of your health plan, you should discontinue it then call Dr.__ and inform him/her of what occurred."*
   - *"Treatments with other physicians or healthcare providers are not necessarily to be discontinued. Please let Dr.__ know if you are being treated by other healthcare providers (physicians, counselors, therapists, etc.). Consult your prescribing doctor before discontinuing medications."*
6. **Test responsibly.**
7. **Treat responsibly.**
8. **Re-test to document effectiveness of your intervention.**
9. **When in doubt, refer the patient for co-management.** If you are working with a serious life-threatening disease, and *your plan* or *the patient's implementation of it* is unable to produce **documentable results**, then you should refer the patient for allopathic/osteopathic/specialist co-management for the sake of protecting the patient from harm and for protecting yourself from undue liability.
10. **Practice defensively.** You will thereby safeguard your patient and your livelihood.

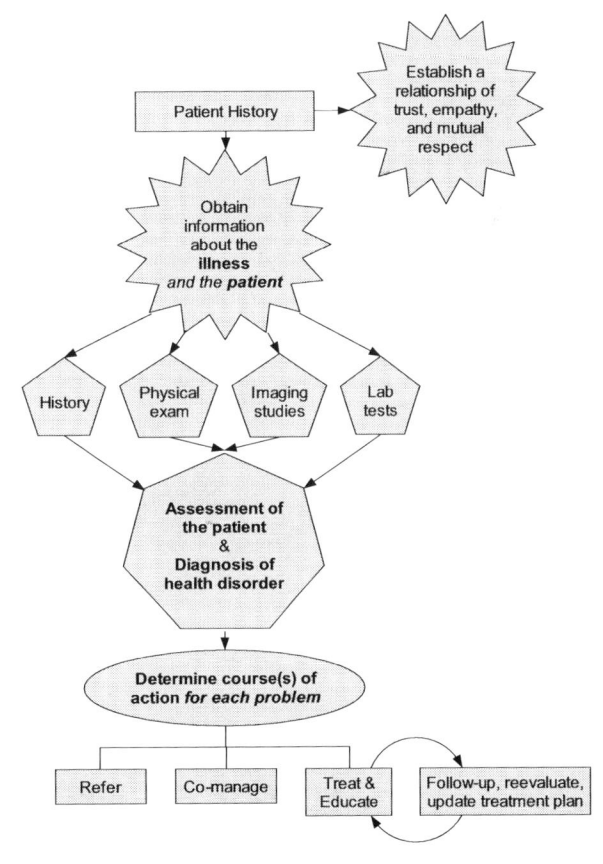

# Musculoskeletal Emergencies

These are some of the "core competencies" that clinicians can never afford to miss, and these are pertinent to patients with musculoskeletal disorders, whether structural/orthopedic or metabolic/rheumatic. With these conditions, clinicians are wise to err on the side of caution— *"When in doubt, refer out"*—and implement the appropriate referral on an expedient basis. These are organized in a clinical/logical manner rather than listed alphabetically.

## Neurovascular Disorders

| *Problem* | *Presentation* | *Assessment* | *Management* |
|---|---|---|---|
| **Neuropsychiatric lupus** | ▪ Psychosis<br>▪ Seizures<br>▪ Transient ischemic attacks<br>▪ Severe depression<br>▪ Delirium, confusion | ▪ Neuropsychiatric manifestations with history of lupus | ▪ Emergency or prompt referral as indicated |
| **Giant cell arteritis, Temporal arteritis**: Considered a medical emergency since it may rapidly progress to blindness due to associated involvement of the ophthalmic artery: *"Loss of vision is the most feared manifestation and occurs quite commonly."* [209] | Presentation typically includes the following:<br>▪ Headache, scalp tenderness<br>▪ Jaw claudication<br>▪ Changes in vision<br>▪ Systemic manifestations of rheumatic disease: fever, weight loss, muscle aches | ▪ Palpation of the temporal artery may reveal a "cord-like" artery<br>▪ Elevated ESR<br>▪ CBC may show anemia<br>▪ Temporal artery biopsy is diagnostic | ▪ Standard medical treatment is with immediate prednisone<br>▪ Implement treatment that is immediately effective or refer patient for medical treatment |
| **Acute red eye**: General term including acute iritis and scleritis; despite the name of this condition, redness may actually be rather minimal, and it is typically accompanied by cloudy changes in region of the iris and lens | ▪ Eye pain and redness<br>▪ May have facial pain<br>▪ May be the presenting manifestation of rheumatic disease | ▪ Red eye<br>▪ Photophobia<br>▪ Reduced vision<br>▪ May have fixed pupil<br>▪ Differential diagnosis includes acute glaucoma, bacterial/amebic/viral conjunctivitis or keratitis, allergy, and irritation due to contact lens | ▪ "The **acute** onset of a **painful, red** eye, even in the absence of visual upset, should be regarded primarily as an ophthalmological emergency." [210]<br>▪ **Granulomatous uveitis** occurs in 15% of patients with sarcoidosis and can result in bilateral blindness—this must be managed as a medically urgent condition |

---

[209] Tierney ML. McPhee SJ, Papadakis MA (eds). <u>Current Medical Diagnosis and Treatment, 41st Edition</u>. New York: Lange Medical Books; 2002. Page 999-1005
[210] McInnes I, Sturrock R. Rheumatological emergencies. *Practitioner*. 1994 Mar;238(1536):220-4

## Neural canal compression

| Problem | Presentation | Assessment | Management |
|---|---|---|---|
| **Atlantoaxial instability**: Excess mobility between the atlas and axis (commonly due to lesion of the dens or transverse ligament) makes the spinal cord vulnerable to compressive injury when the atlas translates anteriorly on the axis especially during cervical flexion; may progress to neurologic compromise including respiratory and somatic paralysis | ▪ Post-traumatic neck injury<br>▪ Down's syndrome<br>▪ May present spontaneously (without trauma) in patients with inflammatory rheumatic disease, especially rheumatoid arthritis and ankylosing spondylitis<br>▪ May have gradual or sudden onset of myelopathy: upper motor neuron lesion (UMNL) signs (e.g., spastic weakness), changes in bowel-bladder function, numbness | ▪ Clinical suspicion is followed by lateral cervical and APOM (anteroposterior open mouth) radiographs to assess ADI (atlantodental interval) and dens<br>▪ MRI should be performed in patients with suspected myelopathy<br>▪ Neurologic examination of the upper and lower extremities<br>▪ Do not force neck flexion; do not perform the Soto Hall test | ▪ **Urgent neurosurgical consultation is recommended; stabilizing surgery is the best option for the prevention of neurologic catastrophes**[211]<br>▪ Onset of myelopathy mandates referral to ER and/or neurosurgeon; immobilize with spine board or hard cervical collar and transport appropriately<br>▪ Asymptomatic and mild increases in ADI (< 5mm) might be managed conservatively with activity restriction, exercises, and bracing/collars)<br>▪ PAR discussion and referral for surgical consultation is necessary for informed consent and safe management |
| **Myelopathy, spinal cord compression or lesion**: May occur due to infection, edema, tumor, spinal fracture, stenosis, or inflammatory disease | ▪ **Spastic weakness**<br>▪ **Bowel-bladder dysfunction**<br>▪ **Numbness**<br>▪ **Problems are distal to cord lesion** | ▪ Hyperreflexia<br>▪ Rigidity<br>▪ Muscle weakness<br>▪ MRI (with and without contrast) should be performed in patients with suspected myelopathy; CT may also be indicated | ▪ Obtain MRI to confirm diagnosis<br>▪ Immobilize spine and transport if necessary<br>▪ Acute myelopathy is a medical emergency that can result in rapid-onset paralysis |
| **Cauda equina syndrome**: Compression of the sacral nerve roots due to lumbar disc herniation<br><br>**Cauda equina syndrome is a surgical emergency.** | ▪ History of sciatic low back pain<br>▪ Urinary retention, perineal numbness, and fecal incontinence are common<br>▪ May have lower extremity weakness | ▪ Assess for bladder distention<br>▪ Assess anal sphincter strength with rectal exam<br>▪ Lower extremity neurologic examination | ▪ Urgent referral for CT/MRI to confirm diagnosis<br>▪ If diagnosis is confirmed or strongly suspected clinically, urgent referral for surgical decompression is mandatory |

---

[211] "When atlantoaxial stability is lost...it is thought that surgical stabilisation of the atlantoaxial joint is more reasonable and beneficial than conservative management. Minimal trauma of an unstable atlantoaxial joint can lead to serious neurological injury." Moon MS, Choi WT, Moon YW, Moon JL, Kim SS. Brooks' posterior stabilization surgery for atlantoaxial instability: review of 54 cases. *J Orthop Surg* (Hong Kong). 2002 Dec;10(2):160-4. http://www.josonline.org/PDF/v10i2p160.pdf

## Acute peripheral nerve compression

| Problem | Presentation | Assessment | Management |
|---|---|---|---|
| **Acute compartment syndrome**: acute onset of *potentially irreversible* muscle and/or nerve compression injury due to inflammation, swelling, or bleeding within a fascial compartment<br><br>**Acute compartment syndrome is a surgical emergency.** | ▪ Most commonly occurs in the anterior leg; may also occur in the posterior leg as well as forearm—these are the areas most notable anatomically for the investment of muscle in tight and resilient fascial sheaths<br>▪ Onset generally follows strenuous exercise that leads to reactive hyperemia and secondary edema<br>▪ May occur following trauma or fracture | Assess for:<br>▪ Pulselessness<br>▪ Palor<br>▪ Painful passive stretch<br>▪ Weakness<br>▪ **Numbness**<br>▪ Assessment and treatment should be performed on an emergency basis since irreversible nerve damage begins within 6 hours of intracompartmental hypertension | ▪ Decompressive fasciotomy is the standard treatment for acute compartment syndrome that could result in permanent muscle necrosis and/or permanent nerve death<br>▪ Acute compartment syndrome can be fatal if rhabdomyolysis precipitates renal failure[212] |

## Musculoskeletal infections

| Problem | Presentation | Assessment | Management |
|---|---|---|---|
| **Septic arthritis**: intraarticular bacterial infection; complications of septic arthritis are 1) articular destruction and 2) **death in 5-10% of patients**[213]<br><br>**Septic arthritis is a medical emergency** | ▪ **Febrile** patient has **acute/subacute mono/oligo-arthritis**<br>▪ Some patients may not have fever<br>▪ Other possible findings: Immuno-suppression due to medications, concomitant disease (RA, DM), elderly<br>▪ In some patients with concomitant disease or medications, the clinical picture can be blurred | ▪ **Warm, swollen, tender joint**<br>▪ Clinical assessment with **immediate referral for joint aspiration**, which reveals manifestations of infection such as WBC's and bacteria<br>▪ Differential diagnosis includes trauma, gout, CPPD, hemochromatosis | ▪ **Immediate referral for joint aspiration**<br>▪ **An aggressive and prolonged course of IV and oral antimicrobials**<br>▪ "Immune support" such as vitamin A and glutamine and general measures to improve health and prevent recurrence |
| **Osteomyelitis, infectious discitis**: considered a medical emergency[214]<br><br>**Osteomyelitis—especially vertebral osteomyelitis—is a medical emergency** | ▪ Febrile patient with bone pain<br>▪ Assess for constitutional manifestations such as weight loss, night sweats, and malaise | ▪ Exacerbation of bone pain when stress/percussion is applied to the bone<br>▪ Lab: CRP & WBC may be elevated<br>▪ MRI is more sensitive than CT, bone scan, or radiography[215] | ▪ Emergency referral for vertebral osteomyelitis, since **up to 15% of patients will develop nerve lesions or cord compression**[216]<br>▪ Urgent referral for other types of osteomyelitis |

---

[212] Paula R. Compartment Syndrome, Extremity. *eMedicine* June 22, 2006 http://www.emedicine.com/emerg/topic739.htm Accessed November 26, 2006
[213] Tierney ML. McPhee SJ, Papadakis MA. Current Medical Diagnosis and Treatment. 35th edition. Stamford: Appleton & Lange, 1996 page 759
[214] American College of Rheumatology Ad Hoc Committee on Clinical Guidelines. Guidelines for the initial evaluation of the adult patient with acute musculoskeletal symptoms. *Arthritis Rheum.* 1996;39(1):1-8
[215] Tierney ML. McPhee SJ, Papadakis MA (eds). Current Medical Diagnosis and Treatment 2002, 41st Edition. New York: Lange Medical; 2002. p 883
[216] King RW, Johnson D. Osteomyelitis. Updated July 13, 2006. *eMedicine* http://www.emedicine.com/emerg/topic349.htm Accessed Dec 24, 2006

# Acute Nontraumatic Monoarthritis and Septic Arthritis

- "Acute monoarthritis is a potential medical emergency that must be investigated and treated promptly."[217]
- "Monoarthropathies should initially be investigated to exclude sepsis. ... Diagnostic joint aspiration ... should be carried out immediately."[218]
- "In acute monoarthritis, it is essential that infection of a joint be diagnosed or excluded, and this can only be done by joint aspiration and synovial fluid culture."[219]
- "Acute monoarthritis should be considered infectious until proven otherwise."[220]

### Clinical Pearl
The primary goal of this section is to solidify your awareness of septic arthritis, its differential diagnoses, and the method and importance of assertive diagnosis and management.

Septic arthritis is a medical emergency, and some authoritative textbooks report a mortality rate of 5-10%.

Septic arthritis must be diagnosed urgently with joint aspiration, and it must be treated with antibiotics in order to preserve the joint and prevent spread of the infection.

## Clinical presentations:
- Patient presents with acute joint pain in one joint (occasionally more than one joint may be involved).
- May or may not have fever and other systemic manifestations of infection.

## Major Differential Diagnoses for Nontraumatic Monoarthritis

| Problem | Presentation | Assessment & Management |
|---|---|---|
| **Septic arthritis**: intraarticular bacterial infection; complications of septic arthritis are 1) articular destruction and 2) **death in 5-10% of patients**[221] | • **Febrile** patient has **acute/subacute mono/oligo-arthritis**<br>• **Onset over hours or days**<br>Other possible findings:<br>• Immuno-suppression due to medications, concomitant disease (RA, DM), elderly<br>• Some patients may not have fever<br>• In some patients with a previous or concomitant disease process, the clinical picture can be blurred | • **Warm, swollen, red, painful joint**<br>• Clinical assessment with **immediate referral for joint aspiration**, which reveals characteristic manifestations of infection such as WBCs and bacteria<br>• **Immediate joint aspiration**<br>• An aggressive and prolonged course of IV and oral antimicrobials<br>• "Immune support" and general measures to improve health and prevent recurrence |
| | | "Septic arthritis is still a life-threatening disease with a mortality of 2–5% and high morbidity."<br><br>Zacher J, Gursche A. Regional musculoskeletal conditions: 'hip' pain. *Best Practice & Research Clinical Rheumatology*. 2003 Feb;17:71-85 |

---

[217] Cibere J. Rheumatology: 4. Acute monoarthritis. CMAJ (*Canadian Medical Association Journal*). 2000;162(11):1577-83 http://www.cmaj.ca/cgi/content/full/162/11/1577 January 24, 2004
[218] McInnes I, Sturrock R. Rheumatological emergencies. Practitioner. 1994 Mar;238(1536):220-4
[219] American College of Rheumatology Ad Hoc Committee on Clinical Guidelines. Guidelines for the initial evaluation of the adult patient with acute musculoskeletal symptoms. *Arthritis Rheum*. 1996 Jan;39(1):1-8
[220] Cibere J. Rheumatology: 4. Acute monoarthritis. CMAJ (*Canadian Medical Association Journal*). 2000;162(11):1577-83 http://www.cmaj.ca/cgi/content/full/162/11/1577 January 24, 2004
[221] Tierney ML. McPhee SJ, Papadakis MA. Current Medical Diagnosis and Treatment. 35th edition. Stamford: Appleton and Lange, 1996 page 759

## Major differential diagnoses for non-traumatic monoarthritis—*continued*

| Problem | Presentation | Assessment & Management |
|---|---|---|
| **Osteochondritis dissecans**: A disorder of unclear etiology (trauma and/or avascular necrosis) which results in the death and subsequent fragmentation of subchondral bone[222] | <ul><li>Primarily affects ages 10-30 years</li><li>**Most common in the knees and elbows**</li><li>Locking and crepitus due to intraarticular loose bodies ("joint mice")</li><li>Some patients are almost asymptomatic, while others have acute pain</li><li>Swelling of the affected joint</li></ul> | <ul><li>Radiographs—consider to assess both knees as the condition is bilateral in 30%</li><li>MRI is used to assess severity and need for surgical intervention</li><li>Stable and nondisplaced lesions may be managed nonsurgically; larger and displaced fragments require surgical repair to reduce long-term complications[223]</li></ul> |
| **Transient synovitis, irritable hip**: Non-specific short-term inflammation and effusion of the hip joint | <ul><li>Acute onset of painful hip and limp</li><li>Decreased pain with hip in flexion and abduction</li><li>Considered the most common cause of hip pain in children[224]</li><li>More common in boys, age 3-6 years and generally younger than 10 years</li><li>May have recent history of viral infection, and some children (1.5-10%) eventually manifest RA or AVN[225]</li></ul> | <ul><li>May have slight elevation of ESR</li><li>Normal WBC</li><li>No fever; the child appears healthy</li><li>"…radiography is indicated to exclude osseous pathological conditions…"[226]</li><li>**Joint aspiration is indicated if septic arthritis is suspected**[227]</li><li>Conservative treatment, restricted exertion and weight-bearing for several weeks</li></ul> |
| **Legg-Calve-Perthe's disease**: Idiopathic ischemic necrosis of the femoral head occurring in children **Avascular necrosis (AVN) of the femoral head, osteonecrosis**: Ischemic necrosis of the femoral head | Perthe's disease:<ul><li>80% occur in children generally between ages of 4-9 years; more common in boys; may present with hip pain or knee pain</li></ul>AVN:<ul><li>Ages 20-40 years</li><li>Unilateral hip pain</li><li>May have knee pain</li><li>History of trauma is common</li></ul>AVN associations:<ul><li>Steroid use, prednisone</li><li>Hyperlipidemia</li><li>Alcoholism</li><li>Pancreatitis</li><li>Hemoglobinopathies</li><li>Smoking</li><li>Fatty liver disease: "fat globules from the liver"[228]</li></ul> | <ul><li>Limited ROM</li><li>**Radiographs**; if normal and clinical suspicion is high order MRI or bone scan</li><li>**Crutches**</li><li>**Orthopedic referral is recommended** although not all patients will require surgery and some may be managed conservatively[229]</li></ul> |

---

[222] Tatum R. Osteochondritis dissecans of the knee: a radiology case report. *J Manipulative Physiol Ther* 2000 Jun;23(5):347-51
[223] Browne RF, Murphy SM, Torreggiani WC, Munk PL, Marchinkow LO. Radiology for the surgeon: musculoskeletal case 30. Osteochondritis dissecans of the medial femoral condyle. *Can J Surg*. 2003 Oct;46(5):361-3 http://www.cma.ca/multimedia/staticContent/HTML/N0/l2/cjs/vol-46/issue-5/pdf/pg361.pdf
[224] Maroo S. Diagnosis of hip pain in children. *Hosp Med* 1999 Nov;60(11):788-93
[225] Souza TA. Differential Diagnosis for the Chiropractor: Protocols and Algorithms. Gaithersberg, Maryland: Aspen Publications. 1997 page 265
[226] Maroo S. Diagnosis of hip pain in children. *Hosp Med* 1999 Nov;60(11):788-93
[227] Maroo S. Diagnosis of hip pain in children. *Hosp Med* 1999 Nov;60(11):788-93

## Review of Clinical Assessments and Concepts

### Major differential diagnoses for non-traumatic monoarthritis—continued

| Problem | Presentation | Assessment & Management |
|---|---|---|
| **Gout** | • **Febrile** patient has **acute/subacute mono/oligo-arthritis**<br>• **Onset over hours or days**<br>• "A history of discreet attacks, usually affecting one joint, that precede the onset of fixed symmetric arthritis is the major clue."[230]<br>• May have fever, chills, tachycardia, leukocytosis—just like septic arthritis | • Clinical presentation may be sufficient for DX; however septic arthritis should be excluded<br>• Serum uric acid is generally meaningless for the diagnosis of gout since many gout patients will have normal serum uric acid<br>• Medical treatment is rest, NSAID's, and allopurinol<br>• Fluid loading: >3 liters per day; monitor for electrolyte imbalances and hyponatremia as needed<br>• Integrative assessment and treatment for insulin resistance, hormonal imbalances, and nutritional deficiencies |
| **CPPD**: Calcium pyrophosphate dihydrate deposition disease | • Idiopathic<br>• May be caused by iron overload in some patients<br>• Presentation may be acute or subacute | • Medical diagnosis is by synovial biopsy<br>• Radiographs reveal chondrocalcinosis<br>• Allopathic treatment is NSAIDs; phytonutritional anti-inflammatory treatments may also be used (see chapter 3 of *Integrative Orthopedics/Rheumatology*)<br>• Oral colchicine 0.5 to 1.5 mg per day prevents attacks[231] |
| **Hemarthrosis**: Generally associated with trauma, anticoagulation (i.e., coumadin), leukemia, hemophilia | • Monoarthralgia with limited motion<br>• May follow direct trauma<br>• Nontraumatic hemarthrosis may be due to anticoagulation, leukemia, hemophilia | • Synovial fluid analysis reveals blood<br>• Treatment of underlying disorder; refer as indicated |
| **Slipped capital femoral epiphysis (SCFE)**: The most common cause of hip pain in adolescents[232] | • Seen in adolescents generally 8-17 years of age<br>• Classic presentation is a tall overweight boy with **hip pain**, knee pain, and/or a painful limp: "*Slipped femoral capital epiphysis is a developmental injury that must be considered in any adolescent who presents with hip pain.*"[233] | • **Radiographs** of both hips (bilateral SCFE in 40%): "<u>AP and frog lateral views are recommended in all children over age of 9 years with hip pain</u>."[234]<br>• Orthopedic referral—"*...the patient should be referred immediately to an orthopedist for surgical stabilization.*"[235] |

---

[228] Skinner HB, Scherger JE. Identifying structural hip and knee problems. Patient age, history, and limited examination may be all that's needed. *Postgrad Med* 1999;106(7):51-2, 55-6, 61-4
[229] Souza TA. <u>Differential Diagnosis for the Chiropractor: Protocols and Algorithms</u>. Gaithersberg, Maryland: Aspen Publications. 1997 page 263
[230] Hardin JG, Waterman J, Labson LH. Rheumatic disease: Which diagnostic tests are useful? *Patient Care* 1999; March 15: 83-102
[231] Beers MH, Berkow R (eds). <u>The Merck Manual. Seventeenth Edition</u>. Whitehouse Station; Merck Research Laboratories 1999 Page
[232] Maroo S. Diagnosis of hip pain in children. *Hosp Med* 1999 Nov;60(11):788-93
[233] O'Kane JW. Anterior hip pain. *Am Fam Physician* 1999 Oct 15;60(6):1687-96
[234] Maroo S. Diagnosis of hip pain in children. *Hosp Med* 1999 Nov;60(11):788-93
[235] O'Kane JW. Anterior hip pain. *Am Fam Physician* 1999 Oct 15;60(6):1687-96

Clinical assessment:
- History and orthopedic assessment of the joint
- Laboratory tests must be performed if you have a suspicion of infection

History/subjective:
- Acute or subacute joint pain with or without systemic manifestations and fever.
- History or may not be significant; other than the obvious risk factor of immunosuppression, septic arthritis can occur with impressive spontaneity and randomness

Differential physical examination and objective findings:
- **Septic arthritis**: pain and limitation of motion, swelling, redness; patient may have systemic symptoms of fever and malaise
- **Gout**: pain and limitation of motion, swelling, redness; patient may have systemic symptoms of fever and malaise
- **Pseudogout and calcium pyrophosphate dihydrate deposition disease (CPDD/CPPD)**: pain and limitation of motion, swelling, redness; patient may have systemic symptoms of fever and malaise
- **Ischemic necrosis**: pain and limitation of motion; swelling, redness and systemic symptoms are less likely.
- **Hemarthrosis**: pain and limitation of motion; often associated with trauma, use of anticoagulant medications[236], or hemophilia and other hematologic abnormalities[237]
- **Tumor**: assess with history, imaging, and biopsy if possible
- **Injury**: Meniscal injury, fracture, ligament injury; physical examination procedures are described in the chapters that follow

Imaging and laboratory assessments:
- **Septic arthritis**: joint aspiration; STAT CBC (for WBC count) and CRP
- **Gout**: joint aspiration; CBC (for WBC count) and CRP
- **Pseudogout and PPDD**: rule out septic arthritis with joint aspiration, CBC, and CRP; radiographs often show chondrocalcinosis
- **Ischemic necrosis**: radiographs are diagnostic
- **Hemarthrosis**: joint aspiration and assessment for underlying disease or medication, especially if the condition was not trauma-induced
- **Tumor**: assess with radiographs
- **Injury**: rule out infection; consider imaging with radiography or MRI.

Establishing the diagnosis:
- The aforementioned examinations and lab assessments should establish the exact diagnosis. **The priorities are 1) first exclude life-threatening illness (i.e., septic arthritis), then 2) to exclude serious injury or illness,** and finally 3) to help manage the exact problem.

Complications:
- **Septic arthritis can result in death 5-10% of patients. "Five to 10 percent of patients with an infected joint die, chiefly from respiratory complications of sepsis. The mortality rate is 30% for patients with polyarticular sepsis. Bony ankylosis and articular destruction**

---

[236] Riley SA, Spencer GE. Destructive monarticular arthritis secondary to anticoagulant therapy. *Clin Orthop*. 1987 Oct;(223):247-51
[237] Jean-Baptiste G, De Ceulaer K. Osteoarticular disorders of haematological origin. *Baillieres Best Pract Res Clin Rheumatol*. 2000 Jun;14(2):307-23

commonly also occur if the treatment is delayed or inadequate."[238]   Complications vary per location, infecting organism, severity, and patient.

Clinical management:
- Suspected septic arthritis requires referral for joint aspiration and antimicrobial drugs.
- Referral if clinical outcome is unsatisfactory or if serious complications are evident.
- Treatment of other conditions that cause acute monoarthritis (such as gout and calcium pyrophosphate dihydrate deposition disease) is based on the problem and individual patient.

Treatments:
- **Septic arthritis requires IV/oral antimicrobial drugs:** Intravenous antibiotics are generally started before culture results are available. After results and culture from synovial fluid analysis have been considered, the dose, combination, and administration of antibiotics can be fine-tuned. Frequently, antibiotics are administered intravenously for at least 3-4 weeks. Surgical/endoscopic drainage/debridement and immobilization during the acute phase may also be implemented.[239]
- **Immunonutrition considerations:** Immunonutritional considerations are listed below; doses listed are for adults. Although studies have not been performed specifically in patients with bone/joint infections, general benefits derived from the use of immunonutrition are reductions in severity/frequency/duration of major infections, abbreviated hospitalization (i.e., early discharge due to expedited healing and recovery), reductions in the need for medications, significant improvements in survival, and hospital savings.[240,241,242,243,244,245,246]
    o Paleo-Mediterranean diet: as detailed later in this text and elsewhere[247,248]
    o Vitamin and mineral supplementation: anti-infective benefits shown in elderly diabetics[249]

---

[238] Tierney ML. McPhee SJ, Papadakis MA. Current Medical Diagnosis and Treatment. 35th edition. Stamford: Appleton & Lange, 1996 page 759
[239] Brusch JL. Septic Arthritis (Last Updated: October 18, 2005). *eMedicine*. http://www.emedicine.com/med/topic3394.htm  Accessed November 25, 2006
[240] "To evaluate the metabolic and immune effects of dietary arginine, glutamine and omega-3 fatty acids (fish oil) supplementation, we performed a prospective study... CONCLUSIONS: The feeding of Neomune in critically injured patients was well tolerated as Traumacal and significant improvement was observed in serum protein. Shorten ICU stay and wean-off respirator day may benefit from using the immunonutrient formula." Chuntrasakul C, Siltham S, Sarasombath S, Sittapairochana C, Leowattana W, Chockvivatanavanit S, Bunnak A. Comparison of a immunonutrition formula enriched arginine, glutamine and omega-3 fatty acid, with a currently high-enriched enteral nutrition for trauma patients. *J Med Assoc Thai*. 2003 Jun;86(6):552-6
[241] "CONCLUSIONS: In conclusion, arginine-enhanced formula improves fistula rates in postoperative head and neck cancer patients and decreases length of stay." de Luis DA, Izaola O, Cuellar L, Terroba MC, Aller R. Randomized clinical trial with an enteral arginine-enhanced formula in early postsurgical head and neck cancer patients. *Eur J Clin Nutr*. 2004;58(11):1505-8
[242] "In this prospective, randomised, double-blind, placebo-controlled study, we randomly assigned 50 patients who were scheduled to undergo coronary artery bypass to receive either an oral immune-enhancing nutritional supplement containing L-arginine, omega3 polyunsaturated fatty acids, and yeast RNA (n=25), or a control (n=25) for a minimum of 5 days... Intake of an oral immune-enhancing nutritional supplement for a minimum of 5 days before surgery can improve outlook in high-risk patients who are undergoing elective cardiac surgery." Tepaske R, Velthuis H, Oudemans-van Straaten HM, Heisterkamp SH, van Deventer SJ, Ince C, Eysman L, Kesecioglu J. Effect of preoperative oral immune-enhancing nutritional supplement on patients at high risk of infection after cardiac surgery: a randomised placebo-controlled trial. *Lancet*. 2001 Sep 1;358(9283):696-701
[243] "The feeding of IMMUNE FORMULA was well tolerated and significant improvement was observed in nutritional and immunologic parameters as in other immunoenhancing diets. Further clinical trials of prospective double-blind randomized design are necessary to address the so that the necessity of using immunonutrition in critically ill patients will be clarified." Chuntrasakul C, Siltharm S, Sarasombath S, Sittapairochana C, Leowattana W, Chockvivatanavanit S, Bunnak A. Metabolic and immune effects of dietary arginine, glutamine and omega-3 fatty acids supplementation in immunocompromised patients. *J Med Assoc Thai*. 1998 May;81(5):334-43
[244] "enteral diet supplemented with arginine, dietary nucleotides, and omega-3 fatty acids (IMPACT, Sandoz Nutrition, Bern, Switzerland)" Senkal M, Mumme A, Eickhoff U, Geier B, Spath G, Wulfert D, Joosten U, Frei A, Kemen M. Early postoperative enteral immunonutrition: clinical outcome and cost-comparison analysis in surgical patients. *Crit Care Med* 1997;25(9):1489-96
[245] "supplemented diet with glutamine, arginine and omega-3-fatty acids... It was clearly established in this trial that early postoperative enteral feeding is safe in patients who have undergone major operations for gastrointestinal cancer. Supplementation of enteral nutrition with glutamine, arginine, and omega-3-fatty acids positively modulated postsurgical immunosuppressive and inflammatory responses." Wu GH, Zhang YW, Wu ZH. Modulation of postoperative immune and inflammatory response by immune-enhancing enteral diet in gastrointestinal cancer patients. *World J Gastroenterol*. 2001 Jun;7(3):357-62 http://www.wjgnet.com/1007-9327/7/357.pdf
[246] "using a formula supplemented with arginine, mRNA, and omega-3 fatty acids from fish oil (Impact)... CONCLUSIONS: Immune-enhancing enteral nutrition resulted in a significant reduction in the mortality rate and infection rate in septic patients admitted to the ICU. These reductions were greater for patients with less severe illness." Galban C, Montejo JC, Mesejo A, Marco P, Celaya S, Sanchez-Segura JM, Farre M, Bryg DJ. An immune-enhancing enteral diet reduces mortality rate and episodes of bacteremia in septic intensive care unit patients. *Crit Care Med*. 2000 Mar;28(3):643-8
[247] Vasquez A. A Five-Part Nutritional Protocol that Produces Consistently Positive Results. *Nutritional Wellness* 2005 September http://www.nutritionalwellness.com/archives/2005/sep/09_vasquez.php
[248] Vasquez A. Implementing the Five-Part Nutritional Wellness Protocol for the Treatment of Various Health Problems. *Nutritional Wellness* 2005 November. http://www.nutritionalwellness.com/archives/2005/nov/11_vasquez.php

- High-dose vitamin A: Vitamin A shows potent immunosupportive benefits, and vitamin A stores are depleted by the stress of infection and injury. Consider 200,000-300,000 IU per day of retinol palmitate for 1-4 weeks, then taper; reduce dose or discontinue with onset of toxicity symptoms such as skin problems (dry skin, flaking skin, chapped or split lips, red skin rash, hair loss), joint pain, bone pain, headaches, anorexia (loss of appetite), edema (water retention, weight gain, swollen ankles, difficulty breathing), fatigue, and/or liver damage.
- Arginine: Dose for adults is in the range of 5-10 grams daily.
- Fatty acid supplementation: In contrast to the higher doses used to provide an anti-inflammatory effect in patients with autoimmune/inflammatory disorders, doses used for immunosupportive treatments should be kept rather modest to avoid the *relative* immunosuppression that has been controversially reported in patients treated with EPA and DHA. Reasonable doses are in the following ranges for adults: EPA+DHA: 500-1,500, and GLA: 300-500 mg.
- Glutamine: Glutamine enhances bacterial killing by neutrophils[250], and administration of 18 grams per day in divided doses to patients in intensive care units was shown to improve survival, expedite hospital discharge, and reduce total healthcare costs.[251] Another study using glutamine 12-18 grams per day showed no benefit in overall mortality but significant benefits in terms of reduced healthcare costs (-30%) and significantly reduced need for medical interventions.[252] After administering glutamine 26 grams/d to severely burned patients, Garrel et al[253] concluded that glutamine reduced the risk of infection by 3-fold and that oral glutamine "may be a life-saving intervention" in patients with severe burns. A dose of 30 grams/d was used in a recent clinical trial showing hemodynamic benefit in patients with sickle cell anemia.[254] The highest glutamine dose that the current author is aware of is the study by Scheltinga et al[255] who used 0.57 gm/kg/day in cancer patients following chemotherapy administration; for a 220-lb-pt, this would be approximately 57 grams of glutamine per day.
- Melatonin: 20-40 mg hs (*hora somni*—Latin: sleep time). Immunostimulatory anti-infective action of melatonin was demonstrated in a small clinical trial wherein septic newborns administered 20 mg melatonin showed significantly increased survival over nontreated controls.[256]

---

[249] "CONCLUSIONS: A multivitamin and mineral supplement reduced the incidence of participant-reported infection and related absenteeism in a sample of participants with type 2 diabetes mellitus and a high prevalence of subclinical micronutrient deficiency." Barringer TA, Kirk JK, Santaniello AC, Foley KL, Michielutte R. Effect of a multivitamin and mineral supplement on infection and quality of life. A randomized, double-blind, placebo-controlled trial. *Ann Intern Med.* 2003 Mar 4;138(5):365-71 http://www.annals.org/cgi/reprint/138/5/365

[250] Furukawa S, Saito H, Fukatsu K, Hashiguchi Y, Inaba T, Lin MT, Inoue T, Han I, Matsuda T, Muto T. Glutamine-enhanced bacterial killing by neutrophils from postoperative patients. *Nutrition* 1997;13(10):863-9. *In vitro* study.

[251] Griffiths RD, Jones C, Palmer TE. Six-month outcome of critically ill patients given glutamine-supplemented parenteral nutrition. *Nutrition* 1997;13(4):295-302

[252] "There was no mortality difference between those patients receiving glutamine-containing enteral feed and the controls. However, there was a significant reduction in the median postintervention ICU and hospital patient costs in the glutamine recipients $23 000 versus $30 900 in the control patients." Jones C, Palmer TE, Griffiths RD. Randomized clinical outcome study of critically ill patients given glutamine-supplemented enteral nutrition. *Nutrition*. 1999 Feb;15(2):108-15

[253] The glutamine dose in this study was "a total of 26 g/day" administered in four divided doses. CONCLUSION: "The results of this prospective randomized clinical trial show that enteral G reduces blood culture positivity, particularly with P. aeruginosa, in adults with severe burns and may be a life-saving intervention." Garrel D, Patenaude J, Nedelec B, Samson L, Dorais J, Champoux J, D'Elia M, Bernier J. Decreased mortality and infectious morbidity in adult burn patients given enteral glutamine supplements: a prospective, controlled, randomized clinical trial. *Crit Care Med*. 2003 Oct;31(10):2444-9

[254] Niihara Y, Matsui NM, Shen YM, Akiyama DA, Johnson CS, Sunga MA, Magpayo J, Embury SH, Kalra VK, Cho SH, Tanaka KR. L-glutamine therapy reduces endothelial adhesion of sickle red blood cells to human umbilical vein endothelial cells. *BMC Blood Disord*. 2005 Jul 25;5:4 http://www.biomedcentral.com.proxy.hsc.unt.edu/1471-2326/5/4

[255] "Subjects with hematologic malignancies in remission underwent a standard treatment of high-dose chemotherapy and total body irradiation before bone marrow transplantation. After completion of this regimen, they were randomized to receive either standard parenteral nutrition (STD, n = 10) or an isocaloric, isonitrogenous nutrient solution enriched with crystalline L-glutamine (0.57 g/kg/day, GLN, n = 10)." Scheltinga MR, Young LS, Benfell K, Bye RL, Ziegler TR, Santos AA, Antin JH, Schloerb PR, Wilmore DW. Glutamine-enriched intravenous feedings attenuate extracellular fluid expansion after a standard stress. *Ann Surg*. 1991 Oct;214(4):385-93; discussion 393-5 http://www.pubmedcentral.nih.gov/articlerender.fcgi?tool=pubmed&pubmedid=1953094 For additional review, see Ziegler TR. Glutamine supplementation in cancer patients receiving bone marrow transplantation and high dose chemotherapy. *J Nutr*. 2001 Sep;131(9 Suppl):2578S-84S http://jn.nutrition.org/cgi/content/full/131/9/2578S

[256] Gitto E, Karbownik M, Reiter RJ, Tan DX, Cuzzocrea S, Chiurazzi P, Cordaro S, Corona G, Trimarchi G, Barberi I. Effects of melatonin treatment in septic newborns. *Pediatr Res*. 2001 Dec;50(6):756-60 http://www.pedresearch.org/cgi/content/full/50/6/756

# Chiropractic: Overview of History and Current Science

"Doctors of Chiropractic are physicians who consider man as an integrated being and give special attention to the physiological and biochemical aspects including structural, spinal, musculoskeletal, neurological, vascular, nutritional, emotional and environmental relationships." *American Chiropractic Association, 2004*[257]

"The human body represents the actions of three laws—spiritual, mechanical, and chemical—united as one triune. As long as there is perfect union of these three, there is health." *Daniel David Palmer, founder of the modern chiropractic profession*[258]

The basic philosophical paradigm which is taught in many chiropractic colleges is to envision health, disease, and patient care from a conceptual model named the "triad of health" which gives its attention to the three fundamental foundations for well-being: namely, the physical/structural, mental/emotional, and biochemical/nutritional/hormonal aspects of health. Revolutionary at the time of its inception in the early 1900's, this model now forms the foundation for the increasingly dominant and very popular paradigm of "holistic medicine." It remains a powerful contrast and an attractive alternative to the reductionistic allopathic approach, which generally approaches the human body as if it were simply a conglomerate of independent organ systems that have little or no functional relationship to each other.[259]

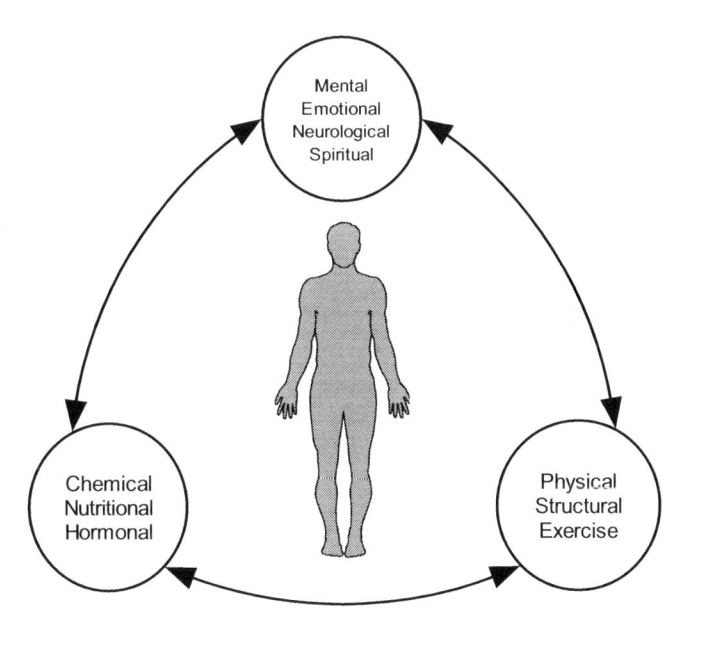

The chiropractic "triad of health"

Using the state of the sciences before the year 1910, chiropractic was founded with a profound appreciation of the integrated nature of health and the therapeutic focus was on spinal manipulation. In describing the chiropractic model of health, DD Palmer[260] wrote, "The human body represents the actions of three laws—spiritual, mechanical, and chemical—united as one triune. As long as there is perfect union of these three, there is health." While the therapeutic focus of the profession has been spinal manipulation, from its inception the chiropractic profession has emphasized a holistic, integrative model of therapeutic intervention, health, and

---

[257] American Chiropractic Association. http://www.amerchiro.org/media/whatis/ Accessed March 13, 2004
[258] Palmer DD. The Science, Art, and Phiosophy, of Chiropractic. Portland, OR; Portland Printing House Company, 1910: 107
[259] Beckman JF, Fernandez CE, Coulter ID. A systems model of health care: a proposal. *J Manipulative Physiol Ther*. 1996 Mar-Apr; 19(3): 208-15
[260] Palmer DD. The Science, Art, and Phiosophy, of Chiropractic. Portland, OR; Portland Printing House Company, 1910: 107

disease, and chiropractic was the first healthcare profession in America to specifically claim that the optimization of health requires attention to spiritual-emotional-psychological, mechanical-physical-structural, and biochemical-nutritional-hormonal-chemical considerations. Accordingly, these cornerstones are fundamental to the modern definition of the chiropractic profession recently articulated by the American Chiropractic Association[261]: "Doctors of Chiropractic are physicians who consider man as an integrated being and give special attention to the physiological and biochemical aspects including structural, spinal, musculoskeletal, neurological, vascular, nutritional, emotional, and environmental relationships."

From its inception, chiropractic was a philosophy of healing that considered the entire health of the patient by addressing the interconnected aspects of our chemical-spiritual-physical being. Later, intraprofessional factions polarized between holistic and vitalistic paradigms; the latter has been presumed to be the philosophy of the entire profession by organizations such as the American Medical Association[262] that have sought to contain and eliminate chiropractic and other forms of natural healthcare[263] by falsifying research[264,265], intentionally misleading the public and manipulating politicians[266,267,268], arriving at illogical conclusions which support the medical paradigm and refute the value of manual therapies[269], and exploiting weaknesses within the profession for its own financial profitability and political advantage.[270] Intentional misrepresentation and defamation of chiropractic continues to occur today, as documented by the 2006 review by Wenban.[271]

## Chiropractic Training and Clinical Benefits

In addition to the basic sciences and foundational skills of laboratory and clinical diagnosis, chiropractic physicians receive extensive training in manual physical manipulation, rehabilitation, therapeutic exercise, and clinical nutrition. According to data with hundreds of medical students and allopathic clinicians, medical school preparation in musculoskeletal medicine is inadequate, and the vast majority of medical graduates are incompetent in basic musculoskeletal diagnosis and management[272,273,274,275,276,277]; conversely, according to limited

---

[261] American Chiropractic Association. What is Chiropractic? http://amerchiro.org/media/whatis/ Accessed January 9, 2005
[262] American Medical Association. Report 12 of the Council on Scientific Affairs (A-97) Full Text. http://www.ama-assn.org/ama/pub/category/13638.html Accessed September 10, 2005.
[263] Getzendanner S. Permanent injunction order against AMA. *JAMA*. 1988 Jan 1;259(1):81-2 http://www.optimalhealthresearch.com/archives/wilk-ama-judgement.pdf
[264] Terrett AG. Misuse of the literature by medical authors in discussing spinal manipulative therapy injury. *J Manipulative Physiol Ther*. 1995 May;18(4):203-10
[265] Morley J, Rosner AL, Redwood D. A case study of misrepresentation of the scientific literature: recent reviews of chiropractic. *J Altern Complement Med*. 2001 Feb;7(1):65-78
[266] Spivak JL. The Medical Trust Unmasked. Louis S. Siegfried Publishers; New York: 1961
[267] Trever W. In the Public Interest. Los Angeles; Scriptures Unlimited; 1972. This is probably the most authoritative documentation of the illegal actions of the AMA up to 1972; contains numerous photocopies of actual AMA documents and minutes of official meetings with overt intentionality of destroying Americans' healthcare options so that the AMA and related organizations would have a monopoly in healthcare.
[268] Wolinsky H, Brune T. The Serpent on the Staff: The Unhealthy Politics of the American Medical Association. GP Putnam and Sons, New York, 1994
[269] Mein EA, Greenman PE, McMillin DL, Richards DG, Nelson CD. Manual medicine diversity: research pitfalls and the emerging medical paradigm. *J Am Osteopath Assoc*. 2001 Aug;101(8):441-4
[270] Wilk CA. Medicine, Monopolies, and Malice: How the Medical Establishment Tried to Destroy Chiropractic. Garden City Park: Avery, 1996
[271] Wenban AB. Inappropriate use of the title 'chiropractor' and term 'chiropractic manipulation' in the peer-reviewed biomedical literature. *Chiropr Osteopat*. 2006;14:16 http://chiroandosteo.com/content/14/1/16
[272] Freedman KB, Bernstein J. The adequacy of medical school education in musculoskeletal medicine. *J Bone Joint Surg Am*. 1998;80(10):1421-7
[273] Freedman KB, Bernstein J. Educational deficiencies in musculoskeletal medicine. *J Bone Joint Surg Am*. 2002;84-A(4):604-8
[274] Joy EA, Hala SV. Musculoskeletal Curricula in Medical Education: Filling In the Missing Pieces. *The Physician and Sportsmedicine* 2004; 32: 42-45
[275] Matzkin E, Smith ME, Freccero CD, Richardson AB. Adequacy of education in musculoskeletal medicine. *J Bone Joint Surg Am*. 2005 Feb;87-A(2):310-4
[276] Schmale GA. More evidence of educational inadequacies in musculoskeletal medicine. *Clin Orthop Relat Res*. 2005 Aug;(437):251-9
[277] Stockard AR, Allen TW. Competence levels in musculoskeletal medicine: comparison of osteopathic and allopathic medical graduates. *J Am Osteopath Assoc*. 2006 Jun;106(6):350-5

data with 123 chiropractic students and 10 chiropractic doctors, chiropractic training in musculoskeletal medicine is significantly superior to allopathic and osteopathic musculoskeletal training.[278] In accord with this comprehensive training in musculoskeletal management, numerous sources of evidence demonstrate that chiropractic management is much safer and less expensive than allopathic medical treatment, particularly for treatment of low-back pain. In their extensive review of the literature, Manga et al[279] published in 1993 that chiropractic management of low-back pain is superior to allopathic medical management in terms of greater safety, greater effectiveness, and reduced cost; they concluded, "There is an overwhelming body of evidence indicating that chiropractic management of low-back pain is more cost-effective than medical management" and "There would be highly significant cost savings if more management of LBP [low-back pain] was transferred from medical physicians to chiropractors." In a randomized trial involving 741 patients, Meade et al[280] showed, "**Chiropractic treatment was more effective than hospital outpatient management, mainly for patients with chronic or severe back pain**... The benefit of chiropractic treatment became more evident throughout the follow up period. Secondary outcome measures also showed that chiropractic was more beneficial." A 3-year follow-up study by these same authors[281] in 1995 showed, "At three years the results confirm the findings of an earlier report that when chiropractic or hospital therapists treat patients with low-back pain as they would in day to day practice, **those treated by chiropractic derive more benefit and long term satisfaction than those treated by hospitals**." More recently, in 2004 Legorreta et al[282] reported that the availability of chiropractic care was associated with significant cost savings among 700,000 patients with chiropractic coverage compared to 1 million patients whose insurance coverage was limited to allopathic medical treatments. Simple extrapolation of the average savings per patient in this study ($208 annual savings associated with chiropractic coverage) to the US population (295 million citizens in 2005[283]) suggests that, if fully implemented in a nation-wide basis, America could save $61,360,000,000 (more than $61 billion per year) in healthcare annual expenses by ensuring chiropractic for all citizens in contrast to failing to provide such coverage; obviously extrapolations such as this should consider other variables, such as the relatively higher prevalence of injury and death among patients treated with drugs and surgery.[284,285] Furthermore, whether the cost savings associated with chiropractic availability are due to 1) improved overall health and reduced need for pharmacosurgical intervention, 2) greater safety and lower cost of chiropractic treatment versus pharmacosurgical treatment, and/or 3) self-selection by wellness-oriented and higher-income patients, remains to be determined. A literature review by Dabbs and Lauretti[286] showed that spinal manipulation is safer than the use of NSAIDs in the treatment of neck pain. Contrasting the rates of

---

[278] Humphreys BK, Sulkowski A, McIntyre K, Kasiban M, Patrick AN. An examination of musculoskeletal cognitive competency in chiropractic interns. *J Manipulative Physiol Ther*. 2007;30(1):44-9

[279] Manga P, Angus D, Papadopoulos C, et al. The Effectiveness and Cost-Effectiveness of Chiropractic Management of Low-Back Pain. Richmond Hill, Ontario: Kenilworth Publishing; 1993

[280] Meade TW, Dyer S, Browne W, Townsend J, Frank AO. Low-back pain of mechanical origin: randomised comparison of chiropractic and hospital outpatient treatment. *BMJ*. 1990;300(6737):1431-7

[281] Meade TW, Dyer S, Browne W, Frank AO. Randomised comparison of chiropractic and hospital outpatient management for low-back pain: results from extended follow up. *BMJ*. 1995;311(7001):349-5

[282] **Legorreta AP, Metz RD, Nelson CF, Ray S, Chernicoff HO, Dinubile NA. Comparative analysis of individuals with and without chiropractic coverage: patient characteristics, utilization, and costs. *Arch Intern Med*. 2004;164:1985-92**

[283] US Census Bureau http://factfinder.census.gov/home/saff/main.html?_lang=en Accessed January 12, 2005

[284] Rosner AL. Evidence-based clinical guidelines for the management of acute low-back pain: response to the guidelines prepared for the Australian Medical Health and Research Council. *J Manipulative Physiol Ther*. 2001;24(3):214-20

[285] Topol EJ. Failing the public health--rofecoxib, Merck, and the FDA. *N Engl J Med*. 2004 Oct 21;351(17):1707-9

[286] Dabbs V, Lauretti WJ. A risk assessment of cervical manipulation vs. NSAIDs for the treatment of neck pain. *J Manipulative Physiol Ther*. 1995;18:530-6

manipulation-associated cerebrovascular accidents to the dangers of medical and surgical treatments for spinal disorders, Rosner[287] noted, "These rates are 400 times lower than the death rates observed from gastrointestinal bleeding due to the use of nonsteroidal anti-inflammatory drugs and 700 times lower than the overall mortality rate for spinal surgery." Similarly, in his review of the literature comparing the safety of chiropractic manipulation in patients with low-back pain associated with lumbar disc herniation, Oliphant[288] showed that, "The apparent safety of spinal manipulation, especially when compared with other [medically] accepted treatments for [lumbar disk herniation], should stimulate its use in the conservative treatment plan of [lumbar disk herniation]."

The clinical benefits and cost-effectiveness of chiropractic management of musculoskeletal conditions is extensively documented, and that spinal manipulation generally shows superior safety to drug and surgical treatment of back and neck pain is also well established.[289,290,291,292,293,294,295] Adjunctive therapies such as post-isometric relaxation[296] and correction of myofascial dysfunction[297] can lead to tremendous and rapid reductions in musculoskeletal pain without the hazards and expense associated with pharmaceutical drugs. Nonmusculoskeletal benefits of musculoskeletal/spinal manipulation include improved pulmonary function and/or quality of life in patients with asthma[298,299,300,301] and improvement or restoration of vision in patients with post-traumatic visual loss.[302,303,304,305,306,307,308,309] More

---

[287] Rosner AL. Evidence-based clinical guidelines for the management of acute low-back pain: response to the guidelines prepared for the Australian Medical Health and Research Council. *J Manipulative Physiol Ther*. 2001;24(3):214-20

[288] Oliphant D. Safety of spinal manipulation in the treatment of lumbar disk herniations: a systematic review and risk assessment. *J Manipulative Physiol Ther*. 2004;27:197-210

[289] Dabbs V, Lauretti WJ. A risk assessment of cervical manipulation vs. NSAIDs for the treatment of neck pain. *J Manipulative Physiol Ther*. 1995;18:530-6

[290] Rosner AL. Evidence-based clinical guidelines for the management of acute low-back pain: response to the guidelines prepared for the Australian Medical Health and Research Council. *J Manipulative Physiol Ther*. 2001 Mar-Apr;24(3):214-20

[291] Oliphant D. Safety of spinal manipulation in the treatment of lumbar disk herniations: a systematic review and risk assessment. *J Manipulative Physiol Ther*. 2004;27:197-210

[292] Meade TW, Dyer S, Browne W, Townsend J, Frank AO. Low-back pain of mechanical origin: randomised comparison of chiropractic and hospital outpatient treatment. *BMJ*. 1990;300(6737):1431-7

[293] Meade TW, Dyer S, Browne W, Frank AO. Randomised comparison of chiropractic and hospital outpatient management for low-back pain: results from extended follow up. *BMJ*. 1995;311(7001):349-5

[294] Manga P, Angus D, Papadopoulos C, et al. The Effectiveness and Cost-Effectiveness of Chiropractic Management of Low-Back Pain. Richmond Hill, Ontario: Kenilworth Publishing; 1993

[295] Legorreta AP, Metz RD, Nelson CF, Ray S, Chernicoff HO, Dinubile NA. Comparative analysis of individuals with and without chiropractic coverage: patient characteristics, utilization, and costs. *Arch Intern Med*. 2004;164:1985-92

[296] Lewit K, Simons DG. Myofascial pain: relief by post-isometric relaxation. *Arch Phys Med Rehabil*. 1984;65(8):452-6

[297] Ingber RS. Iliopsoas myofascial dysfunction: a treatable cause of "failed" low-back syndrome. *Arch Phys Med Rehabil*. 1989 May;70(5):382-6

[298] Nielson NH, Bronfort G, Bendix T, Madsen F, Wecke B. Chronic asthma and chiropractic spinal manipulation: a randomized clinical trial. *Clin Exp Allergy* 1995;25:80-8

[299] Mein EA, Greenman PE, McMillin DL, Richards DG, Nelson CD. Manual medicine diversity: research pitfalls and the emerging medical paradigm. *J Am Osteopath Assoc*. 2001 Aug;101(8):441-4

[300] "There were small increases (7 to 12 liters per minute) in peak expiratory flow in the morning and the evening in both treatment groups,… Symptoms of asthma and use of beta-agonists decreased and the quality of life increased in both groups, with no significant differences between the groups." Balon J, Aker PD, Crowther ER, Danielson C, Cox PG, O'Shaughnessy D, Walker C, Goldsmith CH, Duku E, Sears MR. A comparison of active and simulated chiropractic manipulation as adjunctive treatment for childhood asthma. *N Engl J Med*. 1998 Oct 8;339(15):1013-20

[301] Bronfort G, Evans RL, Kubic P, Filkin P. Chronic pediatric asthma and chiropractic spinal manipulation: a prospective clinical series and randomized clinical pilot study. *J Manipulative Physiol Ther*. 2001 Jul-Aug;24(6):369-77

[302] Stephens D, Pollard H, Bilton D, Thomson P, Gorman F. Bilateral simultaneous optic nerve dysfunction after periorbital trauma: recovery of vision in association with chiropractic spinal manipulation therapy. *J Manipulative Physiol Ther*. 1999 Nov-Dec;22(9):615-21

[303] Stephens D, Gorman F, Bilton D. The step phenomenon in the recovery of vision with spinal manipulation: a report on two 13-yr-olds treated together. *J Manipulative Physiol Ther*. 1997;20(9):628-33

[304] Stephens D, Gorman F. The association between visual incompetence and spinal derangement: an instructive case history. *J Manipulative Physiol Ther*. 1997 Jun;20(5):343-50.

[305] Stephens D, Gorman RF. Does 'normal' vision improve with spinal manipulation? *J Manipulative Physiol Ther*. 1996 Jul-Aug;19(6):415-8

[306] Gorman RF. Monocular scotomata and spinal manipulation: the step phenomenon. *J Manipulative Physiol Ther*. 1996 Jun;19(5):344-9

[307] Gorman RF. Monocular visual loss after closed head trauma: immediate resolution associated with spinal manipulation. *J Manipulative Physiol Ther*. 1995 Jun;18(5):308-14

[308] Gorman RF. The treatment of presumptive optic nerve ischemia by spinal manipulation. *J Manipulative Physiol Ther*. 1995;18(3):172-7

[309] Gorman RF. Automated static perimetry in chiropractic. *J Manipulative Physiol Ther*. 1993 Sep;16(7):481-7

research is required to quantify the potential benefits of spinal manipulation in patients with wide-ranging conditions such as epilepsy[310,311], attention-deficit hyperactivity disorder[312,313], and Parkinson's disease.[314] Given that most pharmaceutical drugs work on single biochemical pathways, spinal manipulation is discordant with the medical/drug paradigm because its effects are numerous (rather than singular) and physical and physiological (rather than biochemical). Thus, when viewed through the allopathic/pharmaceutical lens, spinal manipulation (like acupuncture and other physical modalities), will be viewed as "unscientific" and "does not make sense." In this case, the fault lies with the viewer and the lens, not with the object.

Research documenting the systemic and "nonmusculoskeletal" benefits of spinal manipulation mandates that our concept of "musculoskeletal" must be expanded to appreciate that **musculoskeletal interventions benefit nonmusculoskeletal body systems and physiologic processes**. This conceptual expansion applies also to soft tissue therapeutics such as massage, which can reduce adolescent aggression[315], improve outcome in preterm infants[316], alleviate premenstrual syndrome[317], and increase serotonin and dopamine levels in patients with low-back pain.[318] Studies also suggest benefit in the treatment of non-musculoskeletal complaints[319] with notable research having been performed in the treatment of asthma[320,321], post-traumatic visual loss[322,323,324,325,326,327,328,329], and modulation of immune function.[330,331]

---

[310] Elster EL. Treatment of bipolar, seizure, and sleep disorders and migraine headaches utilizing a chiropractic technique. *J Manipulative Physiol Ther*. 2004 Mar-Apr;27(3):E5

[311] Alcantara J, Heschong R, Plaugher G, Alcantara J. Chiropractic management of a patient with subluxations, low-back pain and epileptic seizures. *J Manipulative Physiol Ther*. 1998;21(6):410-8

[312] Giesen JM, Center DB, Leach RA. An evaluation of chiropractic manipulation as a treatment of hyperactivity in children. *J Manipulative Physiol Ther*. 1989 Oct;12(5):353-63

[313] Bastecki AV, Harrison DE, Haas JW. Cervical kyphosis is a possible link to attention-deficit/hyperactivity disorder. *J Manipulative Physiol Ther*. 2004 Oct;27(8):e14

[314] Elster EL. Upper cervical chiropractic management of a patient with Parkinson's disease: a case report. *J Manipulative Physiol Ther*. 2000 Oct;23(8):573-7

[315] Diego MA, Field T, Hernandez-Reif M, Shaw JA, Rothe EM, Castellanos D, Mesner L. Aggressive adolescents benefit from massage therapy. *Adolescence* 2002 Fall;37(147):597-607

[316] Mainous RO. Infant massage as a component of developmental care: past, present, and future. *Holist Nurs Pract* 2002 Oct;16(5):1-7

[317] Hernandez-Reif M, Martinez A, Field T, Quintero O, Hart S, Burman I. Premenstrual symptoms are relieved by massage therapy. *J Psychosom Obstet Gynaecol* 2000 Mar;21(1):9-15

[318] "RESULTS: By the end of the study, the massage therapy group, as compared to the relaxation group, reported experiencing less pain, depression, anxiety and improved sleep. They also showed improved trunk and pain flexion performance, and their serotonin and dopamine levels were higher." Hernandez-Reif M, Field T, Krasnegor J, Theakston H. Lower back pain is reduced and range of motion increased after massage therapy. *Int J Neurosci* 2001;106(3-4):131-45

[319] Leboeuf-Yde C, Axen I, Ahlefeldt G, Lidefelt P, Rosenbaum A, Thurnherr T. The types and frequencies of improved nonmusculoskeletal symptoms reported after chiropractic spinal manipulative therapy. *J Manipulative Physiol Ther*. 1999 Nov-Dec;22(9):559-64

[320] Mein EA, Greenman PE, McMillin DL, Richards DG, Nelson CD. Manual medicine diversity: research pitfalls and the emerging medical paradigm. *J Am Osteopath Assoc*. 2001 Aug;101(8):441-4

[321] "There were small increases (7 to 12 liters per minute) in peak expiratory flow in the morning and the evening in both treatment groups,... Symptoms of asthma and use of beta-agonists decreased and the quality of life increased in both groups, with no significant differences between the groups." Balon J, Aker PD, Crowther ER, Danielson C, Cox PG, O'Shaughnessy D, Walker C, Goldsmith CH, Duku E, Sears MR. A comparison of active and simulated chiropractic manipulation as adjunctive treatment for childhood asthma. *N Engl J Med*. 1998 Oct 8;339(15):1013-20

[322] Stephens D, Pollard H, Bilton D, Thomson P, Gorman F. Bilateral simultaneous optic nerve dysfunction after periorbital trauma: recovery of vision in association with chiropractic spinal manipulation therapy. *J Manipulative Physiol Ther*. 1999 Nov-Dec;22(9):615-21

[323] Stephens D, Gorman F, Bilton D. The step phenomenon in the recovery of vision with spinal manipulation: a report on two 13-yr-olds treated together. *J Manipulative Physiol Ther*. 1997;20(9):628-33

[324] Stephens D, Gorman F. The association between visual incompetence and spinal derangement: an instructive case history. *J Manipulative Physiol Ther*. 1997 Jun;20(5):343-50

[325] Stephens D, Gorman RF. Does 'normal' vision improve with spinal manipulation? *J Manipulative Physiol Ther*. 1996 Jul-Aug;19(6):415-8

[326] Gorman RF. Monocular scotomata and spinal manipulation: the step phenomenon. *J Manipulative Physiol Ther*. 1996 Jun;19(5):344-9

[327] Gorman RF. Monocular visual loss after closed head trauma: immediate resolution associated with spinal manipulation. *J Manipulative Physiol Ther*. 1995 Jun;18(5):308-14

[328] Gorman RF. The treatment of presumptive optic nerve ischemia by spinal manipulation. *J Manipulative Physiol Ther*. 1995;18(3):172-7

[329] Gorman RF. Automated static perimetry in chiropractic. *J Manipulative Physiol Ther*. 1993 Sep;16(7):481-7

[330] Brennan PC, Triano JJ, McGregor M, Kokjohn K, Hondras MA, Brennan DC. Enhanced neutrophil respiratory burst as a biological marker for manipulation forces: duration of the effect and association with substance P and tumor necrosis factor. *J Manipulative Physiol Ther*. 1992 Feb;15(2):83-9

[331] Brennan PC, Kokjohn K, Kaltinger CJ, Lohr GE, Glendening C, Hondras MA, McGregor M, Triano JJ. Enhanced phagocytic cell respiratory burst induced by spinal manipulation: potential role of substance P. *J Manipulative Physiol Ther*. 1991 Sep;14(7):399-408

## Spinal Manipulation: Mechanistic Considerations

Applied to either the spine or peripheral joints, high-velocity low-amplitude joint manipulation appears to have numerous physical and physiological effects, including but not limited to the following:

1. Releasing entrapped intraarticular menisci and synovial folds,
2. Acutely reducing intradiscal pressure, thus promoting replacement of decentralized disc material,
3. Stretching of deep periarticular muscles to break the cycle of chronic autonomous muscle contraction by lengthening the muscles and thereby releasing excessive actin-myosin binding,
4. Promoting restoration of proper kinesthesia and proprioception,
5. Promoting relaxation of paraspinal muscles by stretching facet joint capsules,
6. Promoting relaxation of paraspinal muscles via "postactivation depression", which is the temporary depletion of contractile neurotransmitters,
7. Temporarily elevating plasma beta-endorphin,
8. Temporarily enhancing phagocytic ability of neutrophils and monocytes, and
9. Activation of the diffuse descending pain inhibitory system located in the periaqueductal gray matter—this is an important aspect of nociceptive inhibition by intense sensory/mechanoreceptor stimulation, which will be discussed in a following section for its relevance to neurogenic inflammation.
10. Improving neurotransmitter balance and reducing pain (soft-tissue manipulation).[332]

While the above list of mechanisms-of-action is certainly not complete, for purposes of this paper it is sufficient to have established that, indeed, joint manipulation in general and spinal manipulation in particular have objective mechanistic effects that correlate with their clinical benefits. Additional details are provided in numerous published reviews and primary research[333,334,335,336,337,338,339] and by Leach[340], whose extensive description of the mechanisms of action of spinal manipulative therapy is unsurpassed. Given such a wide base of experimental and clinical support published in peer-reviewed journals and widely-available textbooks, denigrations directed toward spinal manipulation on the grounds that it is "unscientific" or "unsupported by research" are unfounded and are indicative of selective ignorance.

---

[332] "RESULTS: By the end of the study, the massage therapy group, as compared to the relaxation group, reported experiencing less pain, depression, anxiety and improved sleep. They also showed improved trunk and pain flexion performance, and their serotonin and dopamine levels were higher." Hernandez-Reif M, Field T, Krasnegor J, Theakston H. Lower back pain is reduced and range of motion increased after massage therapy. *Int J Neurosci* 2001;106(3-4):131-45

[333] Maigne JY, Vautravers P. Mechanism of action of spinal manipulative therapy. *Joint Bone Spine*. 2003;70(5):336-41

[334] Brennan PC, Triano JJ, McGregor M, Kokjohn K, Hondras MA, Brennan DC. Enhanced neutrophil respiratory burst as a biological marker for manipulation forces: duration of the effect and association with substance P and tumor necrosis factor. *J Manipulative Physiol Ther*. 1992 Feb;15(2):83-9

[335] Brennan PC, Kokjohn K, Kaltinger CJ, Lohr GE, Glendening C, Hondras MA, McGregor M, Triano JJ. Enhanced phagocytic cell respiratory burst induced by spinal manipulation: potential role of substance P. *J Manipulative Physiol Ther*. 1991 Sep;14(7):399-408

[336] Heikkila H, Johansson M, Wenngren BI. Effects of acupuncture, cervical manipulation and NSAID therapy on dizziness and impaired head repositioning of suspected cervical origin: a pilot study. *Man Ther*. 2000 Aug;5(3):151-7

[337] Rogers RG. The effects of spinal manipulation on cervical kinesthesia in patients with chronic neck pain: a pilot study. *J Manipulative Physiol Ther*. 1997;20(2):80-5

[338] Bergman, Peterson, Lawrence. Chiropractic Technique. New York: Churchill Livingstone 1993. An updated edition is now availabe published by Mosby.

[339] Herzog WH. Mechanical and physiological responses to spinal manipulative treatments. *JNMS: J Neuromuskuskeltal System* 1995; 3: 1-9

[340] Leach RA. (ed). The Chiropractic Theories: A Textbook of Scientific Research, Fourth Edition. Baltimore: Lippincott, Williams & Wilkins, 2004

## Mechanoreceptor-Mediated Inhibition of Neurogenic Inflammation: A Possible Mechanism of Action of Spinal Manipulation

Neurogenic inflammation causes catabolism of articular structures and thus promotes joint destruction[341,342], a phenomena that the current author has termed "neurogenic chondrolysis."[343] The biologic and scientific basis for this concept rests on the following sequence of events which ultimately form a self-perpetuating and multisystem cycle:

1. Using joint pain as an example, we know that acute or chronic joint injury results in the release of inflammatory mediators in local tissues as **immunogenic inflammation,**
2. Nociceptive input is received centrally and results in release of inflammatory mediators *from sensory neurons* termed **neurogenic inflammation**[344] and results in a neurologically-mediated catabolic effect in articular cartilage[345,346] termed **neurogenic chondrolysis**,
3. As immunogenic and neurogenic inflammation synergize to promote joint destruction, pain from degenerating joints further increases nociceptive afferent transmission to further increase neurogenic and thus immunogenic inflammation. Thus, a *positive feedback* vicious cycle of immunogenic and neurogenic inflammation promotes and perpetuates joint destruction,
4. Further complicating this *regional* cycle of neurogenic-immunogenic inflammation and tissue destruction would be any pain or inflammation *in distant parts of the body*, since pain in one part of the body can exacerbate neurogenic inflammation in another part of the body via **neurogenic switching**[347,348] and immunologic reactivity such as allergy or autoimmunity in one part of the body may be transmitted *via the nervous system* to cause immunogenic inflammation in another part of the body via **immunogenic switching.**[349]

The clinical relevance of neurogenic inflammation and immunogenic switching is that they provide a means *beyond biochemistry* by which to understand how and why inflammation *transmitted and perpetuated by the nervous system* must be treated on a body-wide *holistic* basis.

The current author is the first to propose the concept of **mechanoreceptor-mediated inhibition of neurogenic inflammation**.[350] Since neurogenic chondrolysis is inhibited by interference with C-fiber (type IV) mediated afferent transmission[351] and since chiropractic high-velocity low-amplitude (HVLA) manipulation appears to inhibit C-fiber mediated nociception[352,353], then

---

[341] Gouze-Decaris E, Philippe L, Minn A, Haouzi P, Gillet P, Netter P, Terlain B. Neurophysiological basis for neurogenic-mediated articular cartilage anabolism alteration. *Am J Physiol Regul Integr Comp Physiol.* 2001;280(1):R115-22

[342] Decaris E, Guingamp C, Chat M, Philippe L, Grillasca JP, Abid A, Minn A, Gillet P, Netter P, Terlain B. Evidence for neurogenic transmission inducing degenerative cartilage damage distant from local inflammation. *Arthritis Rheum.* 1999;42(9):1951-60

[343] Vasquez A. *Integrative Orthopedics: Exploring the Structural Aspect of the Matrix.* Applying Functional Medicine in Clinical Practice. Tampa, Florida November 29-December 4, 2004. Hosted by the Institute for Functional Medicine: www.FunctionalMedicine.org

[344] Meggs WJ. Mechanisms of allergy and chemical sensitivity. *Toxicol Ind Health.* 1999 Apr-Jun;15(3-4):331-8

[345] Gouze-Decaris E, Philippe L, Minn A, Haouzi P, Gillet P, Netter P, Terlain B. Neurophysiological basis for neurogenic-mediated articular cartilage anabolism alteration. *Am J Physiol Regul Integr Comp Physiol.* 2001;280(1):R115-22

[346] Decaris E, Guingamp C, Chat M, Philippe L, Grillasca JP, Abid A, Minn A, Gillet P, Netter P, Terlain B. Evidence for neurogenic transmission inducing degenerative cartilage damage distant from local inflammation. *Arthritis Rheum.* 1999;42(9):1951-60

[347] Meggs WJ. Neurogenic Switching: A Hypothesis for a Mechanism for Shifting the Site of Inflammation in Allergy and Chemical Sensitivity. *Environ Health Perspect* 1995; 103:54-56

[348] Meggs WJ. Mechanisms of allergy and chemical sensitivity. *Toxicol Ind Health.* 1999 Apr-Jun;15(3-4):331-8

[349] "…—immunogenic switching—… In this scenario, the afferent stimulation from the cranial vasculature, which is inflamed during a migraine because of neurogenic processes, is rerouted by the CNS to produce immunogenic inflammation at the nose and sinuses." Cady RK, Schreiber CP. Sinus headache or migraine? Considerations in making a differential diagnosis. *Neurology.* 2002;58(9 Suppl 6):S10-4

[350] Vasquez A. *Integrative Orthopedics: Exploring the Structural Aspect of the Matrix.* Applying Functional Medicine in Clinical Practice. Tampa, Florida November 29-December 4, 2004. Hosted by the Institute for Functional Medicine: www.FunctionalMedicine.org

[351] Gouze-Decaris E, Philippe L, Minn A, Haouzi P, Gillet P, Netter P, Terlain B. Neurophysiological basis for neurogenic-mediated articular cartilage anabolism alteration. *Am J Physiol Regul Integr Comp Physiol.* 2001;280(1):R115-22

[352] Gillette, R. A speculative argument for the coactivation of diverse somatic receptor populations by forceful chiropractic adjustments. *Man Med* 1987; 3:1-14

chiropractic HVLA manipulation may reduce neurogenic inflammation and may promote articular integrity by inhibiting neurogenic chondrolysis. Further, mechanoreceptor-mediated inhibition of neurogenic inflammation would, for example, help explain the benefits of spinal manipulation in the treatment of asthma[354,355,356], since asthma is known to be mediated in large part by neurogenic inflammation.[357,358] Thus, spinal manipulation appears to provide a means *in addition to other anti-inflammatory interventions such as diet, lifestyle and phytonutritional interventions* by which pain and inflammation can be treated naturally.

A science-based comprehensive protocol can be implemented against pain and inflammation by using ❶ an anti-inflammatory diet, ❷ frequent exercise, ❸ lifestyle and bodyweight optimization, ❹ nutritional supplementation, ❺ botanical supplementation[359,360] ❻ spinal manipulation (with its kinesthetic, analgesic, *directly* and *indirectly* anti-inflammatory, and *probably* piezoelectric benefits[361]), ❼ stress reduction[362,363], ❽ anti-dysbiosis protocols[364], ❾ hormonal correction ("orthoendocrinology"), and ❿ ancillary treatments such as acupuncture[365,366]; additional details and citations for these interventions are provided throughout the text and especially chapter 2, chapter 3 of *Integrative Orthopedics/Rheumatology*, and the chapter on *Therapeutics*. Pain and inflammation are self-perpetuating vicious cycles, perfectly suited to intervention with comprehensive and multicomponent treatment plans profiled above and detailed in *Integrative Orthopedics* and *Integrative Rheumatology*.

---

[353] Boal RW, Gillette RG. Central neuronal plasticity, low-back pain and spinal manipulative therapy. *J Manipulative Physiol Ther*. 2004;27(5):314-26
[354] Nielson NH, Bronfort G, Bendix T, Madsen F, Wecke B. Chronic asthma and chiropractic spinal manipulation: a randomized clinical trial. *Clin Exp Allergy* 1995;25:80-8
[355] "There were small increases (7 to 12 liters per minute) in peak expiratory flow in the morning and the evening in both treatment groups,... Symptoms of asthma and use of beta-agonists decreased and the quality of life increased in both groups, with no significant differences between the groups." Balon J, Aker PD, Crowther ER, Danielson C, Cox PG, O'Shaughnessy D, Walker C, Goldsmith CH, Duku E, Sears MR. A comparison of active and simulated chiropractic manipulation as adjunctive treatment for childhood asthma. *N Engl J Med*. 1998 Oct 8;339(15):1013-20
[356] Bronfort G, Evans RL, Kubic P, Filkin P. Chronic pediatric asthma and chiropractic spinal manipulation: a prospective clinical series and randomized clinical pilot study. *J Manipulative Physiol Ther*. 2001 Jul-Aug;24(6):369-77
[357] Renz H. Neurotrophins in bronchial asthma. *Respir Res*. 2001;2(5):265-8
[358] Groneberg DA, Quarcoo D, Frossard N, Fischer A. Neurogenic mechanisms in bronchial inflammatory diseases. *Allergy*. 2004 Nov; 59(11): 1139-52
[359] Jancso N, Jancso-Gabor A, Szolcsanyi J. Direct evidence for neurogenic inflammation and its prevention by denervation and by pretreatment with capsaicin. *Br J Pharmacol*. 1967 Sep;31(1):138-51
[360] Miller MJ, Vergnolle N, McKnight W, Musah RA, Davison CA, Trentacosti AM, Thompson JH, Sandoval M, Wallace JL. Inhibition of neurogenic inflammation by the Amazonian herbal medicine sangre de grado. *J Invest Dermatol*. 2001;117(3):725-30
[361] Lipinski B. Biological significance of piezoelectricity in relation to acupuncture, Hatha Yoga, osteopathic medicine and action of air ions. *Med Hypotheses*. 1977;3(1):9-12 See also: Athenstaedt H. Pyroelectric and piezoelectric properties of vertebrates. *Ann N Y Acad Sci*. 1974;238:68-94 See also: Athenstaedt H. "Functional polarity" of the spinal cord caused by its longitudinal electric dipole moment. *Am J Physiol*. 1984;247(3 Pt 2):R482-7
[362] Lutgendorf S, Logan H, Kirchner HL, Rothrock N, Svengalis S, Iverson K, Lubaroff D. Effects of relaxation and stress on the capsaicin-induced local inflammatory response. *Psychosom Med*. 2000;62:524-34
[363] "Couples who demonstrated consistently higher levels of hostile behaviors across both their interactions healed at 60% of the rate of low-hostile couples. High-hostile couples also produced relatively larger increases in plasma IL-6 and tumor necrosis factor alpha…" Kiecolt-Glaser JK, Loving TJ, Stowell JR, Malarkey WB, Lemeshow S, Dickinson SL, Glaser R. Hostile marital interactions, proinflammatory cytokine production, and wound healing. *Arch Gen Psychiatry*. 2005 Dec;62(12):1377-84
[364] Chapter 4 of Integrative Rheumatology and Vasquez A. Reducing Pain and Inflammation Naturally. Part 6: Nutritional and Botanical Treatments Against "Silent Infections" and Gastrointestinal Dysbiosis, Commonly Overlooked Causes of Neuromusculoskeletal Inflammation and Chronic Health Problems. *Nutr Perspect* 2006; Jan http://optimalhealthresearch.com/part6
[365] Joos S, Brinkhaus B, Maluche C, Maupai N, Kohnen R, Kraemer N, Hahn EG, Schuppan D. Acupuncture and moxibustion in the treatment of active Crohn's disease: a randomized controlled study. *Digestion*. 2004;69(3):131-9
[366] "These results demonstrate an unorthodox new type of neurohumoral regulatory mechanism of sensory fibres and provide a possible mode of action for the anti-inflammatory effect of counter-irritation and acupuncture." Pinter E, Szolcsanyi J. Systemic anti-inflammatory effect induced by antidromic stimulation of the dorsal roots in the rat. *Neurosci Lett*. 1996;212(1):33-6

## Special Communication

IN THE UNITED STATES DISTRICT COURT
FOR THE NORTHERN DISTRICT OF ILLINOIS
EASTERN DIVISION

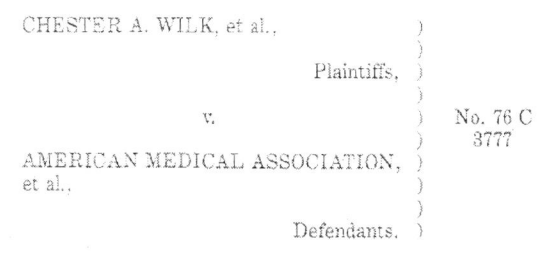

CHESTER A. WILK, et al.,  )
                          )
              Plaintiffs, )
                          )
         v.               )   No. 76 C
                          )   3777
AMERICAN MEDICAL ASSOCIATION, )
et al.,                   )
                          )
              Defendants. )

PERMANENT INJUNCTION ORDER AGAINST AMA

Susan Getzendanner, District Judge

The court conducted a lengthy trial of this case in May and June of 1987 and on August 27, 1987, issued a 101 page opinion finding that the American Medical Association ("AMA") and its members participated in a conspiracy against chiropractors in violation of the nation's antitrust laws. Thereafter an opinion dated September 25, 1987 was substituted for the August 27, 1987 opinion. The question now before the court is the form of injunctive relief that the court will order.

**See also p 83.**

As part of the injunctive relief to be ordered by the court against the AMA, the AMA shall be required to send a copy of this Permanent Injunction Order to each of its current members. The members of the AMA are bound by the terms of the Permanent Injunction Order if they act in concert with the AMA to violate the terms of the order. Accordingly, it is important that the AMA members understand the order and the reasons why the order has been entered.

### The AMA's Boycott and Conspiracy

In the early 1960s, the AMA decided to contain and eliminate chiropractic as a profession. In 1963 the AMA's Committee on Quackery was formed. The committee worked aggressively—both overtly and covertly—to eliminate chiropractic. One of the principal means used by the AMA to achieve its goal was to make it unethical for medical physicians to professionally associate with chiropractors. Under Principle 3 of the AMA's Principles of Medical Ethics, it was unethical for a physician to associate with an "unscientific practitioner," and in 1966 the AMA's House of Delegates passed a resolution calling chiropractic an unscientific cult. To complete the circle, in 1967 the AMA's Judicial Council issued an opinion under Principle 3 holding that it was unethical for a physician to associate professionally with chiropractors.

The AMA's purpose was to prevent medical physicians from referring patients to chiropractors and accepting referrals of patients from chiropractors, to prevent chiropractors from obtaining access to hospital diagnostic services and membership on hospital medical staffs, to prevent medical physicians from teaching at chiropractic colleges or engaging in any joint research, and to prevent any cooperation between the two groups in the delivery of health care services.

Published by order of Susan Getzendanner, US District Judge, Sept 25, 1987.

The AMA believed that the boycott worked—that chiropractic would have achieved greater gains in the absence of the boycott. Since no medical physician would want to be considered unethical by his peers, the success of the boycott is not surprising. However, chiropractic achieved licensing in all 50 states during the existence of the Committee on Quackery.

The Committee on Quackery was disbanded in 1975 and some of the committee's activities became publicly known. Several lawsuits were filed by or on behalf of chiropractors and this case was filed in 1976.

### Change in AMA's Position on Chiropractic

In 1977, the AMA began to change its position on chiropractic. The AMA's Judicial Council adopted new opinions under which medical physicians could refer patients to chiropractors, but there was still the proviso that the medical physician should be confident that the services to be provided on referral would be performed in accordance with accepted scientific standards. In 1979, the AMA's House of Delegates adopted Report UU which said that not everything that a chiropractor may do is without therapeutic value, but it stopped short of saying that such things were based on scientific standards. It was not until 1980 that the AMA revised its Principles of Medical Ethics to eliminate Principle 3. Until Principle 3 was formally eliminated, there was considerable ambiguity about the AMA's position. The ethics code adopted in 1980 provided that a medical physician "shall be free to choose whom to serve, with whom to associate, and the environment in which to provide medical services."

The AMA settled three chiropractic lawsuits by stipulating and agreeing that under the current opinions of the Judicial Council a physician may, without fear of discipline or sanction by the AMA, refer a patient to a duly licensed chiropractor when he believes that referral may benefit the patient. The AMA confirmed that a physician may also choose to accept or to decline patients sent to him by a duly licensed chiropractor. Finally, the AMA confirmed that a physician may teach at a chiropractic college or seminar. These settlements were entered into in 1978, 1980, and 1986.

The AMA's present position on chiropractic, as stated to the court, is that it is ethical for a medical physician to professionally associate with chiropractors provided the physician believes that such association is in the best interests of his patient. This position has not previously been communicated by the AMA to its members.

### Antitrust Laws

Under the Sherman Act, every combination or conspiracy in restraint of trade is illegal. The court has held that the conduct of the AMA and its members constituted a conspiracy in restraint of trade based on the following facts: the purpose of the boycott was to eliminate chiropractic; chiropractors are in competition with some medical physicians; the boycott had substantial anti-competitive effects; there were no pro-competitive effects of the boycott; and the plaintiffs were injured as a result of the conduct. These facts add up to a violation of the Sherman Act.

In this case, however, the court allowed the defendants the opportunity to establish a "patient care defense" which has the following elements:

(1) that they genuinely entertained a concern for what they perceive as scientific method in the care of each person with whom they have entered into a doctor-patient relationship; (2) that this concern is objectively reasonable; (3) that this concern has been the dominant motivating factor in defendants' promulgation of Principle 3 and in the

conduct intended to implement it; and (4) that this concern for scientific method in patient care could not have been adequately satisfied in a manner less restrictive of competition.

The court concluded that the AMA had a genuine concern for scientific methods in patient care, and that this concern was the dominant factor in motivating the AMA's conduct. However, the AMA failed to establish that throughout the entire period of the boycott, from 1966 to 1980, this concern was objectively reasonable. The court reached that conclusion on the basis of extensive testimony from both witnesses for the plaintiffs and the AMA that some forms of chiropractic treatment are effective and the fact that the AMA recognized that chiropractic began to change in the early 1970s. Since the boycott was not formally over until Principle 3 was eliminated in 1980, the court found that the AMA was unable to establish that during the entire period of the conspiracy its position was objectively reasonable. Finally, the court ruled that the AMA's concern for scientific method in patient care could have been adequately satisfied in a manner less restrictive of competition and that a nationwide conspiracy to eliminate a licensed profession was not justified by the concern for scientific method. On the basis of these findings, the court concluded that the AMA had failed to establish the patient care defense.

None of the court's findings constituted a judicial endorsement of chiropractic. All of the parties to the case, including the plaintiffs and the AMA, agreed that chiropractic treatment of diseases such as diabetes, high blood pressure, cancer, heart disease and infectious disease is not proper, and that the historic theory of chiropractic, that there is a single cause and cure of disease is wrong. There was disagreement between the parties as to whether chiropractors should engage in diagnosis. There was evidence that the chiropractic theory of subluxations was unscientific, and evidence that some chiropractors engaged in unscientific practices. The court did not reach the question of whether chiropractic theory was in fact scientific. However, the evidence in the case was that some forms of chiropractic manipulation of the spine and joints was therapeutic. AMA witnesses, including the present Chairman of the Board of Trustees of the AMA, testified that some forms of treatment by chiropractors, including manipulation, can be therapeutic in the treatment of conditions such as back pain syndrome.

### Need for Injunctive Relief

Although the conspiracy ended in 1980, there are lingering effects of the illegal boycott and conspiracy which require an injunction. Some medical physicians' individual decisions on whether or not to professionally associate with chiropractors are still affected by the boycott. The injury to chiropractors' reputations which resulted from the boycott has not been repaired. Chiropractors suffer current economic injury as a result of the boycott. The AMA has never affirmatively acknowledged that there are and should be no collective impediments to professional association and cooperation between chiropractors and medical physicians, except as provided by law. Instead, the AMA has consistently argued that its conduct has not violated the antitrust laws.

Most importantly, the court believes that it is important that the AMA members be made aware of the present AMA position that it is ethical for a medical physician to professionally associate with a chiropractor if the physician believes it is in the best interests of his patient, so that the lingering effects of the illegal group boycott against chiropractors finally can be dissipated.

Under the law, every medical physician, institution, and hospital has the right to make an individual decision as to whether or not that physician, institution, or hospital shall associate professionally with chiropractors. Individual choice by a medical physician voluntarily to associate professionally with chiropractors should be governed only by restrictions under state law, if any, and by the individual medical physician's personal judgment as to what is in the best interest of a patient or patients. Professional association includes referrals, consultations, group practice in partnerships, Health Maintenance Organizations, Preferred Provider Organizations, and other alternative health care delivery systems; the provision of treatment privileges and diagnostic services (including radiological and other laboratory facilities) in or through hospital facilities; association and cooperation in educational programs for students in chiropractic colleges; and cooperation in research, health care seminars, and continuing education programs.

An injunction is necessary to assure that the AMA does not interfere with the right of a physician, hospital, or other institution to make an individual decision on the question of professional association.

### Form of Injunction

1. The AMA, its officers, agents and employees, and all persons who act in active concert with any of them and who receive actual notice of this order are hereby permanently enjoined from restricting, regulating or impeding, or aiding and abetting others from restricting, regulating or impeding, the freedom of any AMA member or any institution or hospital to make an individual decision as to whether or not that AMA member, institution, or hospital shall professionally associate with chiropractors, chiropractic students, or chiropractic institutions.

2. This Permanent Injunction does not and shall not be construed to restrict or otherwise interfere with the AMA's right to take positions on any issue, including chiropractic, and to express or publicize those positions, either alone or in conjunction with others. Nor does this Permanent Injunction restrict or otherwise interfere with the AMA's right to petition or testify before any public body on any legislative or regulatory measure or to join or cooperate with any other entity in so petitioning or testifying. The AMA's membership in a recognized accrediting association or society shall not constitute a violation of this Permanent Injunction.

3. The AMA is directed to send a copy of this order to each AMA member and employee, first class mail, postage prepaid, within thirty days of the entry of this order. In the alternative, the AMA shall provide the Clerk of the Court with mailing labels so that the court may send this order to AMA members and employees.

4. The AMA shall cause the publication of this order in JAMA and the indexing of the order under "Chiropractic" so that persons desiring to find the order in the future will be able to do so.

5. The AMA shall prepare a statement of the AMA's present position on chiropractic for inclusion in the current reports and opinions of the Judicial Council with an appropriate heading that refers to professional association between medical physicians and chiropractors, and indexed in the same manner that other reports and opinions are indexed. The court imposes no restrictions on the AMA's statement but only requires that it be consistent with the AMA's statements of its present position to the court.

6. The AMA shall file a report with the court evidencing compliance with this order on or before January 10, 1988.

It is so ordered.

Susan Getzendanner
United States District Judge

## Competencies and Self-Assessment

These are sample questions and competencies that can be used as example standards of evaluation for students and clinicians. A much more extensive sample is published in each new edition of *Integrative Orthopedics*, *Integrative Rheumatology*, and *Chiropractic and Naturopathic Mastery of Common Clinical Disorders*. To access the most recent complete list of questions and competencies, please go to http://OptimalHealthResearch.com/competencies. For the following questions specific to the clinical management of hypertension, mark the single best answer for each of the following questions.

1) **A hypertensive patient with diabetic nephropathy who is treated with an ACE-inhibitor and spironolactone is most likely to suffer which of the following clinical effects as a result of increased intake of fruits and vegetables:**
   A. Hyper-reflexia and clonus
   B. Seizure or pre-eclampsia
   C. Fatigue or cardiac arrest
   D. Headaches
   E. Water retention and carpal tunnel syndrome

2) **In a patient experiencing musculoskeletal pain as a result of taking an HMG-CoA reductase (3-hydroxy-3-methyl-glutaryl-CoA reductase) inhibiting drug for cardioprotection, which two nutrients are most likely to be of benefit:**
   A. EPA and DHA
   B. Magnesium and pyridoxine
   C. Ubiquinone and cholecalciferol
   D. Boswellia and Willow extract
   E. Vitamin E and vitamin A

3) **Renal artery stenosis typically occurs in which groups:**
   A. Older women and young children
   B. Young adult women and older men and women
   C. Older men and young adult men
   D. Adolescents and young adult men
   E. Older women and young adult men

4) **Which of the following two patient factors would probably contraindicate the initiation of cholecalciferol replacement with a starting dose of 300,000 IU administered as an intramuscular injection:**
   A. Multiple sclerosis and treatment with prednisone
   B. Fibromyalgia and treatment with Lyrica/ pregabalin
   C. Osteoarthritis and treatment with ibuprofen
   D. Sarcoidosis and treatment with hydrochlorothiazide
   E. Rheumatoid arthritis and treatment with methotrexate and sulfasalazine

5) **Which two antihypertensive nutrients are commonly dosed by determination of bowel tolerance:**
   A. Glutamine and arginine
   B. Vitamin E and selenium
   C. Magnesium and vitamin D
   D. Butyric acid and glutamine
   E. Vitamin C and magnesium

6) **Probenicid and allopurinol might be less necessary or unnecessary for hypertensive patients who avoid which of the following:**
   A. Tortillas
   B. Wheat bread
   C. Cheese
   D. Aspartame
   E. Corn syrup

7) **Vitamin D3 deficiency causes a specific biochemical-physiologic effect on ion/mineral imbalance within cells due to elevated levels of parathyroid hormone. Which of the following drugs most directly offsets this imbalance:**
   A. Furosemide
   B. Amlodipine
   C. Spironolactone
   D. Metoprolol
   E. Lisinopril

8) **As an antihypertensive therapy, fasting lowers blood pressure by which mechanism:**
   A. Increased nocturnal production of melatonin
   B. Increased cortisol sensitivity
   C. Reduced estradiol levels
   D. Reduced insulin levels
   E. Elevated prolactin levels

9) **In a young adult unmedicated hypertensive patient with hyperkalemia and a normal serum creatinine, which of the following tests is required in the next step of the evaluation:**
   A. MRI of the pituitary gland
   B. Serum aldosterone and renin
   C. Serum dehydroepiandrosterone sulfate
   D. Serum reverse triiodothyronine
   E. Serum free thyroxine

10) **Your patient with hypertension is found to have a serum creatinine of 1.8 mg/dl. Which of the following treatments must be discontinued:**
    A. Vitamin D3
    B. Furosemide
    C. L-thyroxine
    D. Metformin
    E. Amlodipine

11) **Which of the following conditions is best known for causing pulmonary hypertension and systemic malignant hypertension as a lethal consequence:**
    A. Systemic sclerosis
    B. Dermatomyositis
    C. Fibromyalgia
    D. Rheumatoid arthritis
    E. Eosinophilic fascitis

12) **Upper cervical spine subluxation treated with chiropractic manipulation is causally associated with hypertension via which mechanism:**
    A. Sympathetic activation due to pain
    B. Pain causes sympathetic activation and sodium-water retention
    C. Brainstem compression
    D. Basilar invagination
    E. Tentorial herniation

13) **Accurate determination of thyroid status includes:**
    A. Laboratory measurement of TSH but NOT free T4
    B. Laboratory measurement of TSH along with monitoring response to therapy with triiodothyronine
    C. Laboratory measurement of free T4 and serum cortisol
    D. Laboratory measurement of serum testosterone and serum triiodothyronine
    E. Laboratory measurement of free T4 along with monitoring response to therapy with thyroxine

14) **Which of the following comorbidity patterns suggests vitamin D3 deficiency as a cause of hypertension:**
    A. Peripheral arthropathy and clonus
    B. Generalized musculoskeletal pain, migraine, and insulin resistance
    C. Nonfocal muscle weakness and cardiac arrhythmia
    D. Diarrhea, tachycardia, and exophthalmos
    E. Generalized musculoskeletal pain, hyperreflexia, and constipation

15) **Normal body mass index is:**
    A. 16-21
    B. 17-22
    C. 18-24
    D. 19-27
    E. 20-28

16) **Per published reviews, the optimal range for serum 25-hydroxy-cholecalciferol is:**
    A. 20-80 ng/ml
    B. 20-80 pg/ml
    C. 50-90 pg/ml
    D. 50-100 ng/ml
    E. 50-100 pg/ml

17) **Which components of the Mediterranean diet are not included in the Paleo diet:**
    A. Citrus fruit
    B. Lean meats and fish
    C. Whole grains
    D. Leafy green vegetables
    E. Nuts and seeds

18) **During a water-only fast, if a patient becomes confabulated and does not respond to consumption of a large glass of orange juice, then the problem probably is related to:**
    A. Magnesium
    B. Bicarbonate
    C. Potassium
    D. Sodium
    E. Calcium

19) **Responding to your newspaper advertisement offering headache treatment, a 75-yo type-2 diabetic new patient in your outpatient office on Friday afternoon has a blood pressure of 170/120 mm Hg, anisocoria, papilledema, and is alert and oriented x2. Prior-to-visit lab tests show a hemoglobin a1c 10%, serum creatine 1.8 mg/dL, and serum BNP (brain natriuretic peptide) 600 pg/ml. Prior medical and social history reveals widower x6 months, hypothyroidism, and no other prior surgical or medical history. What is the best management strategy:**
    A. Implement the Paleo-Mediterranean diet and appropriate manipulative and mind-body treatments
    B. Implement the Paleo-Mediterranean diet and mind-body treatments, but defer manipulative treatment
    C. Return office visit on Monday to see if the blood pressure is starting to show improvement and if the anisocoria is resolved
    D. Call for an ambulance; admit to hospital urgent care department
    E. Perform appropriate laboratory tests and review with patient (perhaps via phone or brief office visit) later that same day before the end of the work week
    F. Arrange for nursing care at home
    G. Transfer the patient to a skilled nursing facility

20) **Given that effective nondrug treatment for chronic hypertension can involve lifestyle modification, diet optimization, exercise prescription, nutritional supplementation, manual manipulation of articular structures and soft tissues, and mind-body therapies, which of the following professional groups is LEAST TRAINED to provide nondrug care.**
    A. Allopathic doctors (MD)
    B. Osteopathic doctors (DO)
    C. Chiropractic doctors (DC)
    D. Naturopathic doctors (ND)

# Index

2,4-dichlorophenol, 146
2,5-dichlorophenol, 146
25(OH) vitamin D - testing in patients with pain, 196
Abducens, 185
Acetyl-L-carnitine, 56
Acupuncture, 65
Acute nontraumatic monoarthritis, 219
Acute red eye, 216
Adipokines, 112
Adipose, 112
Affirmation and Re-Birth of the Chiropractic Profession, 18
African American, 71
Aldosterone:renin ratio, 39
Algorithm for the comprehensive management of iron status, 195
Alkalinization, 64
Alternative, 90
ANA - interpretation, 198
ANA - overview, 188
Angiotensin-I-converting enzyme, 66
Anti-CCP antibodies, 201
Anticitrullinated protein antibodies, 201
Anticyclic citrullinated peptide, 201
Antihistorical, 103
Antinuclear antibody - interpretation, 198, 199
Antioxidant capacity of fruits and vegetables, 115
Aortic coarctation, 31
Arachidonate avoidance, 51
Arginine, 58
Arthroscopic knee surgery, 100
Artificial sweeteners, colors and other additives, 119
Ascorbic acid, 63
Aspartame, 119
Atherosclerosis, 88
Atlantoaxial instability, 217, 218
Atlas vertebra realignment, 61
Authentic living, 131
Autointoxication, 153
Autonomization, 87, 135
Avascular necrosis of the femoral head, osteonecrosis, 220
Beta-glucuronidase, 204
Biochemical Individuality - overview, 126
Biochemical individuality, 102
Blood pressure measurement, 34
Body Mass Index, 111
Bowel function, 152
Bradycardia, 71
Caffeine, 120
calcium pyrophosphate dihydrate deposition disease, 221, 222
Canadian Hypertension Education Program recommendations, 46
Carbohydrate loading for supercompensation, 119
Cardiopulmonary examination, 35
Carnitine Insufficiency Caused by Aging and Overnutrition, 119
Carrageenan, 119
Carson, Rachel (author of Silent Spring), 145
Casokinins, 66
Cauda equina syndrome, 169, 170, 217
CBC – overview, 187
CBC: complete blood count - interpretation, 191
CCP, 201
Cervical spine dysfunction, 33
Chemistry panel – overview, 187
Chemistry/metabolic panel - interpretation, 192
Chemistry/metabolic panel, 37
Chiropractic model of illness and healing, 225
Chiropractic spinal manipulative therapy, 61
Chlorpyrifos, 146
Chocolate, 67
Clinical Assessments for HTN, 34
Clinical Management, 41
Clinical practice involves much more than "diagnosis and treatment", 214
Cocaine, 31
Cocoa, 67
Coenzyme Q10 (CoQ10) in cardiac disease, 53
Coenzyme Q-10, 52
Complement, 192
Complements C3 and C4, 192
Complete blood count - interpretation, 191
Complex carbohydrates, 118
Composite seropositivity, 201
Comprehensive parasitology, 204
Comprehensive parasitology, stool analysis, 188
Comprehensive stool analysis and comprehensive parasitology, 204
Conn's syndrome, 32
Conscious living, 103
Consciousness-raising, 135
Consent to treatment, 210
Consistently Positive Results, 157
Contemplation, 98
Controlled breathing, 65
CoQ-10, 52
Corrective experience, 135
CPDD, 222
CPPD, 221, 222
Cranial nerves, 183, 185
C-reactive protein - interpretation, 189
CRP - interpretation, 189
Cushing's disease/syndrome, 31
Cyclic citrullinated protein antibodies, 201
Daily living, 93
Dark Chocolate, 67
DDE, 145
DDT, 145
Dean Ornish, 88
Deep tendon reflexes, 184
Depuration, 148, 150
Detoxification programs are a necessity, 145
Detoxification, 150
Development of CVD, 29
Differential Diagnoses of HTN, 31
Digestion, 152
Disease Complications, 40
Drug class and description, 72
Drug management of hypertension, 12
Drug treatments for chronic HTN, 70
Ear lobe crease, 37
ECG, 39
EKG, 39
Electrocardiography, 39
Emergencies, 216
Emotional literacy, 87, 135
Emotional, mental, and social health, 131
Endocrinologic activity of adipose tissue, 112
Enough, 16
Environmental health, 145
Epicatechin, 67
Erythrocyte sedimentation rate - interpretation, 190
ESR - interpretation, 190
Estrogen, 31
Ethanol, 32

# Index

Exceptional living, 99
Exercise, 108
Exercise, 52
Eye and fundoscopic examination, 37
Facial nerve, 185
Family health history, 179
Fasting (short-term water-only), 47
Fatty acid supplementation, 51
Ferritin - interpretation, 193
Ferritin - overview, 188
Fish oil, 51
Food allergen avoidance, 49
Food allergens, 120
For hypertension, 13
For serious toxicity even at low doses, 129
For the Treatment of Various Health Problems, 161
Foreword by Dr Joe Brimhall, 26
Foundation for Health - introduction, 88
Friction – purpose in physical examination, 181
Fructose avoidance, 50
Fulcrum tests – purpose in physical examination, 181
Functional assessment, 180
Fundoscopic examination, 37
Giant cell arteritis, 216
Glossopharyngeal, 185
Goldhamer, 47
Gout, 221
HIGH-RISK PAIN PATIENTS, 207
History taking, 176
HTN is important clinically for several reasons, 29
HTN patient profile, 71
HTN prevalence, 29
Hydrosoluble coenzyme Q10, 54
Hyperaldosteronism, 32
Hypercalcemia, 32
Hypercalcinosis, 75
Hypercholesterolemia, 88
Hyperinsulinemia, 118
Hyperinsulinemia, 32
Hypertension (integrative model), 69
Hypertension, 88
Hypertension, see also HTN, 27
Hypertensive emergency, 41
Hypertensive urgency, 41
Hyperthyroidism, 33
Hypoglossal nerve, 185
Hypothyroidism, 33
Implementation of Nutritional Supplementation, 165
Implementing the Five-Part Nutritional Wellness Protocol
Individuation, 103
Informed consent, 210
Insulin resistance, 118
Insulin resistance, 32
Internal locus of control, 135
Intestinal health and bowel function, 152
Intracellular Hypercalcinosis, 75
Intracellular Hypercalcinosis, 75
Intradependence, 87, 135
Jared Zeff, N.D., 92
Kidney problems, 129
Laboratory assessments: general considerations of commonly used tests, 187
Laboratory tests in the evaluation of patients with musculoskeletal complaints, 187
Lactoferrin, 204
Lactokinins, 66
Lactulose-mannitol assay, 188
Lactulose-mannitol assay: assessment for intestinal hyperpermeability and malabsorption, 203

L-Arginine, 58
L-carnitine, 56
Lead and HTN, 39
Leaky gut, 203
Lifestyle habits, 95
Low-carbohydrate diet, 47
Magnesium, 55
Malabsorption, 152
ManKind Project, 133
Maximize factors that promote health, 156
Mechanoreceptor-mediated inhibition of neurogenic inflammation, 231
Medical history, 179
Medical procedures - complications from, 151
Medicine, 9
Meditation, 65
Melatonin, 107
Mercury, 147
Metabolic panel - interpretation, 192
Mind-Body Approaches, 65
Minimize factors that promote disease, 156
Monoarthritis, 219
Motivation, 97
Motivation: moving from theory to practice, 98
Muscle strength – grading scale, 184
Musculoskeletal emergencies, 216
Myelopathy, 169, 170, 217
National Heart, Lung, and Blood Institute (NHLBI), 85
Nattokinase, 67
Neurologic assessment, 182
Neurologic examination, 180
Neurologic examination, 36
Neuropsychiatric lupus, 216
Nonsteroidal anti-inflammatory drugs, 32
Nutrigenomics, 127
Nutritional Genomics, 127
Nutritional Treatments for Hypertension, 79
O'Keefe and Cordain in Mayo Clinic Proceedings, 113
Obesity, 111
Oculomotor, 185
Olfactory, 185
Ophthalmic, 185
Oral contraceptives, 31
Ornish, 88
Orthomolecular Medicine - overview, 126
Orthopedic/musculoskeletal examination: concepts and goals, 181
Osteochondritis dissecans, 220
Osteomyelitis, 169, 170, 218
Paleo-Mediterranean Diet, 125
Paleo-Mediterranean Diet, 45
PAR, 210
Paradigms, and their reasonable alternatives, 104
Parasitology, 204
Patients…or for the Drug Companies, 85
Percussion – purpose in physical examination, 181
Pesticide exposure, 146
Phenolic content, 115
Phenotype modulation, 127
Pheochromocytoma, 32
Physical examination, 180
Physical Examination, 34
Physical exertion, 108
Phytochemicals, 114
Phytochemicals, 115
Political and social action, 148
Poor digestion, 152
Possibilities in Health and Healthcare, 83
Pre-contemplation, 98

Predicting amount and duration of weight loss, 35
Preeclampsia, 32
Preparation, 98
Preventive health screening: general recommendations, 154
Price,, 113
Problem management, 91
Protein - calculation of daily intake, 116
Protein Per Pound of Body Weight, 117
Protein supplements, 117
Qigong, 65
Re-establishing the Foundation for Health - details, 92
REFLEXES – grading scale, 184
Reliable indicators of organic neurologic disease, 182
Renal artery (renovascular) stenosis, 32
Renal disease survey, 37
Renal disease, 32
Renal failure, 129
Review of systems, 178
Rheumatoid Factor - interpretation, 200, 202
Rheumatoid factor - overview, 188
Roger J Williams, 102
ROS: review of systems, 178
Safe patient + safe treatment = safe outcome, 210
Scleroderma, 33
Screening laboratory tests in the evaluation of patients with musculoskeletal complaints, 187
Secretory IgA, 204
Septic arthritis, 218, 222, 223
Seropositivity, 201
Serotonin synthesis, 119
Serum 25(OH) vitamin D - a screening test in patients with musculoskeletal pain, 196
Shearing force – purpose in physical examination, 181
Short-chain fatty acids, 204
Sleep apnea, 33
Sleep deprivation, 106
Sleep, 106
Sleep, techniques for improvement, 107
Slipped capital femoral epiphysis, 221
Social history, 179
Sodium benzoate, 119
Sodium chloride, 49
Special considerations in the evaluation of children, 212
Spinal accessory nerve, 185
Spinal cord compression, 169, 170, 217
Spinal manipulation: mechanistic considerations, 230
Stool analysis, 204
Stratification of HTN management, 41
Stress is a "whole body" phenomenon, 132
Stress management and authentic living, 131
Subluxation, 33
Supercompensation, 119
Supplemented Paleo-Mediterranean Diet, 125
Supplements, 129
Systemic sclerosis, 33
Systolic hypertension, 54
Tartrazine, 119
Television, 95
Temporal arteritis, 216
Thyroid disease, 33
Thyroid stimulating hormone - interpretation, 197
Thyroid testing, 38
Tissue, 112
Transcendental meditation, 65
Transient synovitis, irritable hip, 220
Trigeminal, 185
Trochlear, 185
Truncated self, 135
TSH - overview, 188
TSH: thyroid stimulating hormone - interpretation, 197
Unconventional, 90
Unhistorical, 103
Unscientific, 90
Uric acid reduction, 50
Uric acid, 38
Urinalysis (UA), 37
Urinary alkalinization, 64
Urine pH, 38
Vestibulocochlear, 185
Vibration – purpose in physical examination, 181
Visual analog scale, 185
Vitamin C, 63
Vitamin D deficiency - assessment in patients with musculoskeletal pain, 188
Vitamin D status testing, 196
Weight optimization, 52
Wellness promotion, 91
Wellness, 175
Whey peptides, 66
Williams, Roger J,, 102
WomanWithin, 133
Work ethic, 105
Yellow dye #5, 119
Zeff, N.D., 92

---

### Newsletter & Updates
Be alerted to new integrative clinical research and updates to this textbook by signing-up for the free newsletter, sent 6-8 times per year. Contact
newsletter@optimalhealthresearch.com
or
www.OptimalHealthResearch.com/newsletter

Made in the USA
Charleston, SC
30 May 2010